Surgery of the Arteries to the Head

Ramon Berguer   Edouard Kieffer

Surgery of the Arteries to the Head

Color Illustrations by Lorie Manzardo

With 215 illustrations in 341 parts

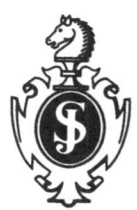

Springer-Verlag

New York Berlin Heidelberg London Paris
Tokyo Hong Kong Barcelona Budapest

Ramon Berguer
Professor of Surgery
Chief, Division of Vascular Surgery
Wayne State University School of Medicine
Harper Hospital
3990 John R
Detroit, MI 48201 USA

Edouard Kieffer
Professor of Surgery
Chief, Division of Vascular Surgery
Pitié-Salpetrière University Hospital
83 Boulevard de l'Hopital
75651 Paris, France

Library of Congress Cataloging-in-Publication Data
Berguer, Ramon.
    Surgery of the arteries to the head / Ramon Berguer, Edouard
Kieffer.
        p. cm.
    Includes bibliographical references and index.
    ISBN-13: 978-1-4612-7706-4   e-ISBN-13: 978-1-4612-2880-6
    DOI: 10.1007/978-1-4612-2880-6

    1. Cerebral arteries--Surgery. 2. Cerebrovascular disease-
-Surgery. I. Kieffer, E. (Edouard) II. Title.
    [DNLM: 1. Cerebral Arteries--surgery. 2. Cerebrovascular
Disorders--surgery. WL 355 B499s]
617.4'81--dc20
DNLM/DLC
for Library of Congress   91-5240

ion managed by Karen Phillips; manufacturing supervised by Jacqui Ashri.
mposed pages prepared from the authors' MultiMate files using PageMaker.

5 4 3 2 1

Foreword

Wesley S. Moore, M.D.
Los Angeles, California

The publication of this book by Drs. Berguer and Kieffer is particularly timely with respect to the development, evolution, and establishment of cerebrovascular surgery as an important strategy for stroke prevention. While the last three decades have resulted in a proliferation in the frequency of operations performed, particularly carotid endarterectomy, the evidence for efficacy has been controversial and often challenged by those with a nihilistic view toward patients with this morbid disorder.

1991 will be remembered as a pivotal year for those advocating a surgical approach to stroke prevention. A portion of the North American Symptomatic Carotid Endarterectomy Trial (NASCET) was brought to an abrupt halt by the Oversight Committee who monitored the study. The committee stopped the study because it was shown that symptomatic patients with carotid bifurcation lesions ranging from 70 to 99% had statistically and dramatically fewer fatal and non-fatal strokes following carotid endarterectomy than those patients treated with medical management alone, including aspirin.

Identical results were also reported in the large European trial (ECSET) and the brief Veterans

Andre Thevenet, M.D.
Montpellier, France

In this book Ramon Berguer and Edouard Kieffer present state-of-the-art information on operations for the extracranial arteries supplying the brain. These two surgeons are recognized authorities in this field, and their dedication and vast personal experience become readily apparent as one reads these pages.

Surgery of the Arteries to the Head is not an encyclopedic review of the subject, which can be found in textbooks, nor is it a repetition of what has been previously written with a compilation of references and controversial data.

Written by surgeons for surgeons, it is a practical manual of vascular surgery based on conclusions the authors have drawn from extensive experience. It is an unusual book in many ways: its title, its form, its style, its content. The subject matter of all the chapters is presented in a lively fashion, like a fireside narration of past adventures. The book is concise and easily understood, a clear and personal yet scholarly treatise incorporating traditional statements with new concepts. Because the authors collaborated closely on all chapters, there are no discrepancies, as is generally the rule.

Wesley S. Moore, continued

Administration Symptomatic trial. 1991 also saw the conclusion of the Veterans Administration-sponsored prospective randomized trial for patients with asymptomatic carotid stenosis. Results of that trial demonstrated a clear reduction in neurologic events in the patients treated by carotid endarterectomy.

While all of these reports have been exciting and serve to validate the enthusiasm for those advocating surgery for cerebro-vascular disease, there has also been a common caveat expressed in all of the studies: that surgery will be of benefit only if the operation is done safely, resulting in minimal stroke morbidity and mortality. Drs. Berguer and Kieffer have written a book, specifically for surgeons, to help them achieve this objective.

Unlike many contemporary books, which are multi-authored, this book is written in its entirety by two people who have a wealth of surgical experience and who are world-renowned for their expertise. The result is a work that is authoritative, evenly written, and reads well with a smooth flowing and clear narrative style. The authors' stated objective is to present the variety of surgical options with an emphasis on technique. They have met this objective well, not only in the narrative but, in particular, with the absolutely superb illustrations, which are clear, anatomically accurate, and abundant throughout the text.

All of the various surgical procedures have been covered in appropriate detail, including the unusual approaches to the distal vertebral artery for which the authors are uniquely qualified by their pioneering effort and extensive personal experience. The book offers a wealth of information to the seasoned surgeon as well as those in training. Careful adherence to the principles clearly presented by Berguer and Kieffer should go a long way to achieving safe surgery for those suffering from cerebrovascular disorders. It will represent an important, useful, and frequently reviewed book for the surgeon's library.

Andre Thevenet, continued

In contrast to prior books on carotid and extracranial cerebrovascular surgery, this one concentrates on basic surgical concepts of cerebral circulation and pathologic processes, as well as precise and detailed description of techniques. The fine points of radiologic evaluation and noninvasive testing of these arteries are excluded because they are the province of another discipline and have no place in a surgeon's handbook of surgical techniques. The merits of this atlas are further enhanced by the profusion of top-quality illustrations from a talented, insightful medical artist.

Having been interested in this fascinating and challenging field since the late 1950s, especially surgery of the carotid and vertebral arteries and of the supraaortic trunks, it gives me great pleasure and satisfaction to see how these procedures have developed and are now accepted as commonplace.

I have known both authors for many years as skilled and talented surgeons and have been impressed by their innovations and technical expertise. It is a pleasure for me to recognize them in the different sections of the volume with their logic, clear exposition, lucid and simple style, and unflagging enthusiasm.

Dwight Harken once classified surgeons into three categories: 1) the good surgeon is able to apply standard techniques skillfully; 2) the very good surgeon simplifies, improves, and applies those standard techniques with flexibility; and 3) the great surgeon, in addition to all the qualities of a good and very good surgeon, is creative and passes improved standards and new techniques on to others. The latter definition certainly applies to Drs. Berguer and Kieffer as they transmit their knowledge through this book.

Without a doubt *Surgery of the Arteries to the Head* will enhance the competence of every vascular surgeon and will become a standard in the field as well as a baseline for advances in the years to come.

Preface

This book was written by two friends who, for the last decade, have shared an interest in the repair of the arteries supplying the head. It has a clear surgical bent towards form and function, anatomy and surgical technique and deliberately avoids issues that we do not feel competent to discuss, such as the epidemiology of these diseases or their biochemical basis. It is written in essay form rather than in the "medical/scientific" style with strings of references supporting balanced and often conflicting opinions and tabulation and analysis of all data. It is an opinionated discourse reflecting personal choices drawn from the collective experience of many surgeons and from our own work.

To date we have done 6514 reconstructions in these arteries: 367 transthoracic and 1032 cervical repairs of the supraaortic trunks, 4210 carotid operations, and 905 vertebral reconstructions. We make no effort to cite the original source of every statement made. Only a few selected references are used, usually to support specific data alluded to in the text or to provide historical sources. In the few instances where personal choice has differed, the initials of the author indicate the source.

The illustrations are the work of medical artist Lorie Manzardo.

To avoid fastidious repetition the following abbreviations are used in the text: SAT (supraaortic trunks), IA (innominate artery), CCA (common carotid artery), ICA (internal carotid artery), ECA (external carotid artery), SA (subclavian artery) VA (vertebral artery), TIA (transient ischemic attack), VBI (vertebrobasilar ischemia), and CT (computerized tomography).

Since it has been accepted by general use, the word graft applies to both autologous and prosthetic arterial replacement material. We are grateful to the Elliman Foundation for their grant support. Our thanks to Jeanne Fitzgerald for her editorial assistance and to Betty Greene for transcribing the many versions of the manuscript. We are especially thankful to our publisher, Springer-Verlag, for their help and expertise in the production of this book.

R. Berguer   **E. Kieffer**
Detroit   *Paris*

Contents

1   Historical Notes

During the second century Galen demonstrated that the arteries contained blood and deduced that the brain was nourished by arterial and venous blood. He described a plexus, or *rete mirabile* (marvelous network), at the base of the brain where vessels converged into a network comparable to "a bunched up fisherman's net" where the "animal spirit" was formed. Galen developed this concept while dissecting animal heads. It was to be dogma for many centuries.

In 1544, as the Spanish and French armies faced off for another round of battles, each had a military surgeon that would change our knowledge of the vessels supplying the brain. On the Spanish side, Andrea Vesalius, the Renaissance anatomist, disagreed with the authoritarian teachings of Galen regarding the rete mirabile and, based on his dissection of human brains, stated that the carotid arteries "quite fail to produce such a plexus reticularis as that which Galen accounts." On the French side the extraordinary Ambroise Paré introduced the ligature of vessels during the mid-sixteenth century and performed the first carotid ligation for trauma in a patient, with resulting hemiplegia and aphasia.

In 1793, the year Louis XVI was guillotined, Hebenstreit successfully ligated a carotid artery for hemorrhage. Cooper is credited with the first ligation of a carotid for an aneurysm in 1805. Virchow[1] in 1856 described the findings and relation of carotid thrombosis and blindness. Elschnig,[2] an ophthalmologist, demonstrated in 1893 the collateral pathway of the ECA which, through the orbital connections with the distal ICA, may supply the eye and brain when the ICA is occluded.

Acceptance of the relation between extracranial carotid disease and brain infarction has waxed and waned over the last 150 years. Abercrombie[3] in 1828 identified carotid disease as a disease of the elderly and compared the associated brain deterioration to the gangrene that develops in a limb when the arterial supply fails. However, medical wisdom by the middle of the nineteenth century was that a stroke due to cerebral "softening" (infarct) was the result of thrombosis of a specific intracranial vessel. Giving support to this hypothesis, Cohnheim[4] described the "end-arterie" in the brain, or "terminal artery," an artery with no anastomosis beyond its origin and whose occlusion would result inevitably in the death of the brain tissue supplied by it. We know today that such "terminal arteries" do not exist in the adult human, although Cohnheim's concept can be accepted as a physiologic one (arteries with few collaterals unable to compensate the deficit of flow) rather than an anatomic one (no collaterals at all).

The concept that disease of the distal arteries is

the cause of stroke was also supported by the influential Hughling Jackson, who explained transient ischemic attacks by the development of small infarcts, with other brain areas compensating for the deficits created. The failure of pathologists to find any local arterial disease in cases of cerebral infarction stimulated the propagation of other theories, such as vasospasm, that would accommodate the prevailing notion that brain infarcts must be due to disease of the arteries directly supplying the area of infarction.

The contrary proposition already advanced by Abercrombie, that extracranial disease might be the cause of a stroke, was again given support by Chiari[5] who in 1905 in Prague described the thrombotic deposits forming over carotid plaques and postulated that they were the cause of embolization and stroke. Eight years later Hunt[6] described the relation between hemiplegia and carotid thrombosis and urged examination of neck arteries in patients presenting with symptoms of cerebral ischemia. Many years would pass before these fundamental observations began to percolate into the practice of medicine as clinical considerations.

Broadbent[7] in 1875 described the lack of arm pulses and feeble carotid pulses in a man whose autopsy revealed severe atheromas of the branches of the aortic arch. In 1908 Takayasu[8] described the ischemic retinal changes that develop with the arteritis that bears his name, although the association of these eye changes with absent pulses in the arm was the observation of Onishi in his discussion of Takayasu's paper.

Meanwhile, on the surgical side of things, World War I stimulated interest in the treatment of vascular injuries, and techniques for resection, anastomosis, and lateral repair were reported by von Parczewski, von Haberer, Lexer, and Denck.[9] Discussing firearm injuries to the carotid, Lefevre[10] in 1918 remarked on the poor prognosis of the triple ligature—CCA, ICA, and ECA—and proposed, after ligature of the CCA or of its bifurcation, the performance of a distal arteriorrhaphy or an anastomosis between the ECA and ICA to provide the latter with retrograde flow from the former.

Although some success outlining arteries with roentgenographic dyes had been reported before, credit is due to Moniz et al.[11] for the development of carotid arteriography in 1924, a technique that for the first time allowed study of carotid artery disease in the living person. Moniz, who received a well-deserved Nobel prize (but for the wrong reason—prefrontal leukotomy), used arteriography to investigate brain tumors and carotid artery occlusive disease. He specifically advised including the neck in the brain arteriograms in order to study the carotid bifurcation.

The findings on the association of carotid disease and hemiplegia reported by Chiari and by Hunt went largely unheard by the clinical community, which was still fixated on the concept of local arterial disease as the cause of brain infarction. In 1951 and 1954 Miller Fisher,[12,13] by applying the winning formula of correlating pathologic and clinical findings, defined with impeccable clarity the basic facts underlying cerebrovascular disease and anticipated the surgical treatment that would follow. Fisher insisted on the need to examine the cervical vessels as part of the evaluation of patients with stroke. He suggested the operation with which Carrea and associates would subsequently achieve a breakthrough in carotid reconstructive surgery. He described the peculiarities of the atheromatous plaques of the carotid bulb, the presence of ulceration and subintimal hemorrhage and their potential for distal embolization, the "silent" occlusion of the internal carotid, and the existence and mechanism of watershed infarction. He even ventured to guess (conservatively) that a residual diameter of 0.5 mm in the ICA would cause a "significant decrease in blood flow."

The equivalent of the work done by Fisher on the carotid artery was done on the vertebral artery five years later by Hutchinson and Yates.[14,15] This team, comprised of a clinician and a pathologist, outlined the pathology of the cervical vertebral artery and its consequences to the brain. The lesions described in the VA included atheromas, intraplaque hemorrhage, intramural dissection, external compression by osteophytes, and terminal thrombosis superimposed on a stenosis. For their report they sketched the brain lesions resulting from this extracranial pathology. These clinicopathologic correlations have not yet appreciably changed the concept and clinical approach to infarction in the posterior circulation even in today's neurologic practice.

In 1951 Conley,[16] a pioneer in radical neck

surgery, described a carotid operation he had used successfully in four patients with cancer invading the CCA. The description antedated the first surgical attempts to treat atheroma of the carotid bifurcation. With remarkable insight into the hemodynamics involved, he proposed an end-to-end anastomosis between the divided stumps of the internal and external carotid arteries in cases where the CCA had to be ligated, a solution similar to that proposed by Lefevre in 1918. He stated that the "free movement of blood" through this anastomosis "means additional nourishment of the brain," and "the predisposition to thrombus formation in the [internal carotid] artery is markedly diminished." Years later flow measurements in patients undergoing elective ligation of the CCA for treatment of intracranial aneurysm or cancer proved the effectiveness of Conley's operation by showing that substantial ICA flow may be derived from retrograde ECA flow.

The same year that Conley did his external-internal carotid anastomosis, a trio of Argentinian surgeons, Carrea, Molins, and Murphy,[17] performed the first elective operation on a diseased carotid. The operation was a transposition of the ECA to the ICA with exclusion of the diseased carotid bulb. In a patient operated in 1953 and reported in detail 22 years later, DeBakey[18] did the first endarterectomy of the ICA as we know the technique today.

Eastcott et al. in 1954 published[19] their first report of resection of a diseased carotid bulb (with end-to-end anastomosis of the common and internal carotid arteries). Their patient was cured of her intermittent hemiplegia by this operation. The publication of this account in *Lancet* was most influential in the development of carotid surgery. That same year Davis and associates[20] published the first report of a thromboendarterectomy of the innominate artery, although their description did not suggest a technically successful result. This technique was later formally described and successfully developed by Wylie.[21] Lin et al.[22] reported the first vein graft replacement of the carotid in 1955, an operation that Carrea and his associates had anticipated as a surgical possibility in cases of thrombosis of the carotid bifurcation with a patent distal ICA.

Reconstruction of the subclavian and vertebral arteries by endarterectomy was described by Cate and

Scott in 1957.[23] DeBakey et al.[24] and Bahnson et al.[25] in 1958—1959 described the technique of bypass applied to the supraaortic trunks. Crawford and co-workers[26] in 1958 described the technique of transsubclavian endarterectomy of the vertebral artery. In 1964 Parrot[27] introduced the technique of transposition of the second portion of the SA to the CCA. A transposition technique for the VA was described by Clark and Perry in 1966.[28]

Saphenous vein was used to bypass vertebral artery lesions during the 1970s.[29] Eventually, transposition of the vertebral artery to the CCA[30] became a better solution for proximal vertebral stenosis.

The approach to the distal vertebral artery had been described by Matas[31] and Henry[32] for its ligature during the treatment of traumatic lesions. Venous grafting and transposition procedures to revascularize the distal vertebral artery were developed using a similar approach.[33,34] The combination of cardiopulmonary bypass and hypothermic circulatory arrest described by Thevenet et al[35] allowed transaortic endarterectomy of atheroma of the aortic arch involving the branch orifices.

Today the approach to the arteries supplying the head is resolved at all extracranial levels. Most investigative efforts are directed to the precise definition of the surgical indications and the choice of technique used for the repair.

The Late Development of Vascular Repairs in the Neck

Reconstruction of the arteries to the head did not evolve simultaneously to the repair of the other arteries in the body for a number of reasons. When the techniques for reconstructing the aorta and femoral arteries were developed during the 1950s, there was scanty information on the pathologic nature and patterns of disease of the carotid and vertebral arteries. Some responsibility for this lack lies in the western tradition of autopsy, which precludes dissection of the neck, and some in the traditional view of the mechanisms of infarction in the brain.

It was the fundamental observations of Chiari,[5] Hunt,[6] Fisher,[13] and Hutchinson and Yates[14] that paved the way for the first attempts to reconstruct obstructed arteries in the neck. With these first operations came the realization of problems peculiar to this territory, e.g., ischemic brain damage due to clamping, intraoperative embolization, and the aggravation of strokes due to acute revascularization. The morbidity associated with these early reconstructions was substantial; the refined surgical techniques required by these vessels were not generally available; and the understanding of the pathologic consequences of these lesions on the brain was limited. During the 1960s, arteriography still carried a substantial risk and produced mediocre outlines of the pathology involved. During those years the arteriograms did not routinely survey the neck arteries from the aorta to the intracranial vessels. Therefore the presence of concomitant (and relevant) pathology, e.g., innominate or intracranial arterial disease, was not considered when refining the indications for and contraindications to these operations. The overwhelming importance of coronary artery disease as a risk factor for these operations was not fully appreciated, and today's successful methods for the diagnosis and treatment of coronary artery disease were not generally available. These factors added up to a substantial number of complications and deaths seen during revascularization of the carotid arteries. Because arteriograms seldom outlined the pathology of the supraaortic trunks and vertebral arteries, these vessels received comparatively little attention from clinicians and surgeons.

The duality of medical and surgical expertise that vascular surgeons developed in the diagnosis and treatment of atherosclerotic lesions of the aorta and legs did not extend to the territory of the head and neck. Surgeons during the 1970s, however, contributed substantially to the development of noninvasive methods to study carotid lesions (an intermediate solution between the imprecise search for a bruit and the evaluation of arterial lesions by arteriography) and developed safer operations for the arteries supplying the head. It took some time to learn that surgical techniques that had proved valuable in other areas were not always suited to the arteries supplying the head. Conversely, techniques such as transposition, which have limited use in the periphery, are particularly well suited to the neck because of the anatomic arrangement of arterial trunks, making it easy to switch a stenotic artery to a neighboring trunk. Whereas surgeons embarked on this field with a modest repository of knowledge about the response of the brain to ischemia and to manipulation of its blood supply, neurologists who were skeptical of what they viewed as somewhat simplistic solutions and surgical excesses generally did not have a good first-hand understanding of the local arterial pathology and of the hemodynamics involved. A conceptual divorce in the understanding of the relation between carotid artery disease and strokes took place during the 1970s.[36,37] With the advent of selective arteriography and CT scanning of the brain, valuable information was gained about the distribution of atherosclerotic lesions and their end-organ effects. The first prospective trials got underway during the late 1980s. By 1991 part of the randomized trial of carotid endarterectomy versus medical therapy was stopped following reports of the statistical superiority of surgical treatment amongst symptomatic patients with severe carotid stenosis.[38,39]

The neck is bound by two territories with which vascular surgeons have traditionally had little familiarity: the mediastinum at its lower end and the base of the skull at its upper end. In general, most vascular surgeons during the 1970s stayed outside the chest and did not directly tackle repair of the supraaortic trunks in the mediastinum; rather, they favored indirect repair, using bypasses laid horizontally, often across the midline and awkwardly designated "extraanatomic." The base of the skull was also unfamiliar to vascular surgeons probably because of the rarity of recognizable vascular disease at this level. Eventually, improvements in anesthetic technique, cardiac management, selective arteriography, and CT scanning resulted in the development of safe operative techniques for the supraaortic trunks, the high cervical carotid artery, and the distal vertebral artery during the late 1970s and early 1980s.

2 The Aortic Arch and Its Branches: Anatomy and Blood Flow

The aortic arch gives off its three branches as it curves around the tracheoesophageal axis between the ascending and descending portions of the aorta. The arch has two curvatures, the main one in a frontosagittal plane and a secondary curvature in the transverse plane (Figure 2.1). The IA and left CCA originate close to each other and run in a nearly frontal plane on each side of the trachea and close to the brachiocephalic venous trunk, which crosses in front of their origin and is itself covered by the remnants of the thymus.

The left SA originates as the last branch of the aortic arch behind and slightly to the left of the left CCA. The distance between the origin of these two arteries (about 1 to 2 cm) is greater than the distance between the origins of the IA and the CCA. The left SA runs under the left pleura up to the thoracic outlet. Between the left CCA and SA, the vagus and phrenic nerves cross each other in an elongated X under the pleural cover.

Variations in the anatomy of the branches of an aortic arch include the IA originating to the left side of the trachea. In neonates this situation may have clinical consequences, with the IA compressing the trachea and causing respiratory distress. In adults this disposition predisposes to arterial erosions after prolonged endotracheal intubation or cannulation through a tracheostomy.

The IA and left CCA share a common ostium in 16% of individuals and originate from a common trunk in 8% of the population (Figure 2.2). The left VA originates as a branch of the aortic arch between the left CCA and SA in 8% of individuals or, much

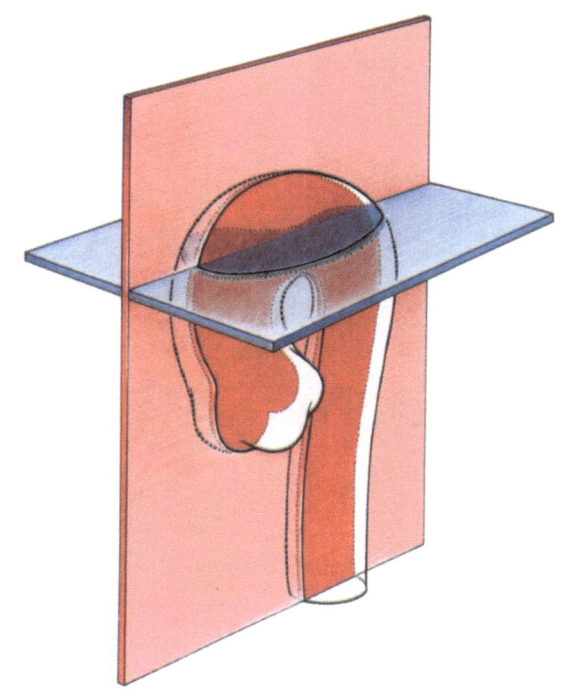

Figure 2.1 Two curvatures of the aortic arch.

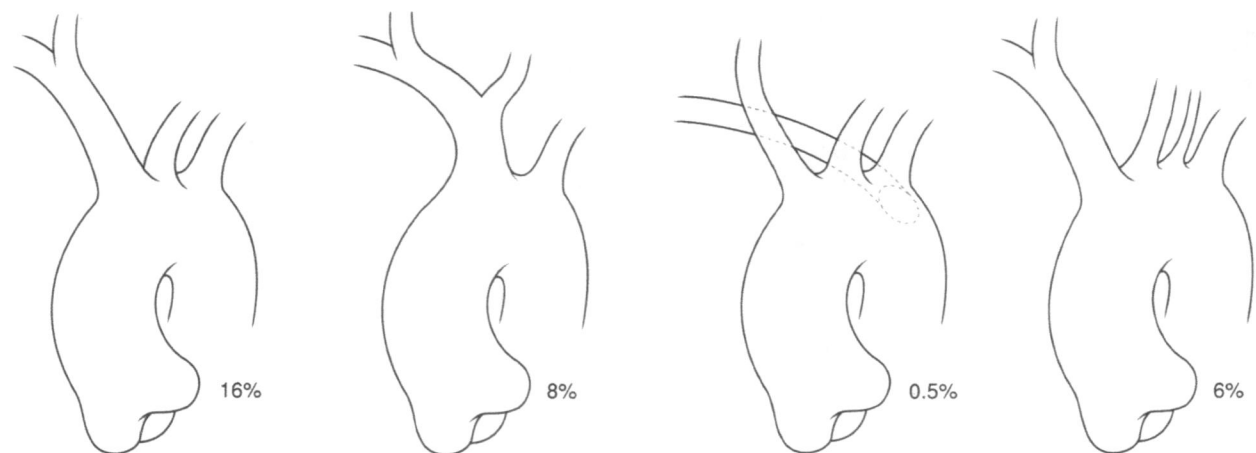

Figure 2.2 Common variations of the aortic arch.

more rarely, behind or distal to the left SA (Figure 2.2).

The most common anomaly of the aortic arch branches is the retroesophageal SA, seen in 0.5% of the population (Figure 2.2). In these cases there is no IA, and the four branches of the arch are, consecutively, the right and left CCA and the left and right SA. One-third of individuals with a RSA have a

common carotid trunk giving off both CCAs, the so-called truncus bicarotidus (Figure 2.3). In patients with an RSA, the right VA may originate directly from the right CCA.

At the takeoff of the RSA there may be a congenital dilatation of the wall called the diverticulum of Kommerel (Figure 2.4), a remnant of the posterior part of the right fourth aortic arch. In

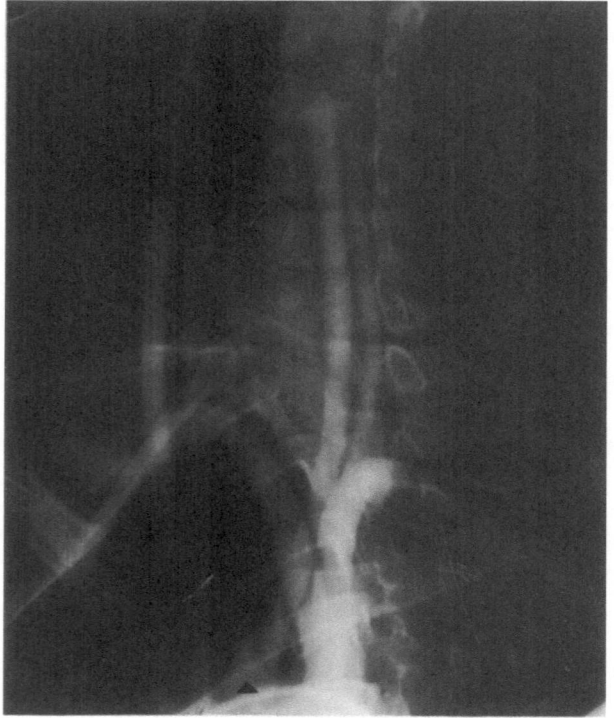

Figure 2.3 Retroesophageal subclavian artery (square) and a truncus bicarotidus (triangle).

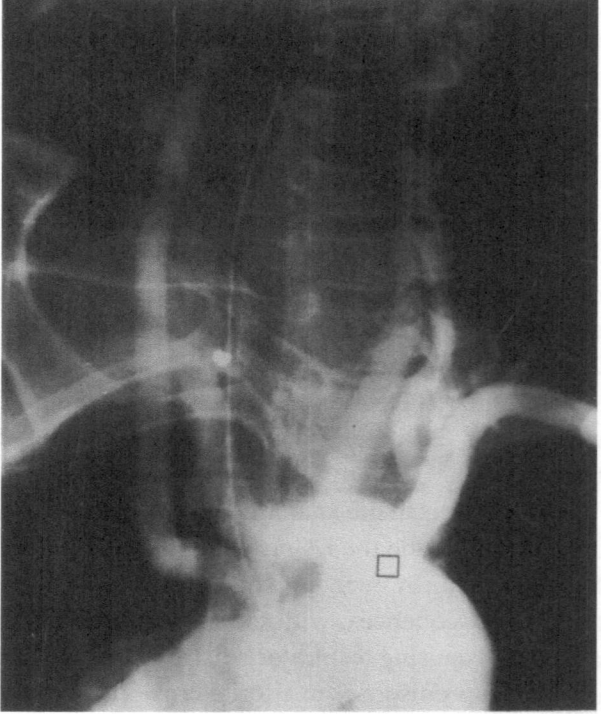

Figure 2.4 Retroesophageal subclavian artery with a diverticulum of Kommerel (box).

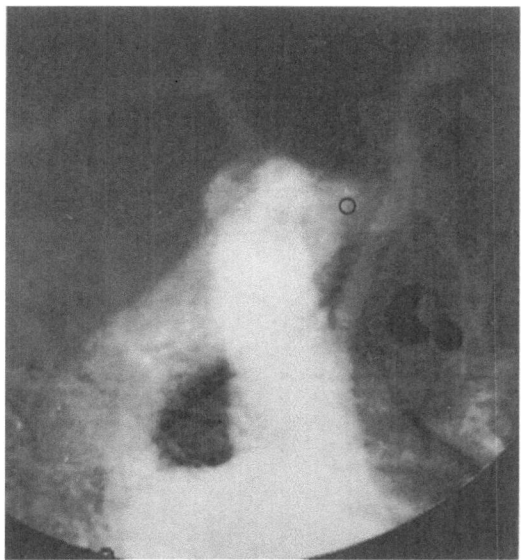 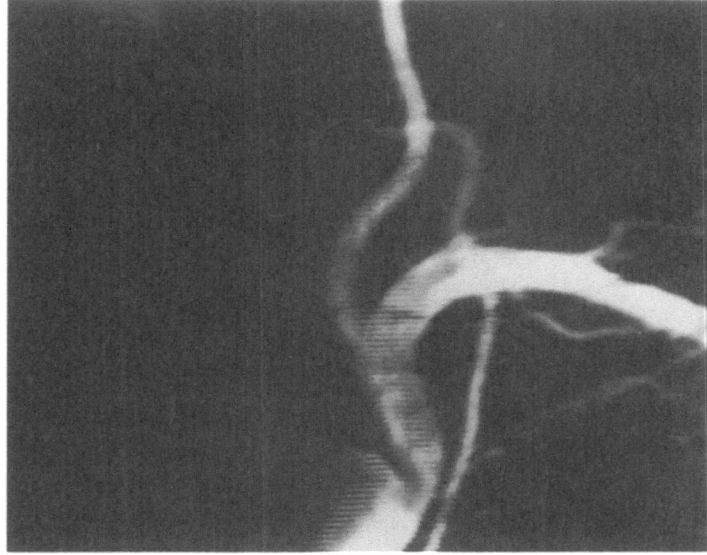

Figure 2.5 Right-sided aortic arch and retroesophageal left subclavian artery with a Kommerel's diverticulum at its origin (circle). Note the plicature of the anomalous left subclavian at the point where its dilated retroesophageal segment joins the normal anatomic course of this vessel.

patients with RSA the right inferior laryngeal nerve does not recur under the SA but, rather, leaves the vagus higher in the neck to go to the larynx, resting on the lateral wall of the right CCA, where it may be injured during carotid dissection. Another frequent anomaly in these patients is the thoracic duct emptying into the right jugulosubclavian confluent.

Anomalies of the branches of the arch are frequent in individuals with a right-sided or double aortic arch. Although these anomalies are usually associated with other congenital cardiac abnormalities, they may occur in isolation as well. Mirror images of the supraaortic branches are seen in patients with a right aortic arch, including a left IA and left RSA (Figure 2.5) A rare anomaly is isolation of the left SA (Figures 2.6 and 2.7), where the first part of the SA is absent and the verte-brosubclavian junction is attached to the pulmonary artery by the ligamentum arteriosus under which the left inferior

laryngeal nerve recurs. In cases with a double aortic arch there is no IA on either side, and both CCA and SA originate directly from each half of the arch.

The measurements of the arch and its branches are not significantly different for men and women.

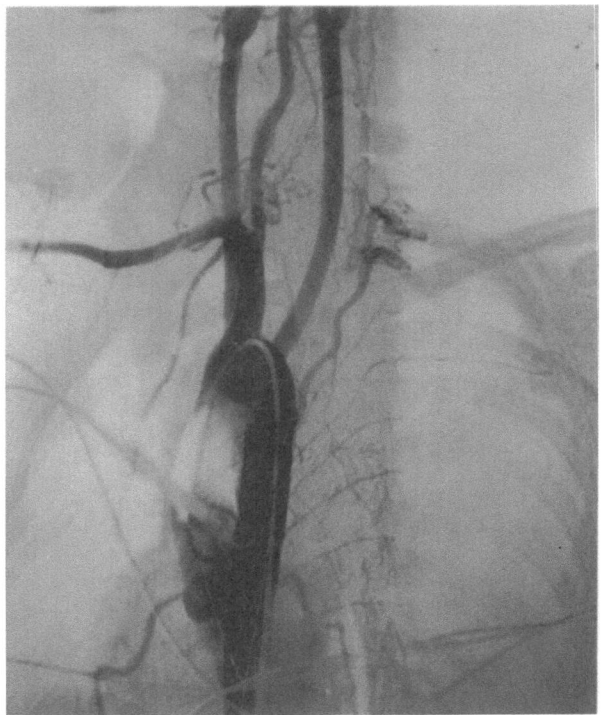

Figure 2.6 Isolation of the left subclavian artery in a patient with a right-sided aortic arch.

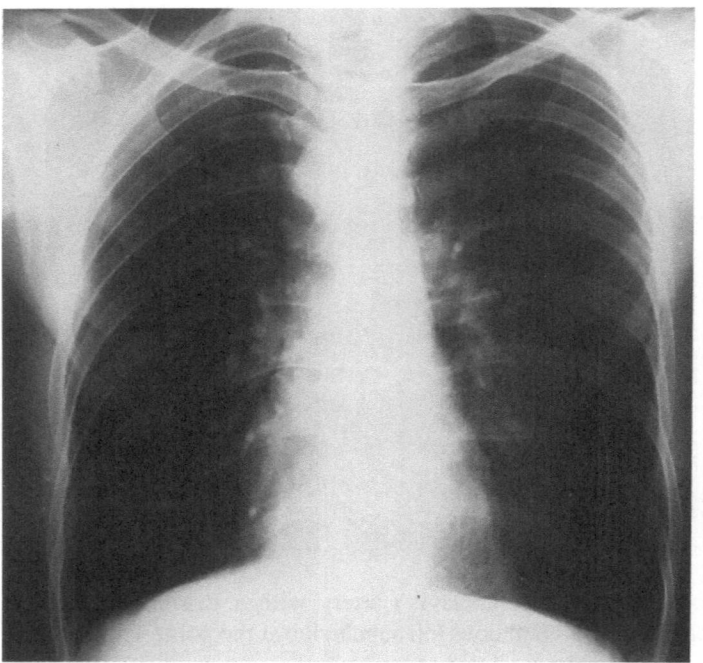 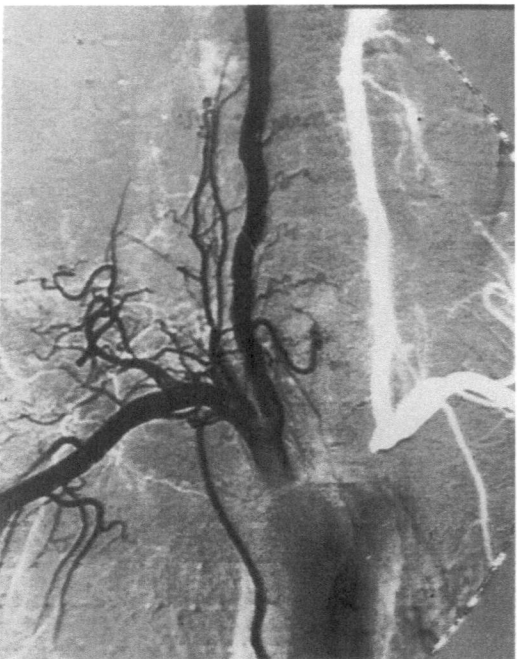

Figure 2.7 (Left) Aortic knob on the right mediastinum identifies the right-sided aortic arch on the chest roentgenogram. **(Right)** A right brachial injection shows the right subclavian and vertebral arteries (in black) and the vertebral steal (in white) on the left side where the subclavian artery is isolated.

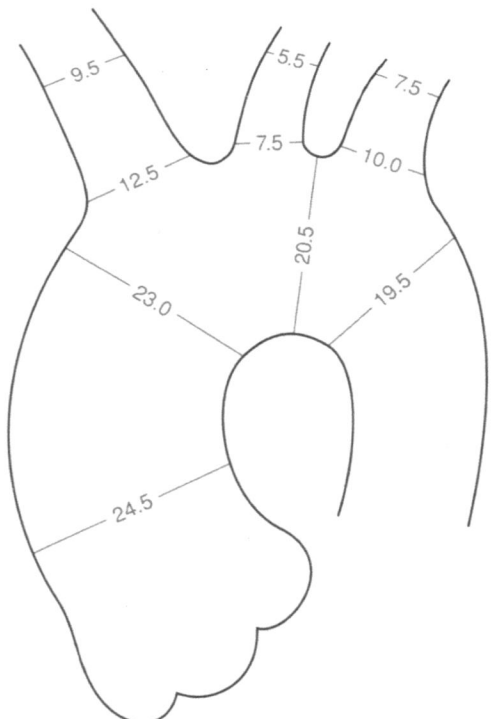

Figure 2.8 shows the measurements obtained by Wright.[40] The diameter and length of the aorta increases slightly in older individuals. Age and hypertension elevate the arch and may induce buckling or kinking, particularly on the right-sided branches.

Figure 2.8 Measurements of the aorta. Diameters are expressed in millimeters. (From Wright.[40])

Figure 2.9 Level of bifurcation of the common carotid artery. (Redrawn from Smith and Larsen.[41])

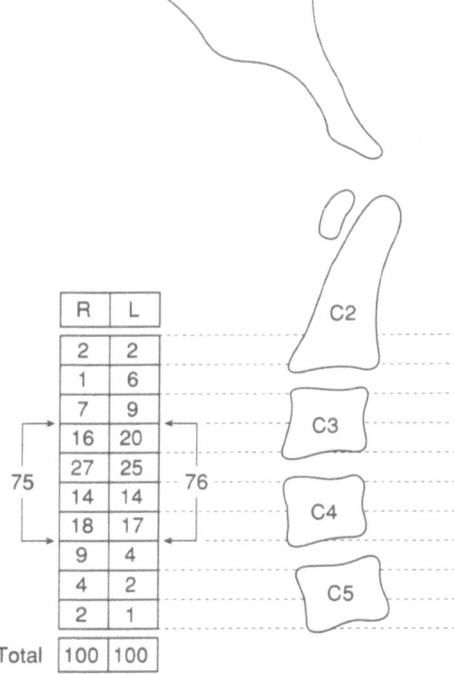

	R	L
	2	2
	1	6
	7	9
	16	20
75	27	25	76
	14	14
	18	17
	9	4
	4	2
	2	1
Total	100	100

C2
C3
C4
C5

Anterior System (Internal Carotid Arteries)

Unlike the vertebral arteries, the carotid arteries are generally symmetric and approximately of the same size. The CCA ascends in the neck behind the strap muscles and the omohyoid. More superficially, the sternomastoid muscle covers the CCA. Within the neurovascular sheath in which they travel, the CCA is in intimate contact with the internal jugular vein, which lies against the posterolateral wall of the artery. The vagus nerve usually lies in the posterior groove formed by the CCA and the internal jugular vein. Posterior to the carotid sheath one finds the sympathetic cervical chain and its ganglia, and medial to it is the thyroid gland and cartilage. In 75% of individuals the CCA bifurcates at the C3–C4 level[41] (Figure 2.9), roughly at the upper border of the thyroid cartilage (in children the carotid bifurcates one vertebral level higher). There is, however, considerable variation in the level of bifurcation, with the highest seen at C1–C2 and the lowest at T1–T2.

The peculiar makeup of the carotid bifurcation, with the dilatation known as the carotid bulb, has attracted interest because of the incidence and importance of atherosclerotic disease in this site. Adams[42] has dated the first reference to this dilatation of the first segment of the ICA back to Allan Burns who in 1811 observed this dilatation "independently of any organic disease of the coats [of the artery]." Luschka in 1862 first recognized the sinus as a normal anatomic feature of the ICA. The fusiform dilatation of the bulb occasionally extends into the distal portion of the CCA (Figure 2.10).

The architecture of the wall of the carotid bulb is different from that of the rest of the ICA: There is more elastic tissue, less smooth muscle, and the ratio of radius to media thickness is high. Heath et al.[43] compared the carotid bulb wall to that of the pulmonary artery.

The diameter of the bulb is equal to or larger than the diameter of the distal CCA. Its bulged-out, thinned wall is more distensible than the adjacent carotid walls. The thinnest part of the wall of the sinus is anteromedial and opposite to the large bulge of the posterolateral wall.

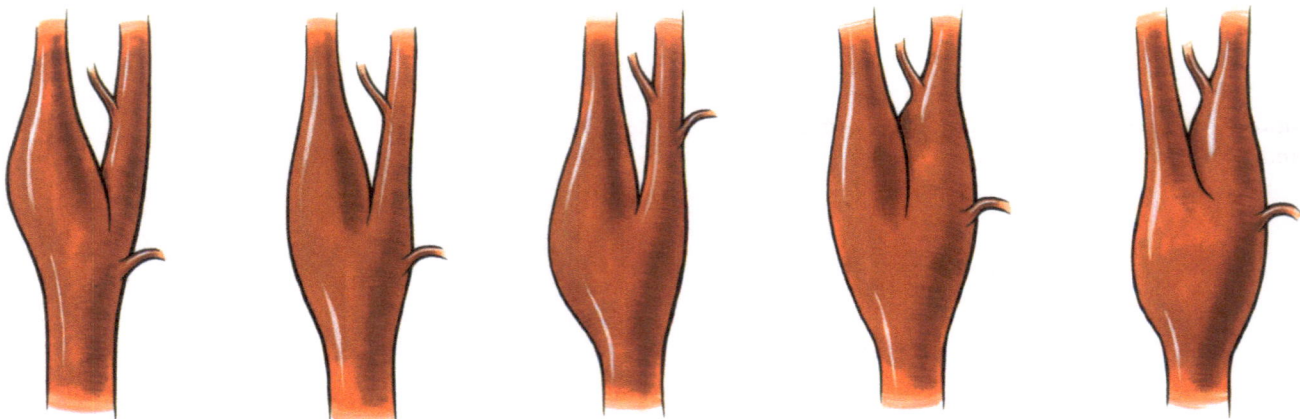

Figure 2.10 Various configurations of the bulbous dilatation of the ICA, and occasionally of the CCA. (Redrawn from Boyd.[44])

Boyd[44] had already concluded in 1937 that "changes in pressure in the general circulation are magnified at the dilatation and, consequently, the nerve-endings of the afferent nerves [in its wall] are able to register these changes in pressure more readily." The stretch sensors are incorporated in the outer layers of its wall. Although physiology textbooks list the carotid as one of several baroceptor sites within the arch of the aorta and its branches, Edwards[45] has reminded us that, to this day, "the existence in man of arterial baroceptor sites other than the carotid sinus is inferred but not demonstrated." If it is the only barocepter site in humans, it makes sense to preserve its function during carotid endarterectomy, particularly if one considers that the operation reestablishes the distensibility of the wall by removing the internal splinting created by the plaque.

The carotid body, an ovoid formation measuring approximately 5x2 mm, is a chemoreceptor and lies in the posterior aspect of the carotid bifurcation. Nerves from both the carotid sinus (baroceptor) and the carotid body (chemoreceptor) form the so-called intercarotid branch of the glossopharyngeal nerve, which travels centrally with the latter.

The geometry of the bifurcation of the carotid artery is shown in Figure 2.11, which incorporates the measurements reported by Forster et al.[46] There is considerable variation in the bifurcation angles and in the absolute measurements of the diameter among individuals.

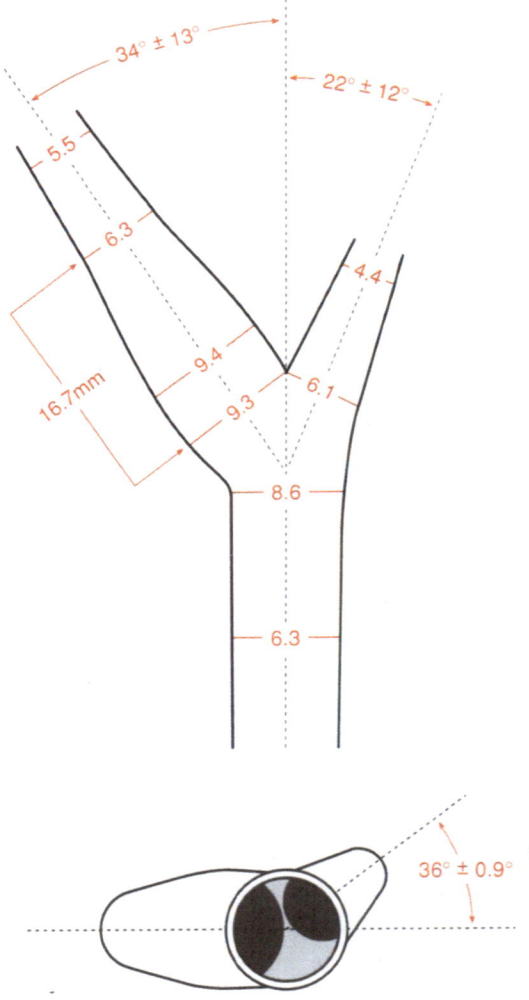

Figure 2.11 Measurements of the diameter and angles of the carotid bifurcation. (Redrawn from Forster et al.[46])

Above the carotid bulb the ICA disappears under an arch formed by the meeting of the hypoglossal and vagus nerves. After it crosses the ICA, the hypoglossal nerve makes a gentle loop, upwardly concave, as it passes in front of the ECA to reach the tongue. This hypoglossal loop is often tented and displaced downward by an early takeoff from an occipital artery or, more often, by an arterial branch of the latter (the sternomastoid artery) supplying the sternomastoid muscle (Figure 2.12). The two branches of the hypoglossal nerve that form the ansa hypoglossi descend in front of and behind the CCA to form a loop anterior to it from where the omohyoid and strap muscles derive their innervation.

The vagus nerve usually courses behind and lateral to the carotid bulb, but it may be found partially covering the cervical portion of the ICA. Above the hypoglossal nerve the ICA is crossed by the digastric muscle, an important boundary when dissections of the ICA are done high in the neck. Behind the digastric muscle the ICA is crossed by the glossopharyngeal nerve. This nerve does not have a single, round trunk like the hypoglossal nerve but, rather, a flat one often splayed in two or three fascicles. Further up, the ICA passes medial to the styloid process and deep to the styloid muscles originating from it. The artery here travels in a narrow boundary formed by the pharynx anteromedially, the ramus of the mandible anteriorly, and the parotid gland (and higher up the mastoid process) posteriorly. The artery rests on the transverse process of C1 and is displaced forward by this process when the head is rotated to the opposite side.

The ICA enters the carotid canal in the temporal bone where it is separated from the middle ear by a thin bony wall. It then leaves this canal to enter the cranium through the foramen lacerum. In its petrous portion the artery is surrounded by a venous plexus that communicates above with the cavernous sinus. At the end of the petrous portion the artery perforates the external layer of the dura and traverses the sinus cavernosus. It then ascends medial to the clinoid process, where it perforates the internal layer of the dura and becomes a short segment known as the supraclinoid ICA, which divides into the anterior and middle cerebral arteries. Other important

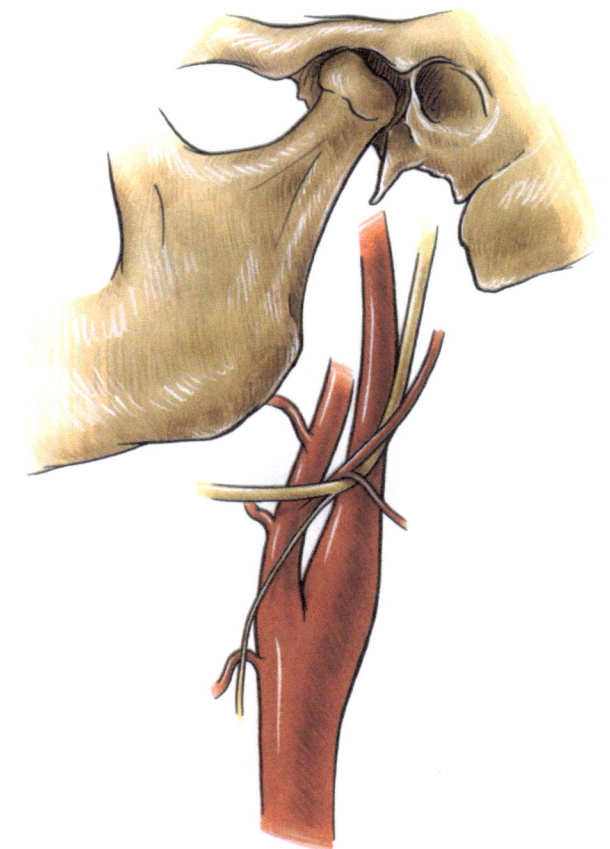

Figure 2.12 Tenting of the hypoglossal nerve by the sternomastoid artery.

branches of the supraclinoid ICA are the ophthalmic, posterior communicating, and anterior choroidal arteries.

The ophthalmic artery supplies the orbit and its contents (Figure 2.13). It is the first branch of the supraclinoid carotid and gives off branches to the lacrimal apparatus, eyelids, ethmoid bone, muscles of the orbit, and eyeball. Two branches of the ophthalmic artery are particularly important when considering ischemic eye symptoms: the central retinal artery and the ciliary arteries. The central retinal artery (0.3 mm diameter) travels within the optic nerve and emerges in the optic disc, dividing into four branches easily seen through an ophthalmoscope. The posterior ciliary arteries (0.5 mm diameter), usually two or three in number, can often be seen on arteriograms.

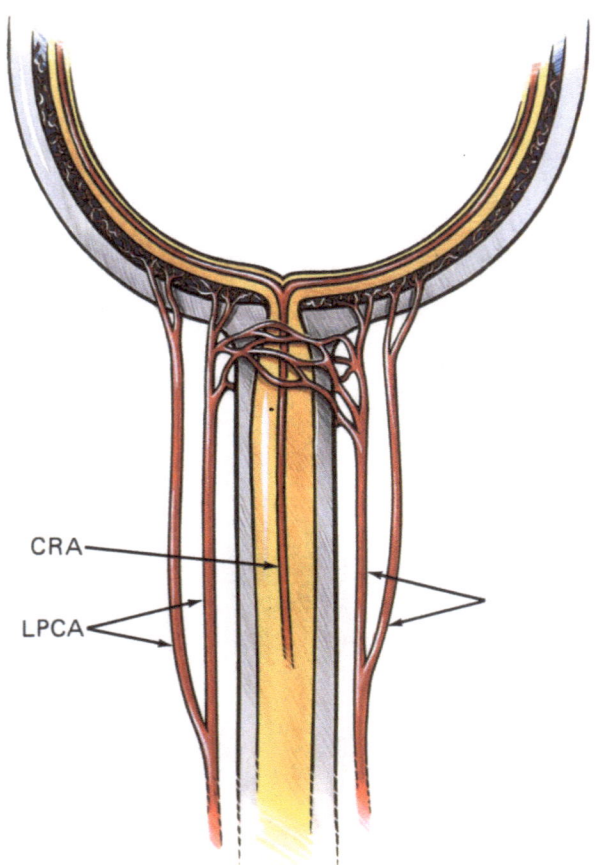

Figure 2.13 Ophthalmic artery supply to the orbit. CRA = central retinal artery; LPCA = long posterior ciliary arteries.

They give off the long and short posterior ciliary arteries, vessels that supply the choroid and the anterior part of the optic nerve. In 15% of individuals a branch of a posterior ciliary artery (cilioretinal branch) supplies a patch of retina.

Some elongation of the ICA and CCA takes place with aging and in the presence of hypertension, although this correlation is denied by some investigators. Nevertheless, it is obvious that the arteries of the young are far straighter than those of the elderly. Because the arteries of the elderly increase in diameter with age, they have to elongate. In addition, as individuals get older they lose height in the cervical spine owing to intervertebral disc atrophy and an increasing anterior spinal curvature. This shortening of the distance between the base of the skull and the thoracic inlet "compresses" the vessels traveling along

the neck. In certain instances, it has been established that coiling of advanced degree is probably congenital, as it can be seen also in children and young adults who do not suffer from hypertension or any known vascular disease.

The development of a sharp kink in an elongated ICA is usually associated with underlying atherosclerotic plaque. Some kinks obstruct blood flow, and the degree of obstruction may increase with rotation of the neck. The development of a kink in an elongated artery as a consequence of plaque has a mechanical analog: an elastic redundant tube with a stiff segment kinks at the junction between the elastic and stiff segments. In the ICA the stiffening is

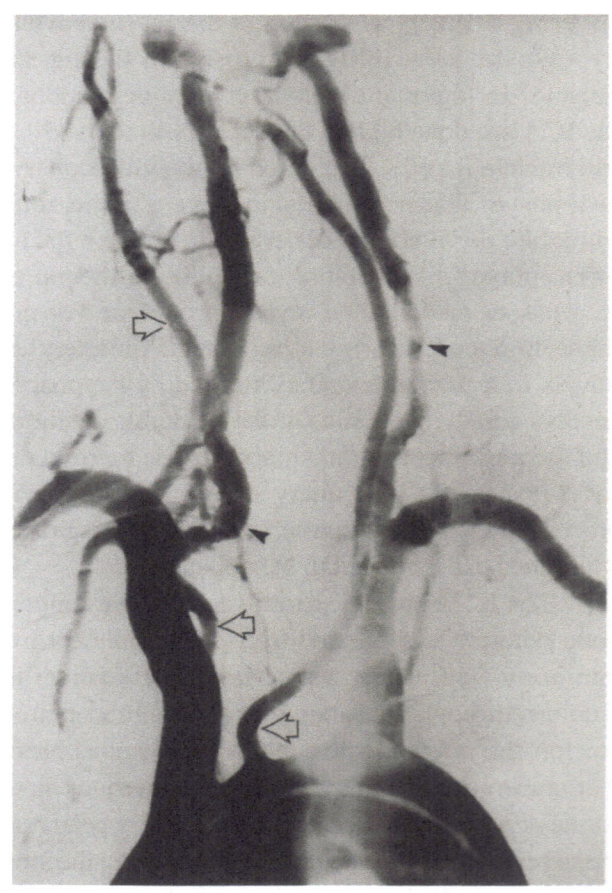

Figure 2.14 Congenital absence of both internal carotid arteries. The right external carotid arises from the innominate artery (top and middle open arrowheads), and the left external carotid arises from the arch of the aorta (bottom open arrowhead). The two large vertebral arteries (solid arrowheads) provide the entire intracranial flow.

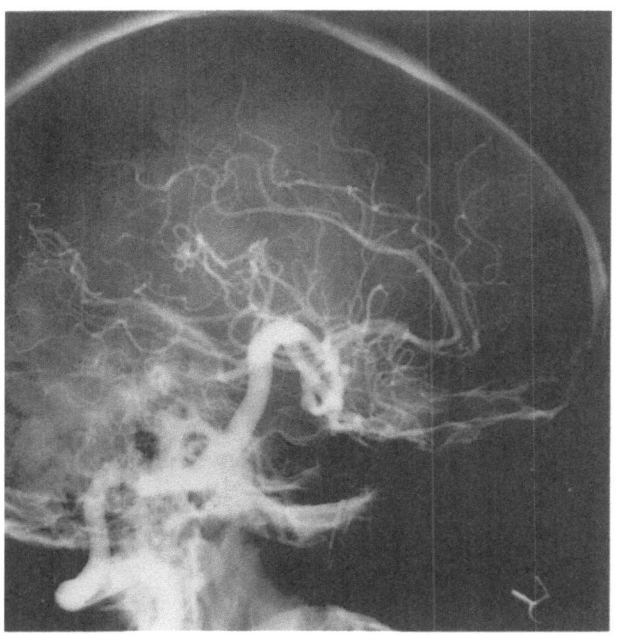

Figure 2.15 Intracranial arteries in the same patient as shown in Figure 2.14. The large basilar artery supplies the entire brain.

caused by the atherosclerotic plaque. The kink occurs only at the distal end of the plaque, where it ends abruptly in the soft, uninvolved wall of the cervical ICA. In the proximal end the plaque usually blends into the atheroma of the thicker wall of the less movable CCA.

The internal and external carotid arteries may be congenitally absent, or they may arise independently from the aorta. When the ECA is absent, the ICA may give off the higher branches normally supplied by the ECA. The ICA may be absent on one or both sides (Figures 2.14 and 2.15). More frequently the ICA is hypoplastic, with the defect involving the entire artery or just a segment of it. We have observed two cases in which the cervical and intracranial ICA lumen was absent but the carotid bulb and CCA were of normal size and appearance (Figure 2.16).

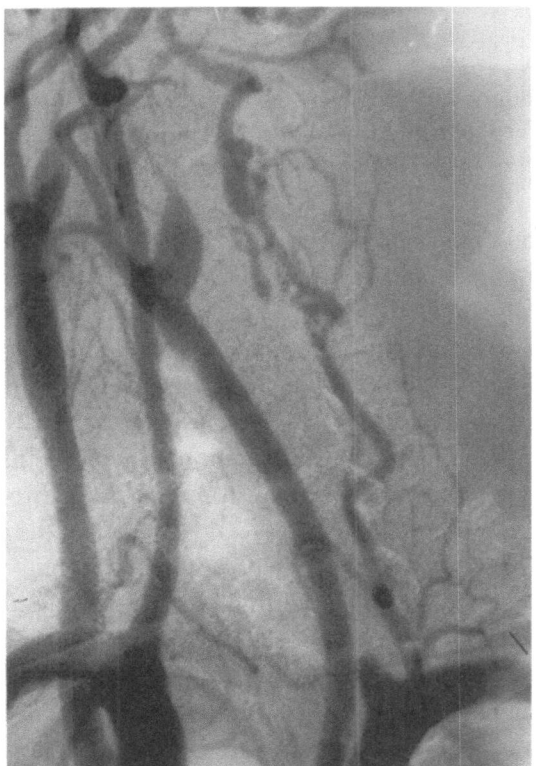

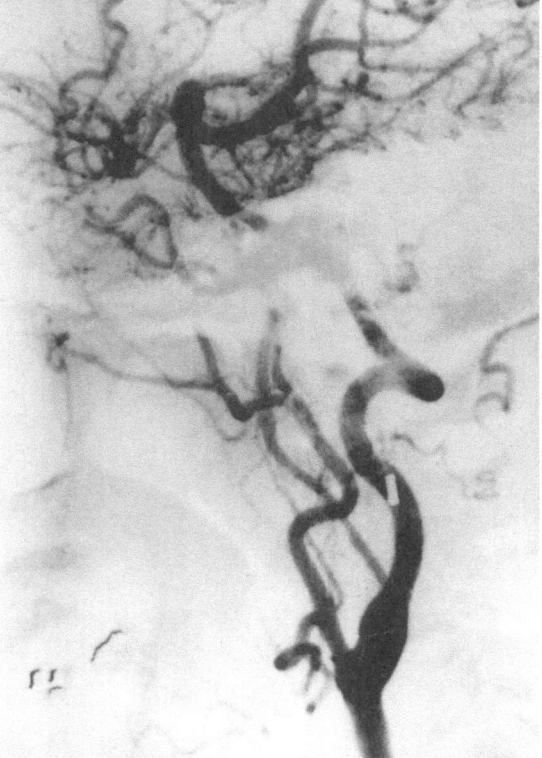

Figure 2.16 (Left) Aplasia of the left internal carotid artery with a normal-appearing carotid bulb. The proximal left vertebral artery was occluded acutely following a head-on automobile collision. At exploration the cervical internal carotid was reduced to thing fibrous cord. **(Right)** The distal vertebral artery was repaired by a bypass from the carotid bulb to the level of C1.

Posterior System (Vertebrobasilar Arteries)

Medical literature has given little detail to the anatomy of the VA. For this reason we have expanded our description of the anatomy of this artery to include relations relevant to understanding its pathology and to the operative techniques used for its reconstruction.

The VA arises from the posterosuperior wall of the SA and, after a short course at the base of the neck, enters the transverse process of the sixth cervical vertebra (Figure 2.17). This length constitutes its first segment. In its second segment the artery ascends in the cervical spine through the transverse process of each vertebra until it exits the foramen of C2. From there the artery curves outward to traverse the gap to

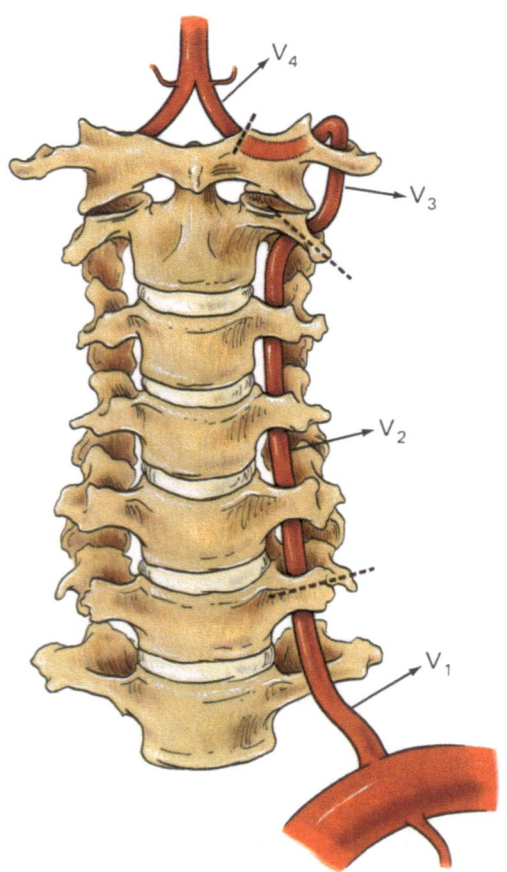

Figure 2.17 Relation of the vertebral artery and cervical spine. The dotted line indicates the level at which the vertebral artery becomes intradural.

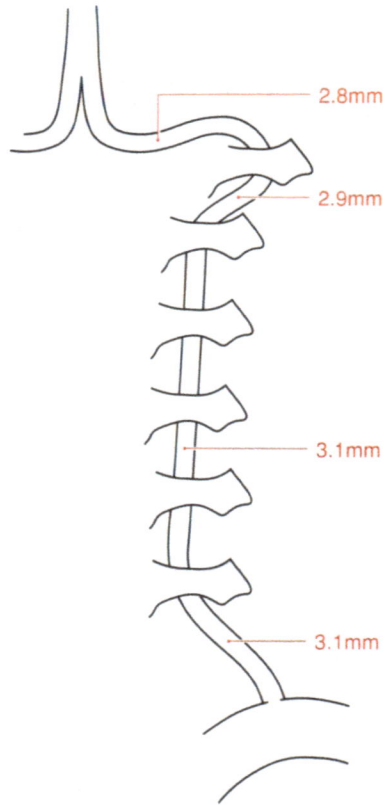

Figure 2.18 Segments of the VA and their dimensions. The diameter of the artery was measured in postmortem, nondistended arteries. (Data from Yates and Hutchinson.[47])

the transverse process of C1, passes through the C1 foramen, and curves back medially, nearly horizontally, in a bony groove of the posterior arch of the atlas to penetrate the atlantooccipital membrane. Conventionally, this point is at the end of its third segment. In its fourth segment the VA, after leaving the atlantooccipital membrane, has a short trajectory inside the rachis, becomes intradural as it passes through the occipital foramen, and ascends in front of the medulla oblongata to the lower end of the pons where it meets the opposite VA to form the basilar artery.

The trajectory of the VA from its origin to the basilar artery is approximately 25 cm in length. Its outside diameter is fairly constant throughout its course: about 5 mm. Figure 2.18 shows the postmortem measurements obtained by Yates and Hutchinson[47] from 100 undiseased VAs.

Vertebral arteries are often asymmetric, with

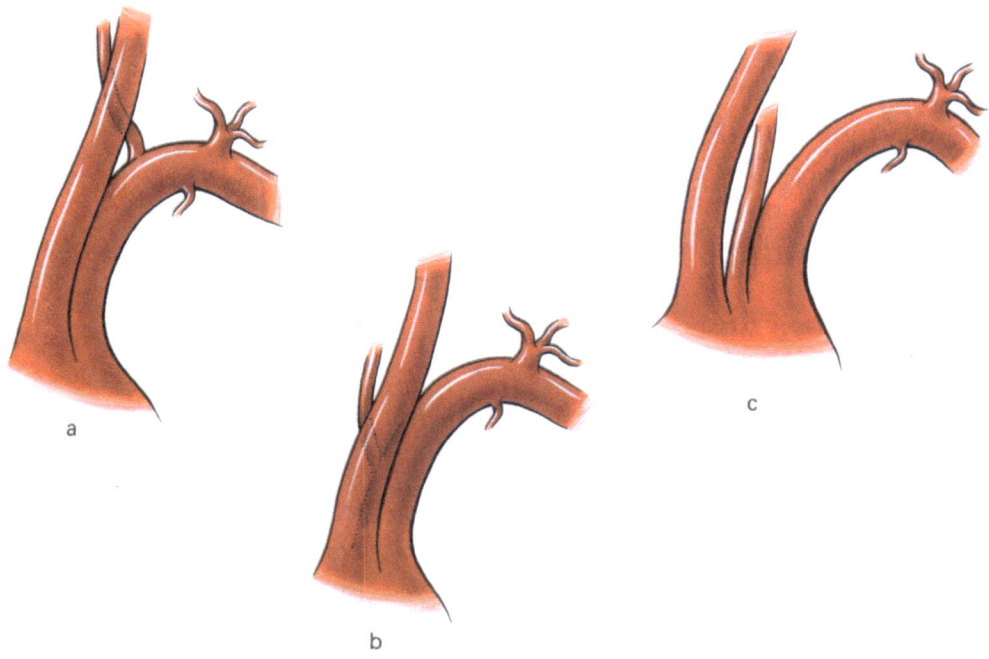

Figure 2.19 The three levels of origin for the left vertebral artery: **(a)** Normal, **(b)** Intrathoracic, **(c)** Aortic arch.

the left side more frequently the larger one. In about 7% of individuals one VA is hypoplastic; it is missing part of its fourth segment and terminates in the posterior inferior cerebellar artery.

In 6% of individuals the VA enters the cervical spine at C7. In another 6% the level of entry into the transverse foramen is at C5 or C4. The most common anomaly of origin (7% of the population) is a left-sided VA arising directly from the aorta. In such cases the artery may enter the cervical spine at the C5 or C4 level. As one might expect, the VA may arise from the left SA at any level between the arch and its normal expected level (Figure 2.19). Vertebral arteries taking origin from the IA or from the CCA are rare, the latter always occurring in association with a retro-esophageal SA (Figure 2.20). Another rare VA anomaly is the bifid origin (Figure 2.21). The extra limb takes origin from the SA or from the arch of the aorta. Both limbs converge into a single trunk before entering the cervical spine.

Normally, the *first segment* of the VA, which lies between the scalenus anticus and the longus colli, has no branches. In rare exceptions one of the vessels

normally arising from the thyrocervical trunk may exit the VA at this level. This first segment of the artery measures approximately 3 to 5 cm in length.

Throughout most of its cervical course the VA is in close relation with its accompanying vein(s). In the first segment, however, a single vertebral vein overlies the artery.

On the left side, the thoracic duct crosses the VA at a superficial level as it emerges behind the carotid to empty into the jugulosubclavian venous confluent. In a deeper plane, the inferior thyroid artery crosses both the VA and the vein toward the end of the first segment of the VA.

Shortly after its origin the VA enters into a relation with the cervical sympathetic chain (Figure 2.22). Variations in the configuration of the lower cervical ganglion and imprecise anatomic nomenclature have been the source of some confusion about this relation. Of the three sympathetic ganglia (superior, middle, and inferior), the position of the middle one is the most variable. It may lie above or below the transverse process of C6. The lower-lying middle ganglion is less common and is often referred to in the

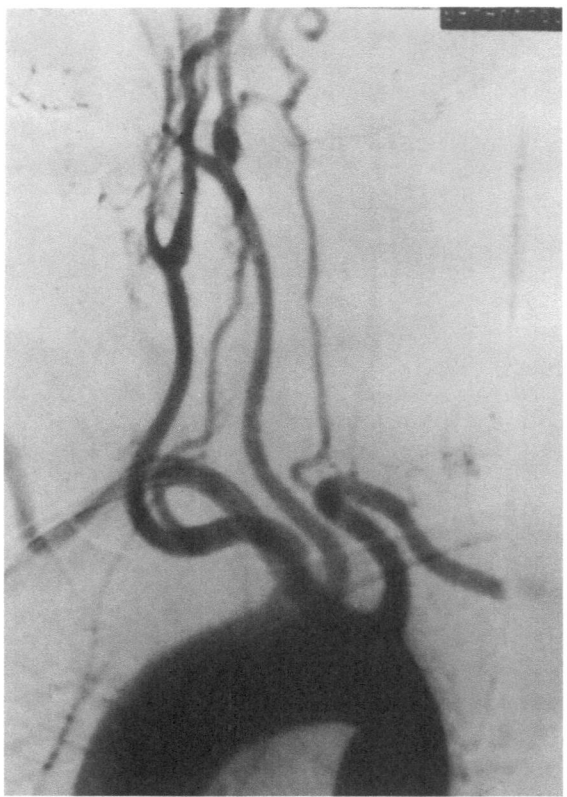

Figure 2.20 Abnormal origin of the vertebral artery from a right common carotid artery in a patient with a retroesophageal right subclavian artery.

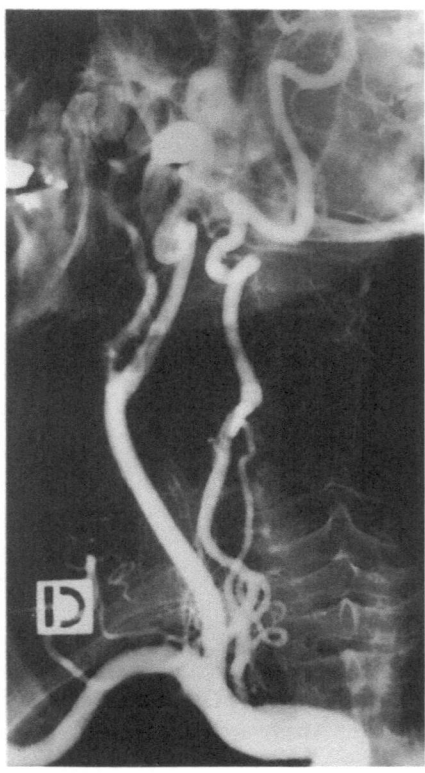

Figure 2.21 Bifid origin of a right vertebral artery from two sites of the right subclavian artery. There is also an abnormal entrance of the vertebral artery at the level of C4 resulting in a localized dissection (arrow).

literature as the "intermediate ganglion." This low-lying ganglion is the one that we find associated with the first segment of the VA in about one-third of cases. The upper ganglion is the largest. The lower ganglion is usually (80% of cases) fused with the first thoracic ganglion and then called the stellate ganglion. The stellate ganglion usually lies over the first thoracic costo-vertebral joint. It is close to the origin of the vertebral artery, most often medial or anteromedial to the takeoff of the VA from the SA. The average distance[48] between the lower pole of the middle ganglion and the upper pole of the stellate ganglion is a mere 15 mm.

In the most common situation (Figure 2.23) the chain, as it leaves the middle ganglion, crosses the inferior thyroid artery at C7 and splits in front of and behind the VA to reach the stellate ganglion. There is an additional twig connecting the middle and stellate ganglia that passes in front of the SA and is called the ansa subclavia.

The fibers that form the vertebral nerve make their exit from the lower cervical ganglion and from the intermediate ganglion. The vertebral nerve adjacent to the posterior wall of the VA accompanies the artery through its foraminal course up to the C2–C1 level. This nerve thins out as the artery ascends in the neck and sends connecting rami to the cervical spinal nerves where the latter exit the vertebrae. The vertebral nerve with its rami is a sympathetic pathway to the somatic cervical nerves that avoids the regular sympathetic route. This situation implies that an anatomically complete sympathetic denervation of the upper extremity and neck requires interruption of the intermediate cervical ganglion and the vertebral nerve, as well as of the two upper thoracic ganglia.

There is also a neural plexus around the VA contiguous with the subclavian plexus and receiving rami from cervical nerves, the vertebral nerve, and the middle cervical sympathetic ganglion. This plexus is thin at the origin of the VA but becomes dense in the distal portion of the artery, where it blends with the plexus surrounding the basilar artery. It is similar to the periarterial nervous plexus found around the mesenteric arteries.

The *second segment* of the VA extends from C6 to the top of the C2 foramen. In this segment the artery travels in a tunnel composed alternately of bony walls (transverse foramina) and muscular walls (anterior and posterior intertransversarium muscles). At each vertebral level (Figure 2.24) the artery crosses and rests on the anterior ramus of each cervical root, often leaving a small, visible impression on the nerve. The

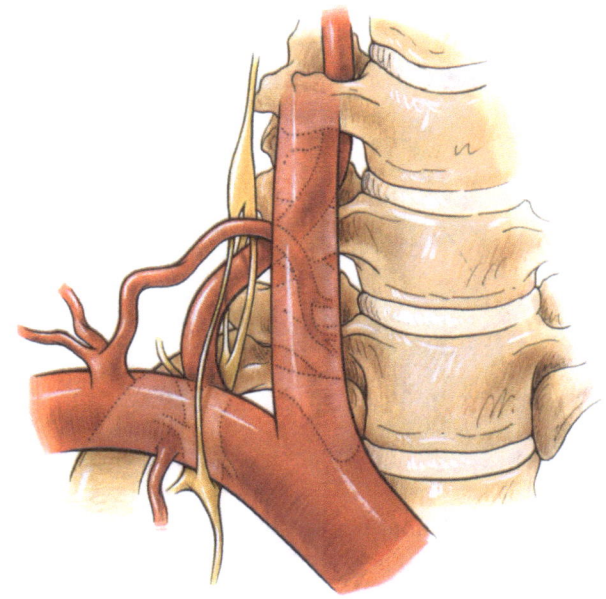

Figure 2.23 Intermediate and stellate ganglia and the first segment of the vertebral artery. The ansa subclavia connects the stellate and middle ganglia in front of the subclavian artery.

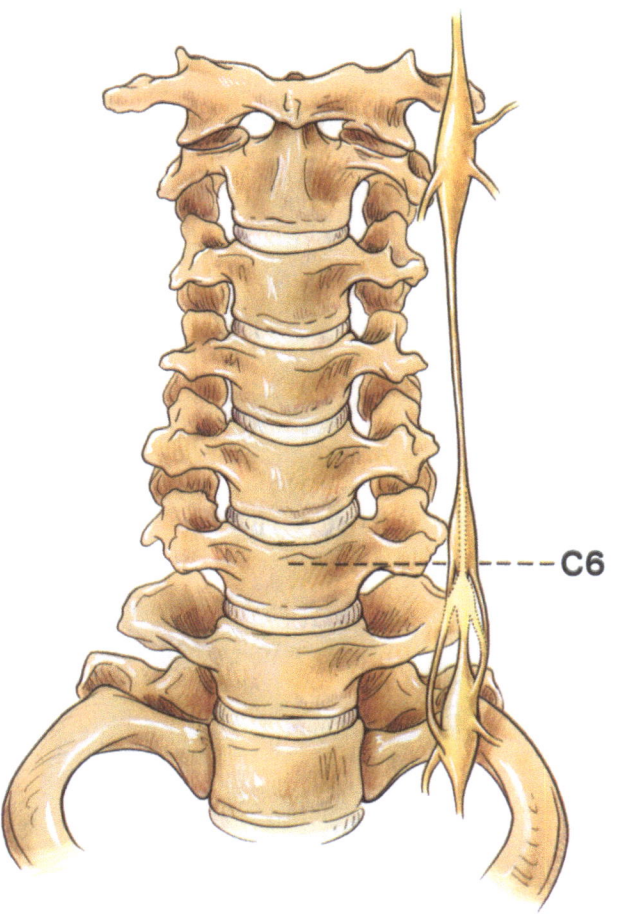

Figure 2.22 Relations of the cervical spine to the sympathetic chain. The middle ganglion may be above or below (colored in light yellow) the transverse process of C6. In the latter case it is often called an "intermediate ganglion."

VA is enveloped by a vertebral venous plexus that, like the artery, adheres to the periosteum of the adjacent bone. At each vertebral level the VA supplies branches to the muscles of the spine, the ligaments and joints of the cervical vertebrae, the vertebral bodies, the meningeal cover of the spine, and the nerve roots. The latter, called radicular arteries, send some radiculomedullary branches to the spinal cord. Some of the latter regress during adult life. Branches of the SA (cervical ascending artery) provide additional arterial "twigs" to the nerve roots and occasionally to the spinal cord. The cervical intervertebral connections (Figure 2.25) that run in front of and behind the vertebral bodies link the two vertebral arteries like the steps of a ladder.

The *third* (suboccipital) *segment* of the VA begins at the exit of the transverse foramen of C2 and ends at the atlantooccipital membrane. The segment of VA between C2 and C1 is the longest between any of the transverse processes. The orifice of C1 is more lateral than that of C2, which sets the artery into an oblique course. In addition, the gap between the transverse processes of C1 and C2 is the widest in the

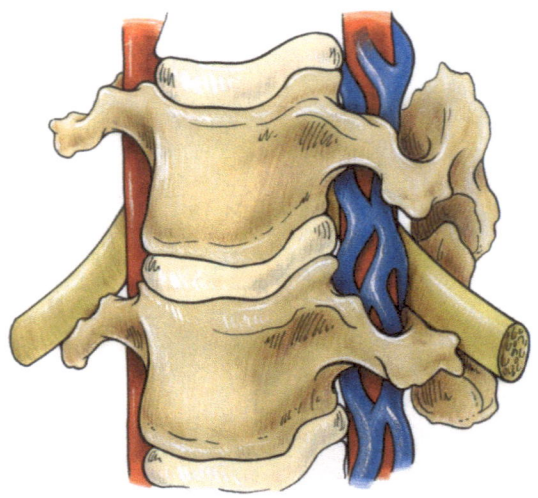

Figure 2.24 Relations between the vertebral artery, vertebrae, and nerve roots in the second segment of the VA (C6–C2).

cervical spine. Finally, the VA is slightly redundant in this segment to allow for the exceptional rotational mobility of the atlantoaxial joint.

In the C2–C1 space the relation between the artery and the anterior ramus of the C2 nerve is different in that the nerve ramus crosses over and closely cinches the artery, whereas in the other cervical segments the root is posterior to the VA. In the C1–C2 interspace segment the artery is also surrounded by veins, although this venous plexus does not cover the surface of the artery as completely as in the lower interspaces. Conversely, the venous plexus surrounding the VA above C1, the suboccipital plexus, is the most dense in the entire course of the VA.

In its third segment, usually as it emerges from the transverse process of C2, the VA receives one or more important anastomotic collaterals from the occipital artery. In cases of occlusion of the second segment of the VA, this occipital anastomosis usually keeps the distal VA patent (Figure 2.26). Less frequently the arterial connection between the occipital and the VA takes place at the C1 or C3 level (Figure 2.27). A branch from the cervical ascending artery may also supply the distal VA at this level. This collateral supply to the distal VA makes possible surgical reconstruction of the artery at this level in cases where its first and second segments are occluded. The occipital contribution to the distal VA is

a prominent feature of the normal anatomy in dogs,[49] where the larger vessel resulting from the fusion of the VA and of the branch from the occipital artery is called the cerebrospinal artery.

Emerging from the transverse process of C1, the artery travels in a bony groove in the posterior arch of the atlas, where it is enveloped by a rich venous plexus and covered by short, deep muscles, making surgical access difficult. The posterior arch of the atlas may form a bony roof over the VA, which is then completely encircled by bone. Rarely, the lateral mass of the atlas does not have a foramen for the VA, in which case the artery loops around the transverse process to regain its course over the posterior arch of the atlas (Figure 2.28).

After exiting the atlantooccipital membrane, the VA penetrates the dura mater, passes through the occipital foramen, and becomes intracranial as it ascends in front of the medulla oblongata to end at the

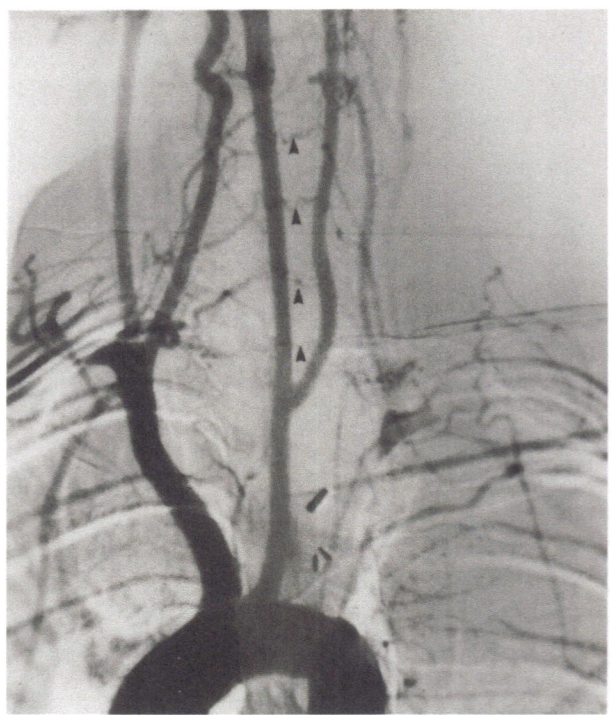

Figure 2.25 Cervical-intervertebral connections (arrowheads) in a young girl in whom the proximal subclavian artery was used as a patch to correct an aortic coarctation. The patient presented with a symptomatic subclavian steal that was corrected by transposition of the vertebral artery into the left common carotid artery.

Figure 2.26 Occipital connection of the vertebral artery. In this patient with an occluded internal carotid artery, the collaterals from the occipital artery fill the vertebral artery anterograde toward the basilar artery and retrogradely toward the base of the neck, where the vertebral artery is occluded.

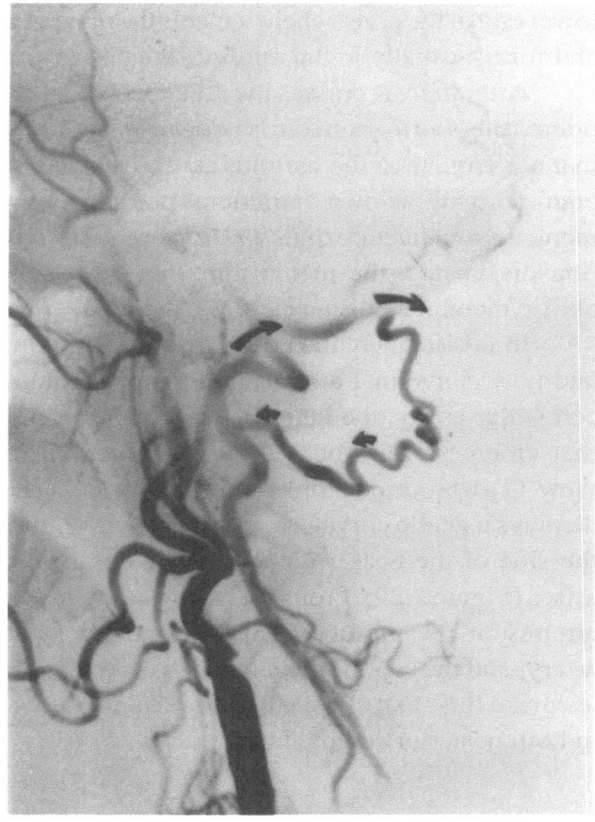

a

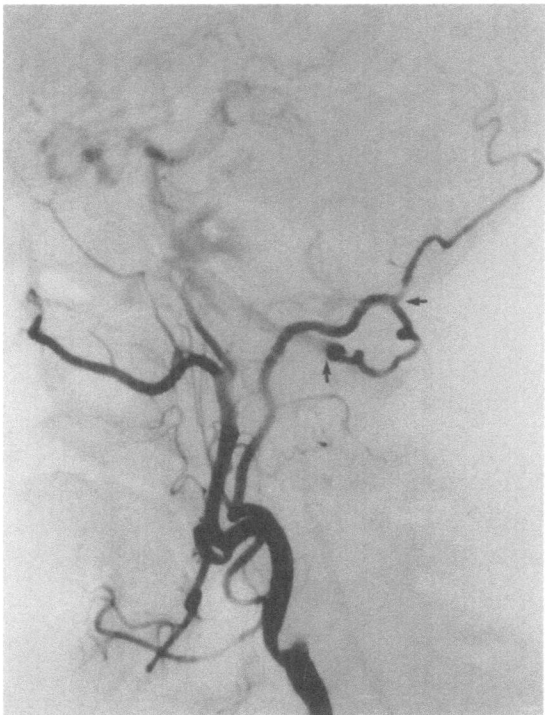

b

Figure 2.27 (a) Occipital collateral may enter the vertebral artery at the level of C1, as seen in this selective external carotid injection. **(b)** The importance of the occipital collateral is seen in this patient with an occluded internal carotid.

lower end of the pons, where it meets the opposite VA and forms, usually in the midline, the basilar trunk.

After the VA crosses the atlantooccipital membrane, the *fourth* (intradural) *segment* begins. In a manner similar to the carotid, as the VA enters the cranium, with its own extramural pressure environment, the architecture of its wall changes. The adventitia disappears, the media thins, and the external elastic membrane disappears.

In this segment the artery gives off the anterior and posterior spinal arteries and the posteroinferior cerebellar artery, the latter being the largest branch that emerges from the VA. In the anteroposterior view (Towne projection) the basilar artery usually displays a gentle curvature with its concavity toward the side of the neck from where the dominant VA arises (Figure 2.29). From the basilar artery itself, the arteries of the protuberance, the internal auditory artery, and the superior and anterior cerebellar arteries make their exit. Typically, the basilar artery ends in both posterior cerebral arteries.

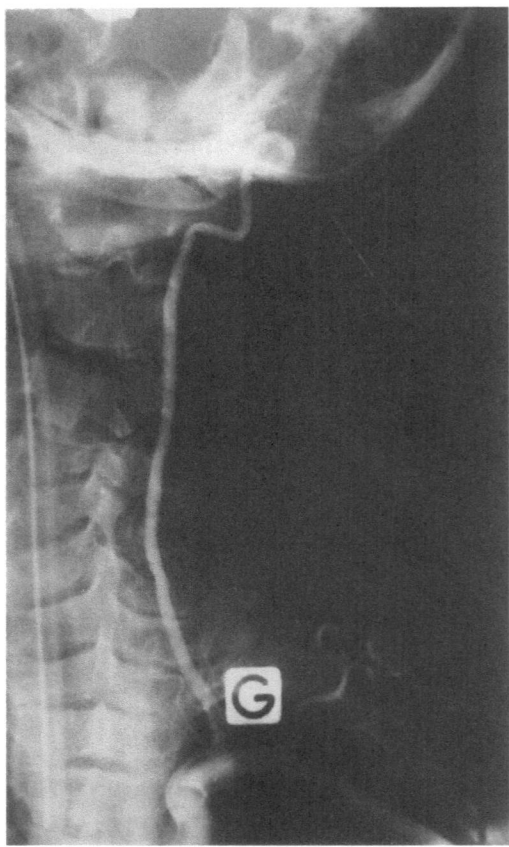

Figure 2.28 Imperforation of the transverse foramen of C1 with the vertebral artery looping around it.

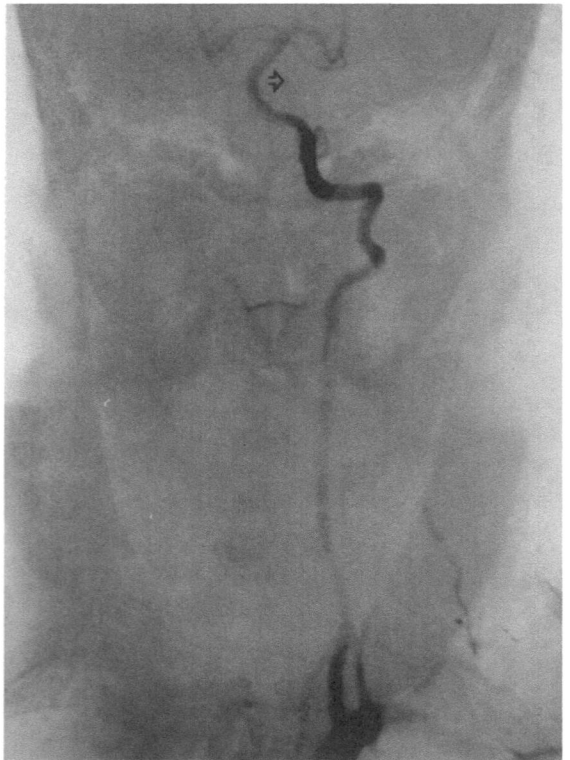

Figure 2.29 Curvature of the basilar artery opens toward the side of the dominant vertebral artery.

Failsafe System (External Carotid Arteries)

The ECA is the smaller of the two branches into which the CCA bifurcates. It supplies the face, neck, scalp, and important meningeal arteries. The ECA has connections to both ICA and VA circulations. Some of its branches share territory with branches of the SA.

As with most muscular arteries the pattern of branching of the ECA is variable. It is beyond our scope, however, to list the many variations that can be found. Because of the rich connections it has with the ICA and VA systems, the ECA is a functional network that can, in specific circumstances, supply either system with blood. The main branches of the ECA (Figure 2.30) are as follows.

1. *Superior thyroid artery*, which may arise as the first branch of the ECA or from the terminal portion of the CCA. Beyond its origin the artery is in close relation to the external branch of the superior laryngeal nerve. Rarely, this nerve branch crosses over the superior thyroid artery at its origin.

2. *Ascending pharyngeal artery*, which gives small branches to the meninges where they anastomose with others coming from the petrosal and cavernous ICA. The origin of the ascending pharyngeal artery may be as low as the flow divider at the bifurcation or may even be a branch of the ICA. Such low origin may result in annoying back-bleeding during carotid endarterectomy after the three components of the carotid bifurcation have been clamped away from the bifurcation, missing the ascending pharyngeal artery. This artery can also connect with the VA through muscular branches.

3. *Facial artery*, which connects, through its terminal branch (the angular artery), with the supraorbital artery, the latter a branch of the ophthalmic artery.

4. *Lingual artery*, which loops around the hypoglossal nerve.

5. *Occipital artery*, which sends important collateral branches to the VA at the C1–C3 level. The sternomastoid artery, which may originate directly from the ECA or may be a branch of the occipital artery, sometimes tents the hypoglossal nerve downward.

6. *Posterior auricular artery*.

7. *Superficial temporal artery*, which anastomoses, by means of the frontal artery, with the supraorbital branch of the ophthalmic artery.

8. *Internal maxillary artery*, which has important meningeal connections with the ICA through its branch, the middle meningeal artery. The vidian artery, another branch of the internal maxillary artery, connects with the ICA through the foramen lacerum. The internal maxillary artery has anastomoses to branches of the ophthalmic artery (ICA) through its infraorbital branch and through its sphenopalatine branches via the meningeal ethmoidal artery.

The ECA trunk is crossed by veins draining the face and tongue. Shortly after its takeoff, the ECA covers the superior laryngeal nerve medially and is crossed over by the hypoglossal nerve. Higher up the ECA slips under the digastric and stylohyoid muscles.

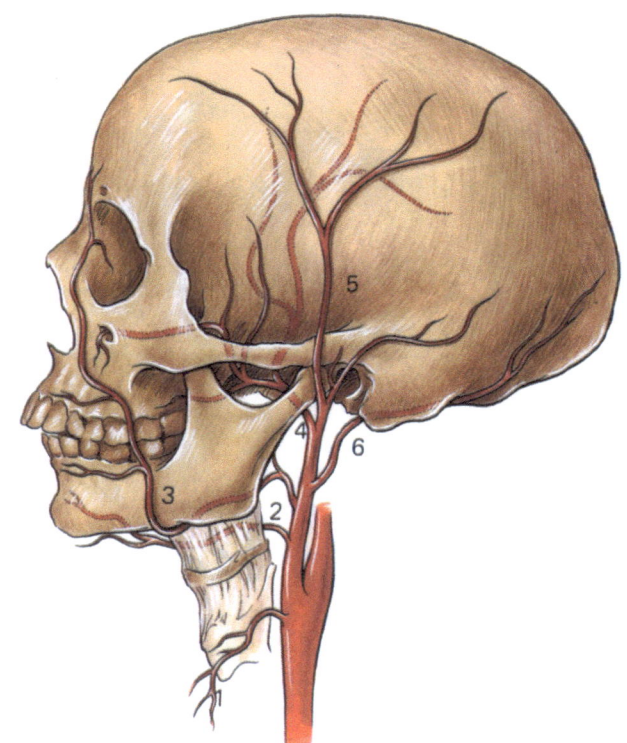

Figure 2.30 Main branches of the external carotid artery. 1, superior thyroid; 2, lingual; 3, facial; 4, internal maxillary; 5, superficial temporal; and 6, occipital.

The glossopharyngeal nerve crosses underneath the artery and medial to it. Higher up, the ECA gives off its two terminal branches, the superficial temporal and internal maxillary arteries close to its penetration into the parotid gland.

Intracranial and Extracranial Connections

Anomalous Persistence of Fetal Connections

Persisting fetal connections between the carotid and vertebral systems may function as an important anas-

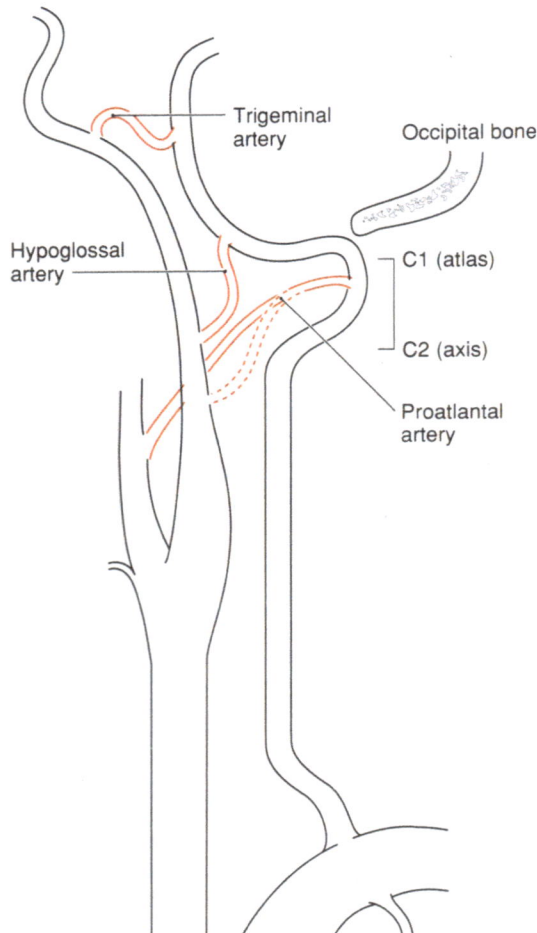

Figure 2.31 Fetal connections between the carotid and vertebrobasilar systems that may persist into adult life. The proatlantal artery may arise from the external or internal carotid arteries.

tomotic bridge between them. When these fetal communications persist, the VA does not develop to a normal size, and it is either small or incomplete; i.e., part of the fourth segment is missing. The persistent fetal connections seen in the adult are the trigeminal, hypoglossal, and proatlantal arteries (Figure 2.31). (An otic artery is often included among this family of anomalous vessels, but it is exceedingly rare, with some neuroradiologists doubting its existence.)

The *trigeminal artery* is the most common of these fetal connections that persists into adult life. It is seen in approximately 1 of 700 individuals. Its name derives from the fact that the intracranial course of this artery follows the sensory root of the trigeminal nerve. The trigeminal artery, which arises from the ICA as the latter enters the cavernous sinus, joins with the basilar artery (Figure 2.32). When there is persistence of these communications that supply the basilar artery, the latter may be hypoplastic proximal to the point of entrance of the abnormal communication or, more commonly, the VA on the side of the persistent trigeminal may be hypoplastic. Blood flows from the ICA to the basilar artery, and embolization of the basilar territory may occur through this abnormal communication during an operation on the ICA.

A *hypoglossal artery*, when present, arises from the cervical ICA anywhere from C1 to C3 and enters the posterior fossa through the anterior condyloid foramen accompanying the hypoglossal nerve. When a hypoglossal artery is present, one or both proximal VAs are hypoplastic, and the posterior communicating arteries are absent (Figures 2.33 and 2.34). A hypoglossal artery is suspected when one encounters a branch from the higher cervical ICA during dissection or when black-bleeding is noted from the ICA after distal clamping.

A persistent *proatlantal artery* connects the carotid and vertebrobasilar systems at the level of the atlas. It may arise from the ICA or ECA (Figure 2.31), and it joins the horizontal segment of the VA as the latter rests on the atlas. The ipsilateral VA is absent or hypoplastic. From a functional point of view this artery can be considered a VA taking origin in the internal or external carotid arteries. We have operated on a patient with severe vertebrobasilar symptoms

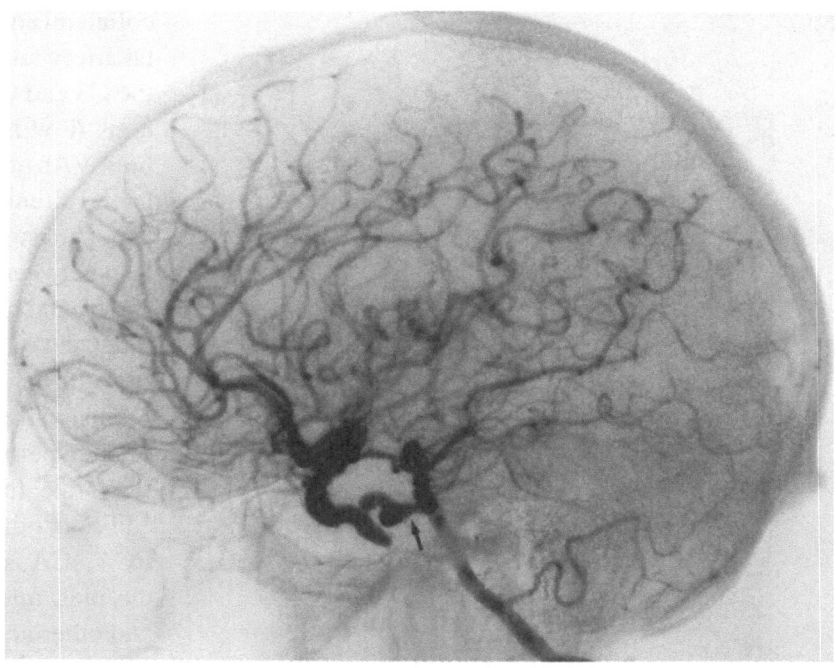

Figure 2.32 Persistent trigeminal artery (arrow). In this patient with an occluded internal carotid artery, the trigeminal artery and to a lesser extent the posterior communicating artery supply the anterior circulation.

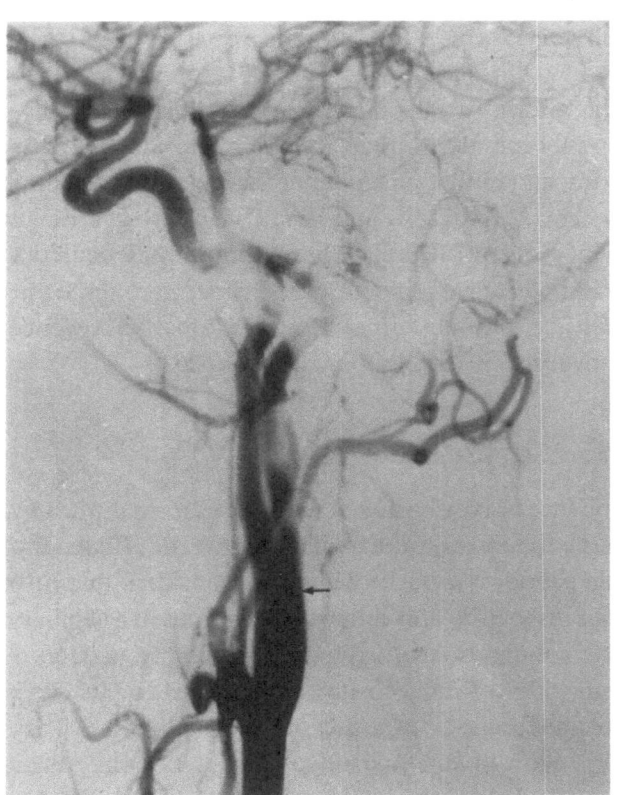

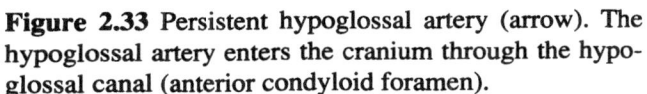

Figure 2.33 Persistent hypoglossal artery (arrow). The hypoglossal artery enters the cranium through the hypoglossal canal (anterior condyloid foramen).

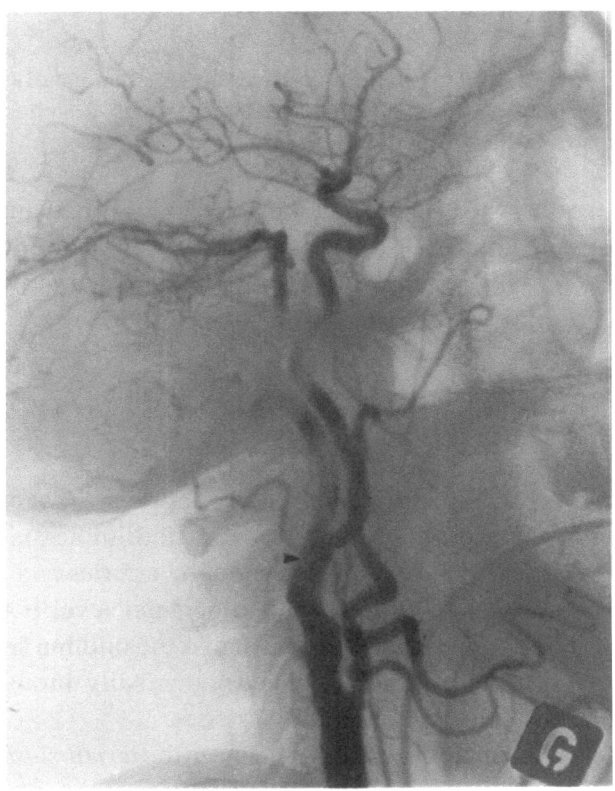

Figure 2.34 Persistent hypoglossal artery (arrrowhead) in this patient resulted in embolization of the vertebrobasilar territory from the ulceration of the internal carotid bulb.

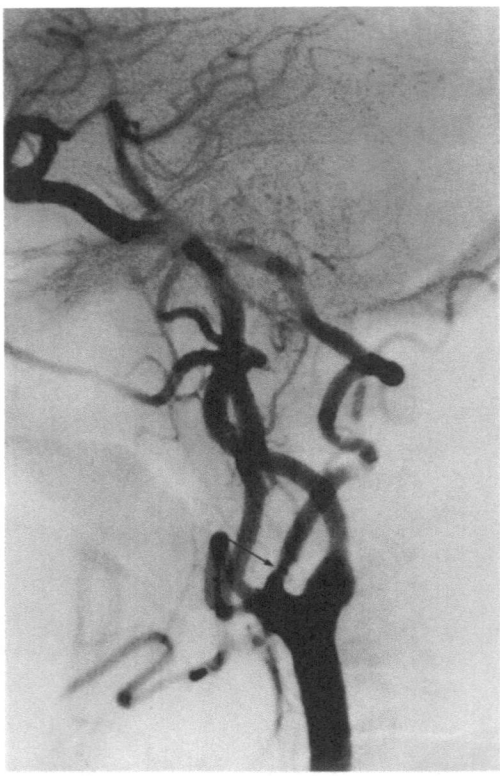

Figure 2.35 This patient with vertebrobasilar insufficiency had a persistent proatlantal artery with a stenosis (arrow) at its origin.

secondary to a stenosis at the takeoff of a proatlantal artery (Figure 2.35). The proximal vertebral arteries were hypoplastic. Symptoms disappeared after an angioplasty of the proatlantal artery origin.

Collateral Pathways and Intertruncal Connections

The most important connections between the *right and left arterial systems* occurs at the intracranial level at the junction of both vertebral arteries and at the circle of Willis. At the extracranial level both ECA territories communicate across the midline and both vertebral arteries are linked segmentally through the intervertebral connecting arteries.

The main connections between the *territories of the internal carotid and basilar arteries* at the intracranial level are the posterior communicating arteries and the posterior loop of the circle of Willis. The ECA and the VA are also connected through one or more

collateral anastomoses occurring between the occipital artery and the distal VA, usually at C2 but also at the C3 and C1 levels. This collateral pathway maintains flow into the distal and basilar arteries when both VAs are occluded. It becomes an essential collateral circuit when both VAs and ICAs are occluded.

Anastomosis through collateral pathways exist also between the ECA and ICA through the angular and frontal branches of the former and the ophthalmic branches of the latter. These anastomoses preserve flow through the supraclinoid ICA by retrograde perfusion through the ophthalmic artery. The latter is often hypertrophic as a consequence of the increased flow rate through it (Figure 2.36). There are, in addition, other smaller pathways communicating the ECA, ICA, and VA territories, including branches of the pial, middle meningeal, ascending pharyngeal, and other arteries.

Flow Patterns in Aortic Arch Branches

The arterial trunks supplying the head travel in a parallel bundle through the neck and are linked by extra- and intracranial connections between the three systems: ICA, ECA, and VA. This network arrangement protects the brain when a major trunk occludes. Within this arrangement we consider here three normal and one abnormal flow patterns: divergence, convergence, oscillation, and reversal.

Flow Divergence

The successive division of the arteries from the heart to the periphery follows a fractal pattern. The efficiency of this pattern is evident when one considers that most cells in the body are within a few microns of a capillary. The volume of such an extensive supply network is surprisingly small, occupying only 3% of the body volume for the arterial side of the circulation.

Flow divergence, or splitting, takes place at the exit of every arterial branch and at bifurcations. The amount of flow going into each branch is determined by the peripheral resistance of the territory supplied by each branch and the geometry of the bifurcation.

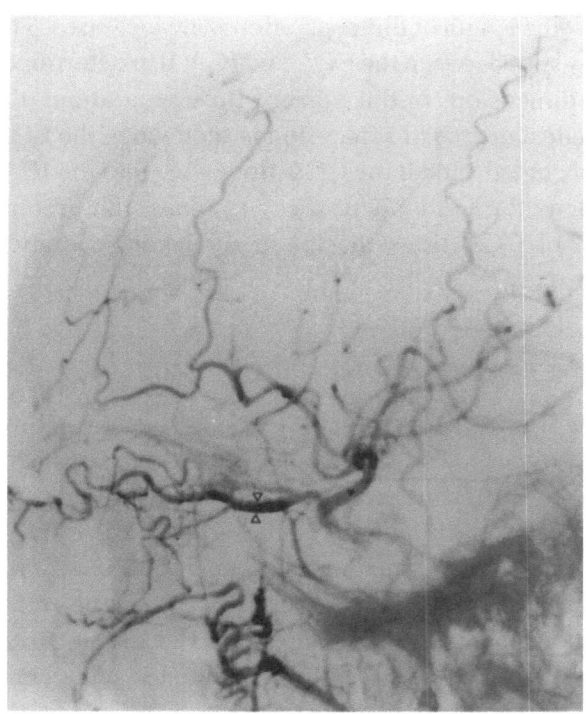

Figure 2.36 Hypertrophic ophthalmic artery (between markers) shunts blood from the external carotid artery to the distal internal carotid artery. The proximal internal carotid artery is occluded.

The general principles governing flow through bifurcations can be studied in simple models that permit isolation and ranking of the variables involved. In these models flow can be considered laminar, with both branches having an identical diameter and the territory supplied by each branch having the same peripheral resistance. Under these circumstances and using a continuity equation, establishing the most efficient geometry for a bifurcation is a straightforward proposition.

An important characteristic of a bifurcation is the ratio of the cross-sectional area of its branches to that of the trunk. This ratio

$$\beta = \frac{2A_1}{A_0}$$

(where A_0 = cross-sectional area of trunk; A_1 = cross-sectional area of each branch) for bifurcations with equal branches determines whether the vascular bed

expands or contracts at a bifurcation and therefore determines the changes in velocity and pressure that will take place in its branches. (Despite its significance the value of β has been disregarded in most commercially available bifurcated arterial prostheses.) From Poiseuille's law, which is applicable to the conditions set above and a continuity equation, it can be shown[50] that for the pressure gradient to remain the same in the trunk as in the branches β must equal $\sqrt{2}$ (~1.4). If it is less than that, as in the case for the first branchings of the supraaortic trunks (β ~1.1), pressure will drop as flow enters the branches of a bifurcation. The value of β increases as the arteries approach the periphery, reaching a value of $\beta = 6$ in some precapillary beds. This expansion of the vascular bed causes considerable slowing of the velocity of the blood.

The β ratio also determines the amount of wave reflection that takes place in a bifurcation. As pressure waves progressing toward the periphery encounter waves reflected back from a bifurcation, a set of nodes and antinodes develops that may result in large pressure fluctuations and cause considerable stresses in the arterial wall. It can be experimentally calculated that, for the bifurcation of the terminal aorta, wave reflection is minimal when $\beta = 1.15$.[51] This is the value found in infants. By age 40 the value of β has already dropped to 0.7.

At bifurcations (and at the takeoff of major branches), important flow changes may determine the localization of atherosclerotic disease. High shear stresses develop on the wall of the flow divider, whereas flow separation and lowshear are found on the opposite wall. In the supraaortic trunks atheroma is most often found at the site of these abnormal flow patterns, where vessels bifurcate at an angle from a trunk. The most notable case of flow divergence in the neck vessels takes place at the carotid bifurcation.

Investigators have looked for mechanical explanations of the prevalent localization of atheroma in the carotid bulb, usually in its posterior aspect opposite to the takeoff of the ECA. The stream of blood in the posterior wall of the CCA curves posteriorly as it enters the bulb. Approximately 70% of the volume flow in the CCA travels up the ICA. In the bulb, this split stream expands to fill a dilation (the bulb) whose diameter is equal to or larger than that of the terminal portion of the CCA. This sudden expansion of the lumen and the change in the direction of flow results in separation of the stream boundary and in the appearance of reverse flow near the wall.[51] Eddies appear in this low-shear area of separation (Figure 2.37).

This phenomenon, which can be seen in flow models, can be demonstrated in human carotid arteries with ultrasonic duplex systems that sample velocity signals from this discrete area. It is suspected that platelet aggregates form in these eddies, but the precise mechanism by which these platelet aggregates contribute to the formation of atheroma is not known. The height (i.e., its intraluminal projection) and the length of the zone of boundary layer separation and recirculation of flow depend on the geometry of the bifurcation and the flow conditions present. At higher flows, as indicated by higher Reynolds numbers, the length of this separation zone increases. The flow split between the ECA and ICA also determines the dimensions of this zone of flow separation: the smallest degree of separation is seen when the ECA is occluded and all the CCA flow goes into the ICA. When the ECA siphons away a substantial proportion of CCA flow, the boundary layer separation increases.

Flow Convergence

The arterial supply to the head also shows flow convergence. The arrangement of two arteries converging into a single one, as seen in the vertebrobasilar confluent, is unique in the arterial anatomy of humans. In this situation the sum of the cross-sectional areas of the two VAs is greater than the cross-sectional area of the basilar artery. Because the total cross section decreases, flow accelerates at the junction as it enters the basilar artery.

This acceleration, however, does not destabilize the flow pattern. McDonald[50] studied this flow convergence in the rabbit. By injecting india ink into one VA he could see through the quasitransparent walls of the vertebrobasilar junction that the dyed stream from one VA remained mostly unmixed with the undyed flow from the opposite VA throughout the length of the basilar artery. The calculated Reynolds number for flow in the basilar artery was only about 100, too low for turbulence to develop. It is highly unlikely that, in humans, the Reynolds number would approach anywhere near 1000 where full turbulence would be expected. These separate streams from each VA are seen in humans in selective arteriograms of a VA: The contribution of each VA remains relatively unmixed (Figure 2.38), and the basilar artery appears thinner than it is because only one-half of its lumen contains dyed blood.

A rare anatomic curiosity, a VA with a double origin converging into a single trunk, is another instance of flow convergence (Figure 2.21). Higher up in the circle of Willis, flow convergence also takes place as the communicating arteries balance the perfusion differences that may exist at the end of the carotid and basilar arteries.

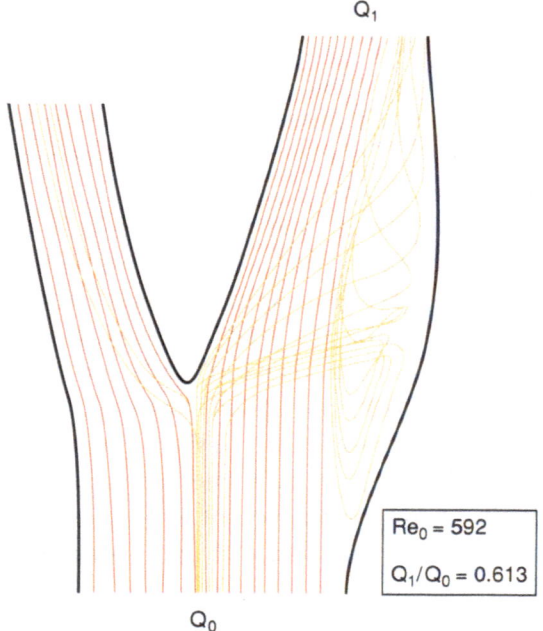

Q_1

$Re_0 = 592$

$Q_1/Q_0 = 0.613$

Q_0

Figure 2.37 Flow patterns in a model of the bifurcation of the common carotid artery. Q_0 and Q_1 represent volume flow through the common and internal carotid arteries, respectively. Re = Reynolds number. (Redrawn from Motomiya and Karino.[52])

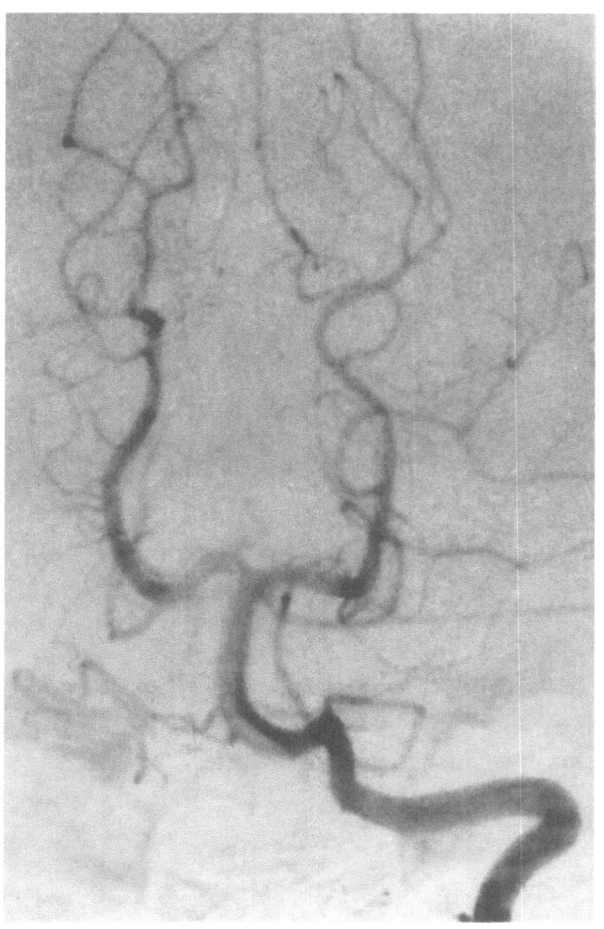

Figure 2.38 Streaming of dye in the basilar artery after selective injection of one vertebral artery may give the appearance of a diminution of caliber in the former.

Flow Oscillation

The direction of flow may alternate in certain boundary areas. The most obvious is the point about the circle of Willis where the carotid and basilar flows meet. As the head and neck go through their range of motion, the inflow through the carotid and vertebral arteries changes (see Chapter 4), and a decrease in flow in one artery is compensated by an increase in the other. The pressures in the terminal carotid and basilar arteries change, as does the point where the flow streams meet. In the presence of VA occlusion (or temporary compression) the injection of dye in the CCA during arteriography may result in opacification of the basilar artery (via the posterior communicating

artery) down to its mid portion. Conversely, with temporary or chronic ICA occlusion, flow from the basilar artery may be seen supplying the anterior or middle cerebral arteries via the posterior communicating artery. Naturally, a complete and well-developed circle of Willis facilitates the movement of this boundary into the carotid or basilar artery territory. The anatomy of the circle of Willis also determines into which territory this boundary moves when compensation of flow is needed. For instance, during hypotension of a carotid system (during clamping of an ICA) in a patient without an anterior communicating artery, a large posterior communicating artery preferentially perfuses the ipsilateral middle cerebral artery with flow from the basilar artery.

Flow Reversal

A third pattern of flow, observed under abnormal conditions, is the reversal of VA blood flow better known as the "subclavian steal." Here, blockage in the first portion of the SA causes the pressure in the second portion to drop below that existing in the vertebrobasilar junction. As a consequence, VA flow is reversed and feeds into the SA to supply the arm (Figures 2.39 and 2.40). The opposite VA is the main contributor to this retrograde flow, but some forward flow continues to supply the basilar artery. As a result, most patients have no symptoms from this reversal of flow in one VA. In a few patients the volume of blood siphoned away from the basilar artery is substantial and results in vertebrobasilar ischemic symptoms.

With the progressive development of SA or IA stenosis that eventually results in a steal, there is a point at which the pressure gradient between the top and bottom of the VA is large enough to reverse the flow but only during the peak of the systolic phase. As the pressure drops to its diastolic level, the pressure differential between the top of the VA and the SA decreases or does not exist at all. This situation results in another form of oscillating flow, the "intermittent steal." Here the reversal of blood flow is temporary and occurs only during part of the systole.

A much rarer reversal of flow may take place when the IA is occluded and the flow in the CCA, and

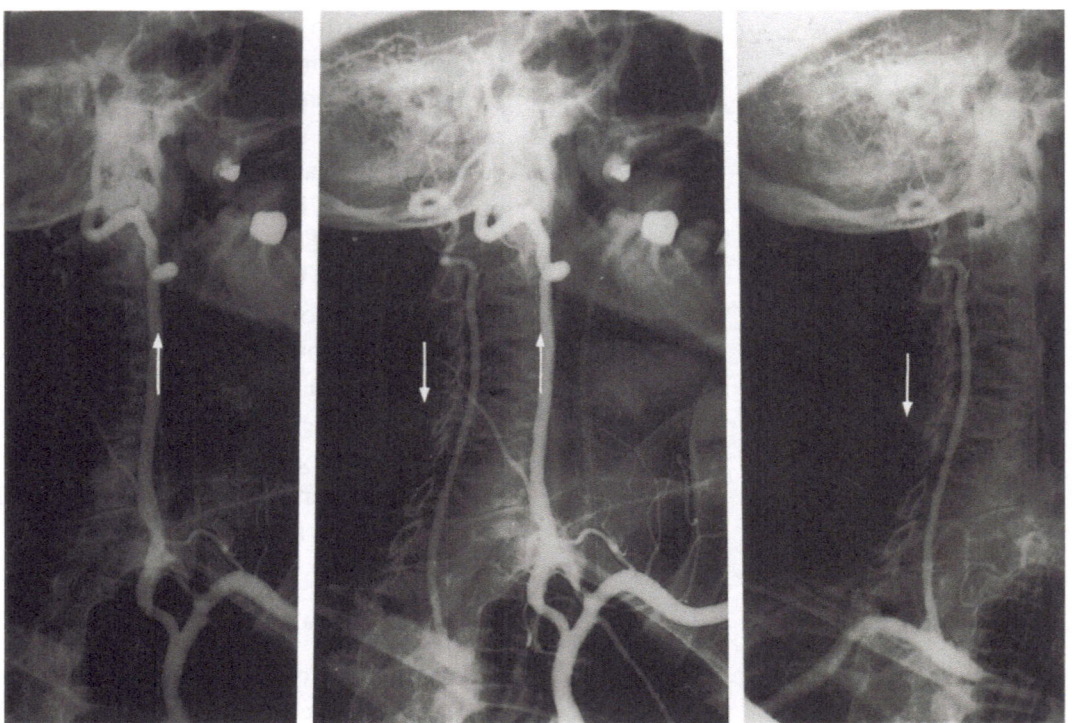

Figure 2.39 Right subclavian steal secondary to occlusion of the first segment of this artery.

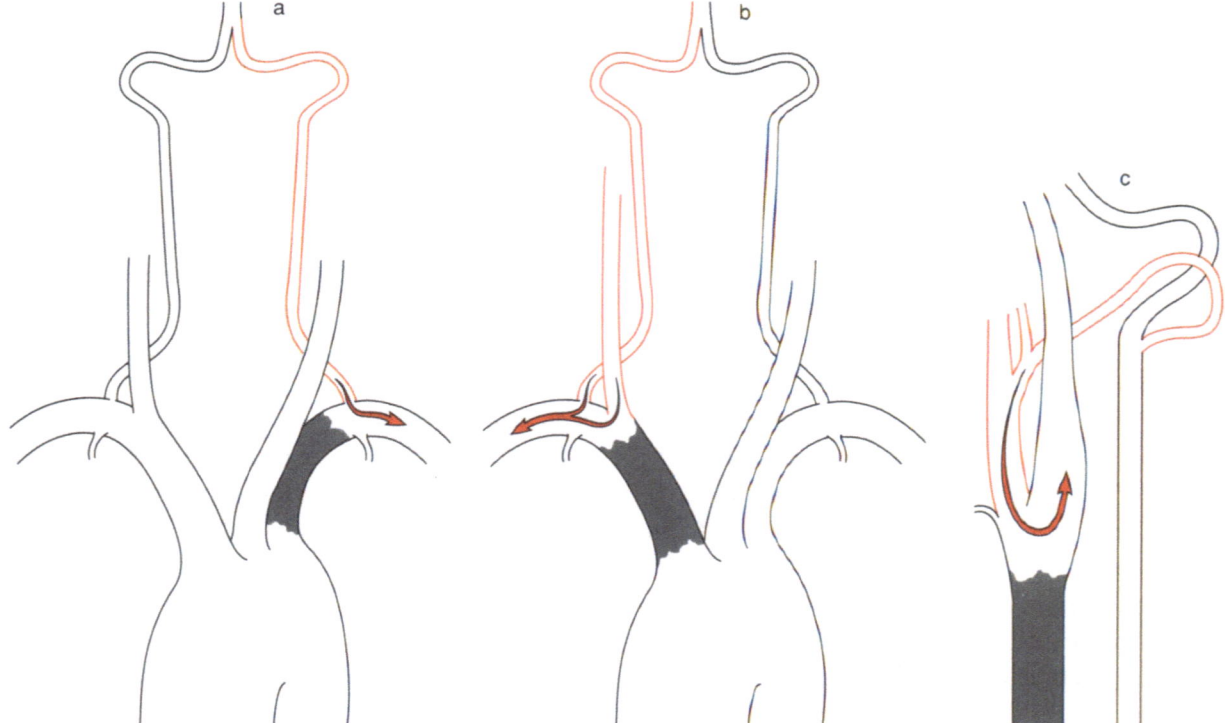

Figure 2.40 Three patterns of flow reversal. (**a**) Subclavian steal distal to an occluded subclavian artery. (**b**) Reversal of flow in the carotid and vertebral arteries distal to an occluded innominate artery (innominate steal). (**c**) Reversal of flow in the occipital artery and proximal external carotid distal to an occluded common carotid artery (carotid steal).

Figure 2.41 In this patient with occluded common and internal carotid arteries, blood is shunted from the vertebral artery via the occipital artery into the external carotid artery territory. The territory of the internal carotid artery is supplied by the posterior communicating artery.

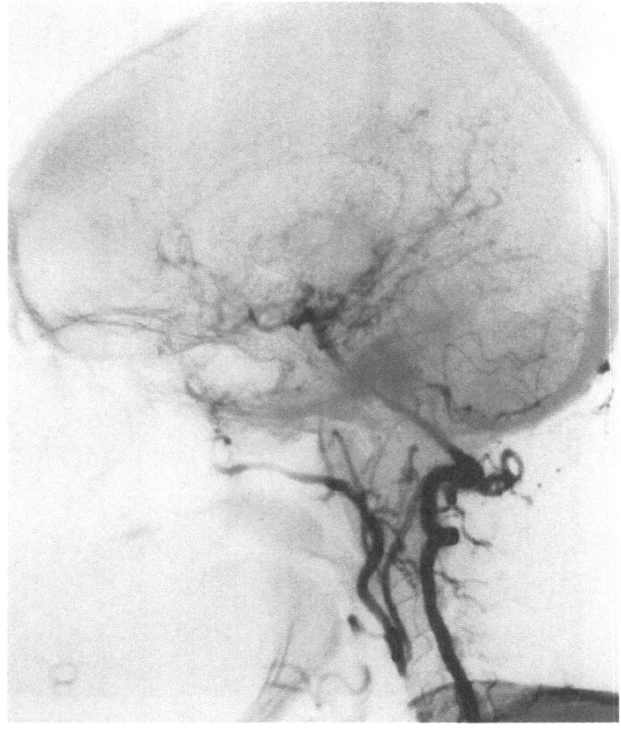

sometimes in the VA, is reversed to supply the subclavian territory (Figure 2.40). Here, with the flow in one ICA reversed, there is greater potential for substantial brain ischemia.

The branches of the occipital artery that anastomose the ECA and VA systems may supply the distal bed of either vessel whose origin is occluded. If the CCA becomes occluded (Figure 2.40) the occipital artery derives blood from the VA and carries reversed flow into the ECA and to the carotid bifurcation, from which point flow progresses normally into the other branches of the ECA (Figure 2.41) and into the ICA if the latter is patent. This reversal of flow in the branches of the ECA is also seen in individuals who have an occluded ECA origin, usually caused by a technical flaw during endarterectomy of the carotid bifurcation. In this circumstance the occipital artery brings reversed flow from the VA to supply the territory of the ECA.

When the proximal VA is occluded, the ipsilateral ECA supplies flow to the distal VA segment through occipital anastomoses that enter the VA at the level of C2. In some cases not only the distal but also the proximal VA, down to the level of occlusion, are perfused by reversed flow supplied by these occipital artery branches (Figure 2.26).

Signatures of the Vertebral and External Carotid Arteries

Each of the three arterial systems supplying the head has a characteristic signature in its blood flow waveform. The signature (Figure 2.42) is determined by the peripheral resistance of the territory supplied by each artery. Because the ICA supplies the tissue with the least resistance, its velocity waveform shows continuous flow forward through systole and diastole. The ECA territory has the highest resistance: Its flow reverses at the end of systole and then moves forward again during the diastolic recoil. The signature of the CCA is a mix of the pattern of its two branches. Because two-thirds of the CCA flow goes into the ICA, its signature more resembles that of the ICA than the ECA. However, when the ICA is severely stenosed, the signature of the CCA takes on the characteristics of the ECA with zero or reversed flow at the end of systole. When the ICA is occluded, the signature of the CCA is identical to that of the ECA.

The territory supplied by the vertebrobasilar system has a higher peripheral resistance than that supplied by the ICA, which is why it is the first to

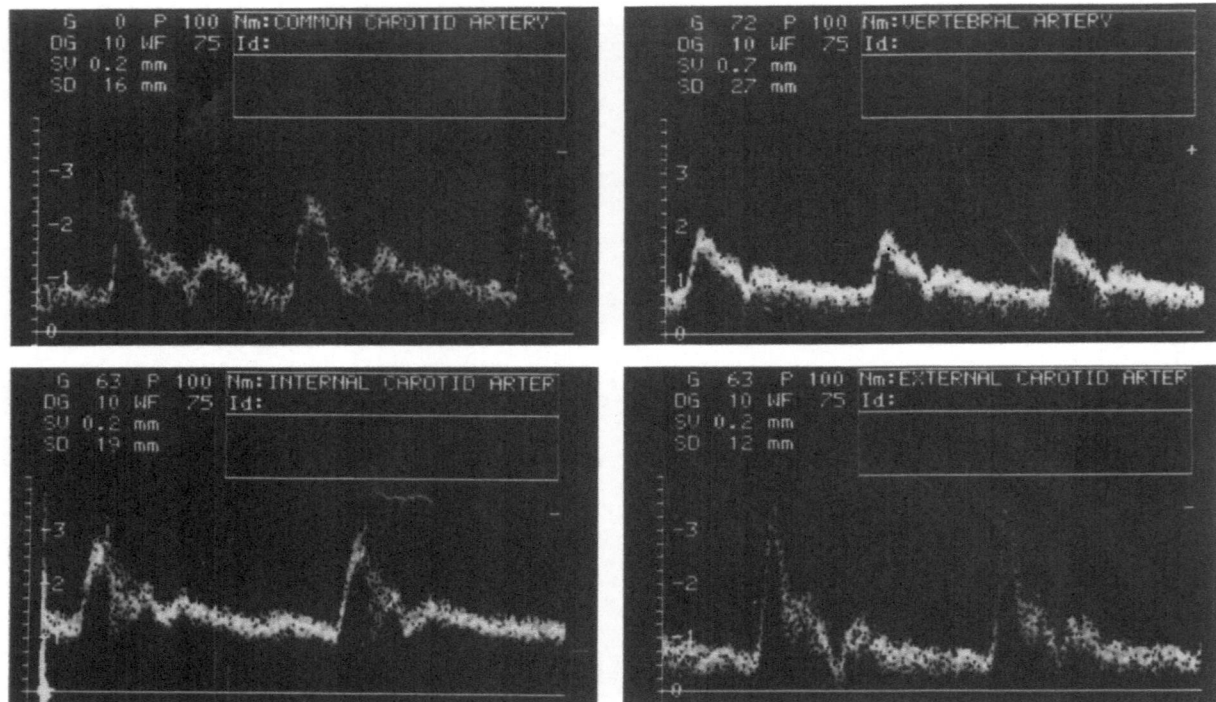

Figure 2.42 Flow velocity signals of the normal common internal and external carotid arteries and the vertebral artery.

show signs of ischemia when there is a systemic drop of pressure resulting in fainting or dizziness. The signature of the VA—like its peripheral resistance—is intermediate between those of the ICA and ECA.

Regulation of Cerebral Blood Flow

Cerebral blood flow stays fairly constant at about 50 ml/100 gm/min throughout the normal activities of a day. Small increases may be measured in discrete areas undergoing activity, such as those noted in the pre- and postcentral gyri when doing work with the contralateral hand or in the temporal lobe while listening. These discrete and proportionately small changes reflect the increase in aerobic metabolism that follows increased cellular activity. At the extremes of this local blood flow regulation is the augmentation of cerebral blood flow seen during epileptic seizures and the decrease that accompanies barbiturate coma.

Changes in pCO_2 and pO_2 also cause alterations in cerebral blood flow. It is likely that both mechanisms act upon the pH of the arteriolar muscle cells. Vasodilatation is observed with elevation of pCO_2 and to a lesser extent with a decrease in pO_2, where vasoconstriction of the cerebral arteries follows a drop in pCO_2 or, also to a lesser extent, an increase in pO_2.

The brain, in addition, has an important mechanism for autoregulating its blood flow driven by the intravascular pressure or, more precisely, by the tension within the walls of its arterioles. Within certain physiologic limits, if the mean arterial blood pressure is raised, the arterioles contract; conversely, if the mean arterial pressure drops, the distal arterioles relax. Because flow to tissue is primarily a function of the mean arterial blood pressure and the state of contraction/relaxation of the arteriolar bed, the result of this autoregulatory loop is to maintain a constant volume of flow (Figure 2.43) in the face of changing mean arterial blood pressure.

This autoregulatory mechanism works only in a

Figure 2.43 Autoregulation of cerebral blood flow in normal (blue line) and chronically hypertensive (red line) subjects.

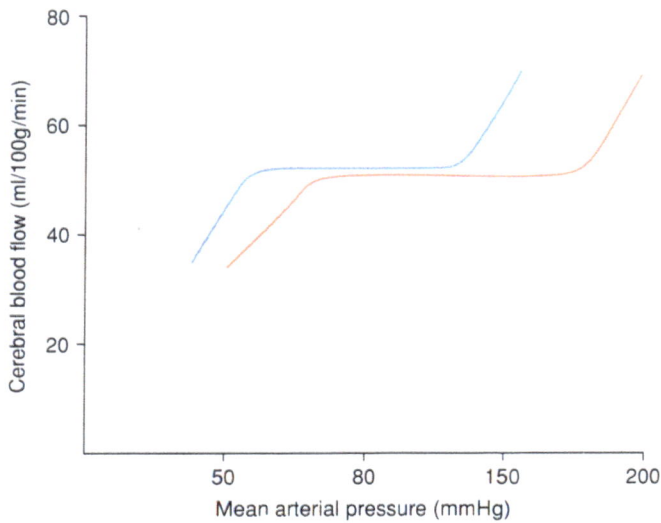

normal environment and within certain parameters of pressure. For normal individuals the latter limits are between 60 and 130 mm Hg of *mean* arterial pressure. Patients with systolic pressures around 200 mm Hg are at the upper limit of autoregulation, where flow may break through the arteriolar constriction with resulting alteration of the blood-brain barrier, edema, and perhaps hemorrhage. At the other end of the scale, patients with systolic pressure below 80 mm Hg have already reached maximum arteriolar dilatation, and an additional drop in pressure results in a drop of their cerebral blood flow. This drop appears first in the watershed areas of the territories supplied by the major arterial branches.

Brain autoregulation is lost after ischemic injury, trauma, and lactic acidosis. Patients with chronic hypertension show an upward shift in the pressure/flow curve of autoregulation (Figure 2.43). The practical corollary is that patients with chronic hypertension are likely to experience a drop in cerebral flow rates and suffer hypoxia due to low systemic pressures that would be innocuous to normal individuals. Diabetics, even those without peripheral neuropathy, may behave as if they have an impaired autoregulatory mechanism, and their brains may be damaged with changes in blood pressure that would not affect normal individuals.

In areas where the brain is edematous it may display "false autoregulation." These areas with edema have a baseline perfusion that is lower than normal. In this situation an increase in perfusion pressure may fail to increase cerebral blood flow probably because tissue pressure has already increased (edema) and the resulting transmural pressure does not change much. In contrast, small drops in blood pressure in an edematous brain can cause dramatic drops in blood flow, sometimes down to zero. In this situation reestablishing the previous blood pressure may not restart flow; this is called the "no reflow" phenomenon.

3 Arterial Lesions and Patterns of Disease

Disease of the branches of the aortic arch most commonly involves the carotid, then the vertebral, and finally the subclavian and innominate arteries. Although their most common disease is atherosclerosis, these arteries are also affected by arteritis, fibromuscular dysplasia (complicated or not), mechanical trauma, radiation injury, extension of aortic dissections, and infected false aneurysms.

Lesions in the Arterial Wall

Atheroma

The evolution of arterial lesions from fatty streaks and intimal thickening to a fully developed atheromatous plaque takes years. A mature plaque contains a core of lipids and cholesterol, as well as calcium deposits and fibrous tissue; it usually continues to grow, developing degenerative features, such as intraplaque hemorrhage or ulceration.

Plaque deposits are usually rated in terms of their relative size, which is expressed as the percentage of obstruction they produce in the lumen of the artery. The percentage of stenosis may refer to the diameter or to the cross-sectional area lost.* Although plaques that cause severe stenosis are gener-

ally associated with more serious clinical findings, the correlation is neither close nor necessarily a consequence of the severe restriction imposed on blood flow through the artery.

Evolution of a Plaque. The study of atheromatous plaques (Figure 3.1) has revealed a number of physical features that contribute to their morbid behavior: hemorrhage within the plaque, a break in the intimal covering and subsequent ulceration, the presence of surface thrombus, and small calcifications on their surface. Plaques presenting these morbid features are often called "complex" and tend to be older and have a larger volume, which is one reason why severe stenoses are associated with serious clinical events. In other words, with time plaques not only grow larger, they develop the morbid features that are likely to result in symptoms. A large plaque responsible for a severe stenosis may cause symptoms because of microembolization (thromboembolic mechanism), progressive critical restriction of blood

---

*Most duplex estimates are based on spectral changes and refer to the cross-sectional area lost. Most radiographic reporting refers to diameter lost. The percent loss of cross-sectional area (s) is calculated from the stenosed/unstenosed diameters

$$s = [1 - (d/D)^2] \times 100$$

where d = diameter of stenosis and D = diameter of unstenosed vessel.

flow (hemodynamic mechanism), or bleeding into its cavity with a sudden increase in size (hemodynamic and possibly thromboembolic mechanisms).

Plaques removed from symptomatic patients have a high incidence of intraplaque hemorrhage. It is not known if this hemorrhage comes from within (caused by a break in the capillaries at the base of the plaque) or from without (caused by a crack in its intimal covering followed by suffusion of blood from the vessel lumen into the plaque cavity). Bleeding into a plaque is associated with a volume increase and sudden aggravation of the vessel blockage. If the hemorrhage has come from the lumen of the vessel into the plaque, some tear or crack on the covering of the plaque must have taken place. If the bleeding comes from within and bursts through the roof of the plaque, it may result in the discharge of loose particles of atheroma into the bloodstream. Whatever the mechanism, the opening between the cavity within the plaque and the lumen permits the egress of atheromatous plaque material into the bloodstream and the deposition of thrombus within the ulcerated plaque. Later, this thrombus may also embolize distally. In plaques with surface thrombus the latter is usually a loosely attached gel-like material covering an intimal ulceration. This thrombus material is another source of embolization.

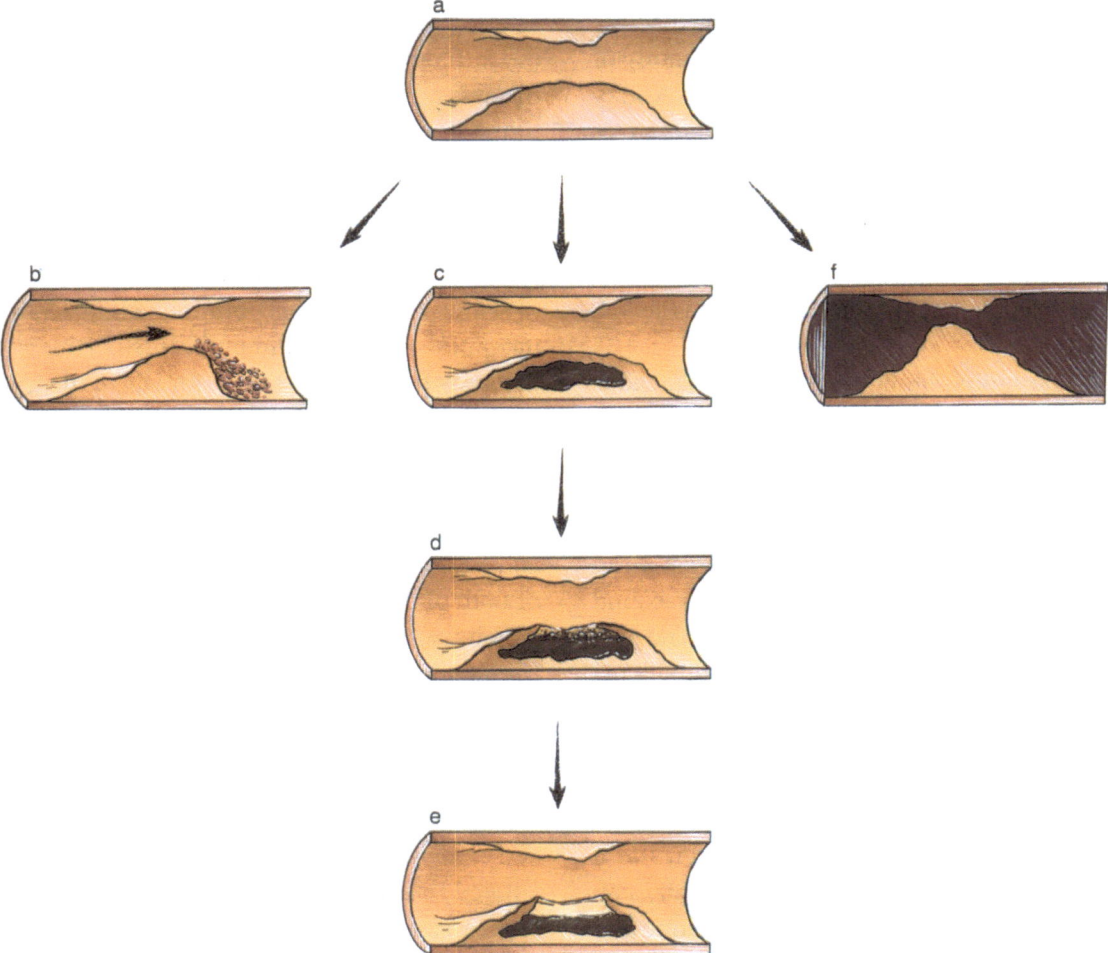

Figure 3.1 Development of pathologic features in a plaque (**a**). (**b**) Partial obstruction created by a plaque may result in accumulation of a fibrin-platelet thrombus downstream from the obstruction. (**c**) The plaque may "soften" in its core. (**d**) This softening may break through to the surface, exposing the contents of the soft core to the bloodstream. (**e**) An ulceration may become covered by a fibrin deposit and even heal. (**f**) The increased size of the obstruction created by the plaque may result in thrombosis of the vessel lumen.

Considering the atheromatous lesions that develop in the arteries supplying the head, we have a disproportionate amount of information relative to carotid bifurcation plaques but little knowledge about those found in the SAT and VA. The lesions removed from the SAT have the same appearance as those taken from the carotid bifurcation and, like them, are associated with a high incidence of degenerative features.

Routine postmortem studies, which could give us information on the nature of these plaque deposits, generally do not include the VA and the proximal SA. Autopsy studies directed toward the VA, such as the seminal work of Yates and associates,[15] have correlated the presence of plaques in the VA with discrete infarctions in the territory supplied by it. The study of Yates et al. also showed that plaques in the VA may display the same morbid features encountered in carotid bifurcation plaques, i.e., intraplaque hemorrhage, ulceration, and surface thrombus. As we shall see later, there is substantive pathologic evidence that microembolization is frequent in the vertebrobasilar territory and that its source is often a lesion of the VA (Figure 3.2).

As we learn more about the features that cause a plaque to become morbid, it is evident that our traditional reliance on arteriographic features is inadequate, just as it would be if we were to evaluate the pathologic features of the tumors of the bowel based on the outline shown during a barium contrast x-ray examination. The images produced by ultrasound echoes permit the identification of "soft" and "fibrous" plaque components. The "soft" components correspond to lipid, cholesterol, and blood elements and connote an increased likelihood of breakdown of the core and roof of the plaque and embolization. The predominantly "fibrous" plaque is less likely to cavitate and break down than a "soft" one and it has a more benign clinical outlook. Ultrasonography can also detect small hemorrhages within the plaque and sometimes a discontinuity in the intimal covering, suggesting an ulceration.

The Question of Ulceration. An ulceration is a break in the intimal covering of a plaque that exposes the media and the atheromatous core of the lesion to the bloodstream. It may be diagnosed preoperatively by ultrasonography or arteriography. With the former technique, an ulceration is usually seen as a discontinuity in the covering of a complex plaque. The ability of ultrasonography to resolve an ulceration depends on the physical composition of the plaque and the orientation of the ultrasound beam with respect to the intimal defect. More often than not an ulceration is suspected rather than seen by ultrasonography.

An arteriogram may show an ulceration as an indentation of dye into the wall of an artery. The depth of this indentation is used to rate ulcerative plaques in the ICA bulb into types A, B, or C, as their depth[53] increases. There is no close correlation between the arteriographic diagnosis of ulceration in a plaque and the intraoperative findings. Blaisdell et al.[54] showed that this correlation is better for large plaques than for those causing a mild degree of stenosis.

The prognosis of ulcerated plaques in the ICA is also a matter of controversy. The two longitudinal studies done on patients with an arteriographic diagnosis of ulceration[53,55] concluded with opposing points of view regarding the clinical significance of an ulceration of the carotid bulb. It is pertinent to recall that with both studies the diagnosis of ulceration was made by arteriography at the time the patient entered the study but not when the clinical outcome was assessed several years later. The lack of simultaneous correlation between the development of symptoms and the actual appearance of the plaque is a drawback of both of these studies. In addition, the arteriogram, which was the point of entry of these patients, is not a reliable indicator of ulceration. An ulceration of the carotid bulb in some instances progresses to become covered with a compact deposit of fibrin and platelets that nearly fills the crater and does not appear to have a high thrombogenic potential. Because their patients had evidence of carotid disease at the time they were entered into the study one cannot attribute to a single feature (the ulcer) diagnosed at the beginning of the study by a fallible method (arteriography) the clinical events that followed years later.

It is often said that plaques found at the origin of the VA are usually fibrous and smooth; therefore if they cause symptoms, it should be by restricting flow rather than by microembolization. The fact is that we

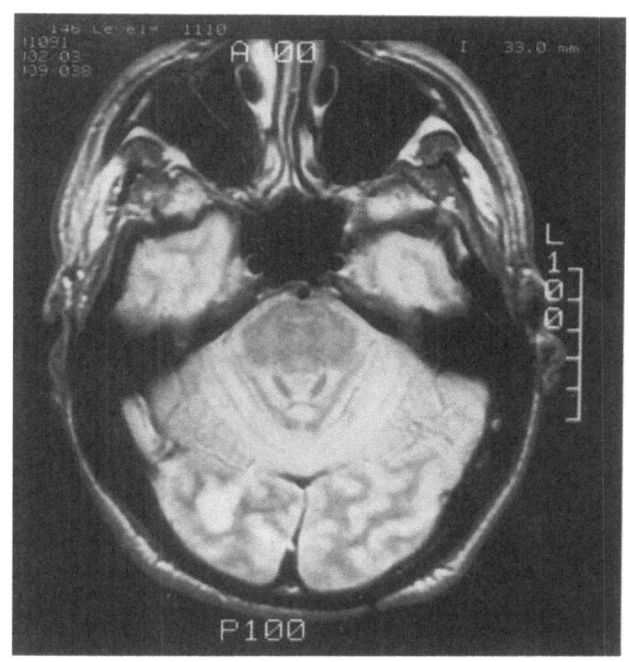

Figure 3.2 (a) Magnetic resonance imaging scan showing a cerebellar infarction. (b) Selected right subclavian arteriogram showing an emboligenous lesion in the vertebral artery at an abnormal point of entrance into the cervical spine (solid arrow). (c) Anteroposterior view shows severe alteration of the right posterior inferior cerebellar artery (open arrow). (d) Intraoperation film obtained after ligation of the right vertebral artery at C2 and carotid-distal vertebral (C1) bypass with saphenous vein.

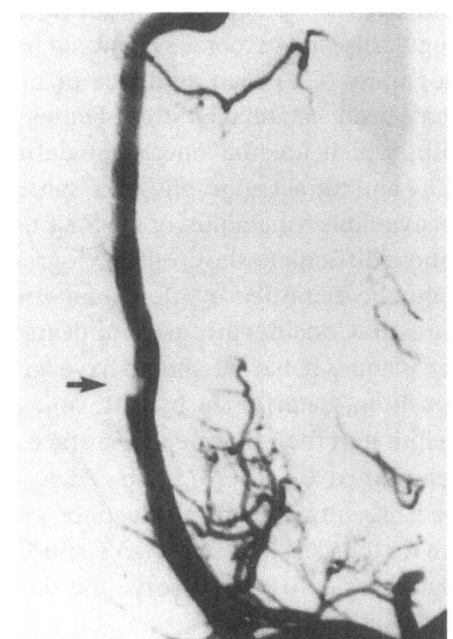
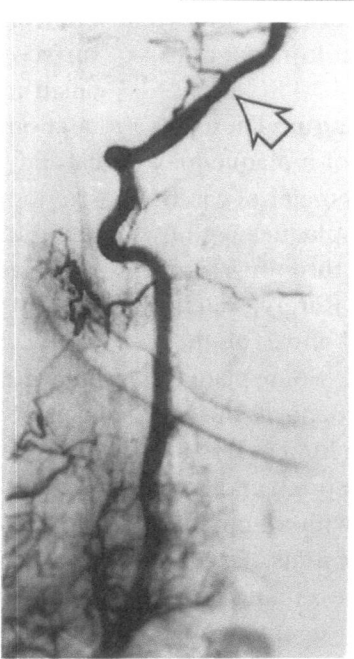
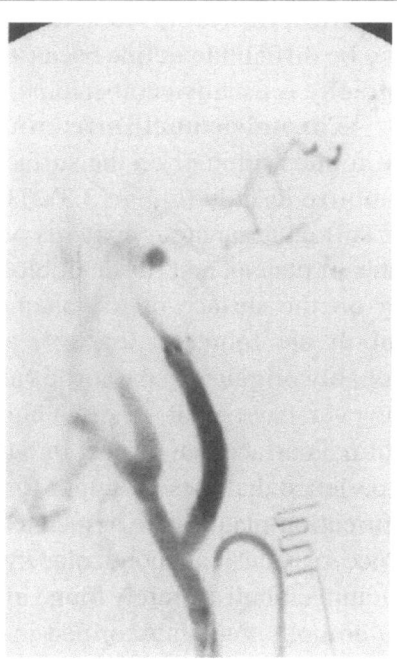

have scanty pathologic information about these VA lesions. Arteriograms are of little help in resolving the topographic features of the plaques found at the ostium of the VA, which are short (3 to 4 mm) and located in an artery of small caliber. It is even difficult to detect their presence because the SA is often superimposed on the origin of the VA. Thus it is unlikely that tiny surface irregularities in them can be identified on an arteriographic film. The gross study of these lesions is further hampered by the fact that most operations done to correct them, e.g., transposition or bypass procedures, leave the plaque excluded and therefore uninspected in the proximal VA stump.

Atheromatous lesions in the IA or SA are often large and complex and may be a source of thromboembolization of the carotid and vertebrobasilar

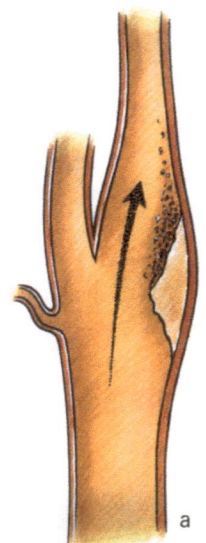 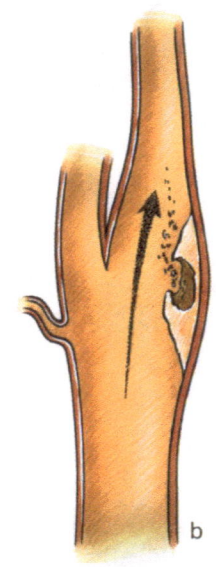 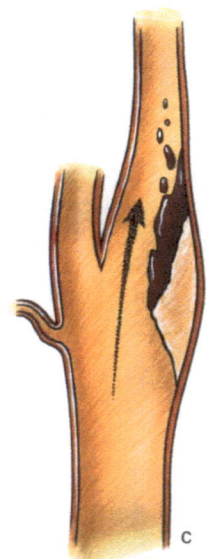

Figure 3.3 Three mechanisms for thromboembolization from an internal carotid plaque. (**a**) Fibrin-platelet aggregates associated with an obstructing plaque. (**b**) Atheromatous contents. (**c**) Thrombus forming on the surface.

territories. However, subtle lesions of these arteries may be difficult to define because multiplanar arteriography is usually cumbersome.

Thromboembolism from a Plaque. The material found within or on the surface of a plaque may embolize distally (Figure 3.3). This material can be the soft, atheromatous contents of a plaque, agglutinates of platelet and fibrin, or blood thrombus forming on the surface of the plaque. Rarely, calcific emboli are found in the eye, and most of them probably originate in the aortic valve. Some plaques, however, have small, sandy calcium deposits on their luminal surface that project into the lumen. It is our experience that these calcium formations in carotid bifurcation plaques are associated with a high incidence of transient monocular symptoms. Because calcium emboli are rarely found in the retinal vessels, the embolic materials formed in these calcium excrescences are probably fibrin-platelet aggregates.

A plaque with a fibrous, glistening surface without discontinuity that does not narrow the lumen of the vessel beyond its critical level generally does not generate thrombus or embolize its contents, and it remains benign. Platelet and whole blood thrombi tend to form on plaques with irregular surfaces, particularly those that present to the bloodstream elements of the tunica media or the core of an atheroma.

The relation between plaque ulceration and gross surface irregularity and cerebral symptoms [or computed tomography (CT) scan evidence of brain infarction] has been established for plaques in the carotid bulb, which are the ones best defined by arteriography and ultrasonography. The same correlation is not available for plaques of the SAT and VA, which are more difficult to show on arteriograms and usually cannot be identified by ultrasound imaging.

Diagnostic Considerations. It appears that to characterize plaques better we should have an idea of their composition, determined by ultrasonography, and a description of their outline and surface irregularities, determined by arteriography. The task is difficult because ultrasonography cannot give this information for those lesions in the SAT and VA, and the arteriogram often cannot resolve the outline of their surfaces.

Although we diagnose ulcerations in arteriographic images when there is an indentation of dye into the artery wall, the minimal dimensions of a step, projection, or crater that has clinical significance are not known. Is a 1.0 mm defect, which approaches the limit of resolution of standard arteriographic films, the smallest irregularity with which we need to be concerned? Why not 0.5 mm? At the other end of the spectrum of arteriographic findings are the large valleys between fibrous ridges of a plaque in the carotid bulb. They are often read as "ulcerations," but in fact under direct examination at operation they are found to be merely "valleys" that may have a smooth intimal surface free of thrombus. Plaques projecting sharply into the lumen are more likely to form thrombus, usually immediately downstream from the projection.

The many configurations that result from this combination of ulcerations and projections on the surface of a plaque make their definition and quantification difficult. On the one hand, their random outline, similar to a coastline, does not lend itself to analysis by traditional euclidean geometry. On the other, their lack of resemblance to one another and the fact that our interest does not extend into the domain of the tiny precludes the use of the modern techniques of fractal geometry to describe them. To further complicate matters, the surface of a plaque is not stable: Craters may be temporarily plugged by thrombus, whereas others may heal and become covered by a fibrous, relatively smooth surface. We still lack a formulation that describes and quantifies the topologic irregularities of a plaque surface.

Fibromuscular Dysplasia

The pathology of fibromuscular dysplasia involves primarily the media of the ICA and VA in their extracranial course. These lesions are found more commonly in women who are generally younger than those seen because of atheromatous disease. However, fibrous dysplasia and atherosclerosis may coexist in the same artery.

In its most common form the media develops annular thickenings separated by segments of normal or thinned artery. The result is an artery that is elongated and has the appearance of a string of beads. Segmental narrowings may create turbulence and a critical stenosis to the flow of blood. Topographically, the most frequently affected segment is the C2–C1 level of the ICA. The ICA and VA affected with fibromuscular dysplasia are usually elongated or tortuous.

Fibromuscular dysplasia of the ICA may be associated with intracranial berry aneurysms and other dysplastic lesions, particularly of the renal arteries but also of the vertebral and external iliac arteries. Concomitant involvement of mesenteric arteries is rare. Associated atheromatous carotid lesions are seen in about 20% of patients.

The fibrodysplastic lesion is typically located in the mid and high cervical segments of the ICA or VA. As at other body locations the fibrodysplastic lesion develops in a relatively long segment of artery that has few or no large branches. Female hormones seem to accelerate the process of fibrous dysplasia.

The most frequent appearance of fibrodysplastic lesions is that of a string of beads, with alternating stenoses and dilatations (Figure 3.4), although concentric tubular narrowing may also occur. Fibrodysplastic lesions of the ICA and VA sometimes underlie "spontaneous" intramural dissection.

If fibrous dysplasia is present in the carotid/vertebral arteries of a patient, the renal arteries should be checked for associated fibrodysplastic lesions (approximate incidence 30%) and the intracranial vasculature for associated berry aneurysms (approximate incidence 15%).

Extrinsic Compression

In their path from the mediastinum to the base of the skull, the walls of the ICA and VA interface with bone, and at these points the artery may attach its adventitia to the periosteum on which it comes to rest. Some segments of the ICA and the VA rest on complete or incomplete bony canals, such as the foramina of the transverse processes, the posterior arch of the atlas, and the petrous segment of the carotid; and in these segments the artery is relatively free of disease. It is speculative if the venous plexus surrounding the artery at this level in any way softens the bone impact against the pulsating arterial wall. For instance, the early lipid deposits seen in the second portion of the VA generally correspond to those segments where the artery is slightly dilated as it runs between two transverse processes. Eventually as atheromatous disease progresses, this pattern is blurred.

At the point of contact between artery and *abnormal* bone there may be inflammation of the adventitial

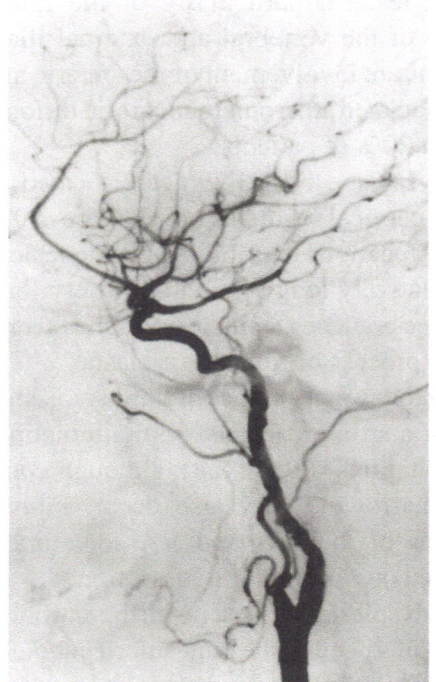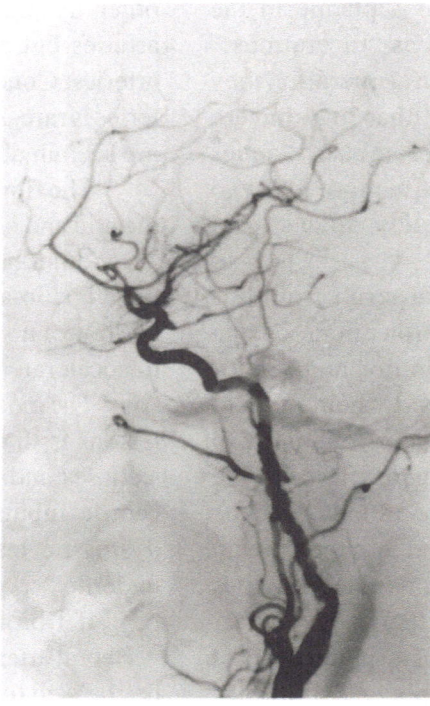

Figure 3.4 Fibromuscular dysplasia of both internal carotid arteries.

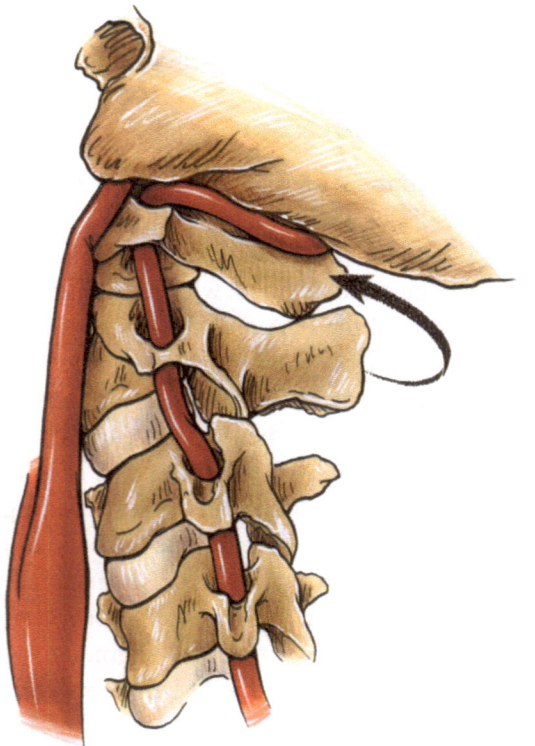

Figure 3.5 Cervical internal carotid is anterior to the large transverse process of C1. The latter can push and displace the artery when the neck is rotated to the opposite side.

coat and development of atheromatous plaque, as seen, for example, at the contact point between the VA and the uncovertebral osteophyte.

The most common point for extrinsic compression of the cervical ICA is where it passes immediately in front of the transverse mass of the atlas (Figure 3.5). This transverse process moves forward with head rotation to the opposite side and may occlude the artery. Additionally, with a brusque deceleration injury, the transverse process thrust forward may inflict a closed injury to the artery, with tearing of the intima, intramural hematoma, and thrombosis or embolization.

The ICA may also be compressed by the hypoglossal nerve, which loops around it. The cinching of the hypoglossal nerve around the artery can be exaggerated by a taut sternomastoid branch (or an occipital artery) pulling the nerve posteroinferiorly and causing a sharp angulation of its course (Figure 3.6). In addition, excessive length of the ICA, such as when the artery has a loop or a lateral origin, exaggerates the detour the hypoglossal nerve must make around the branches of the carotid bifurcation and increases the likelihood of compression of the nerve against the ICA.

The compression of the artery against the nerve

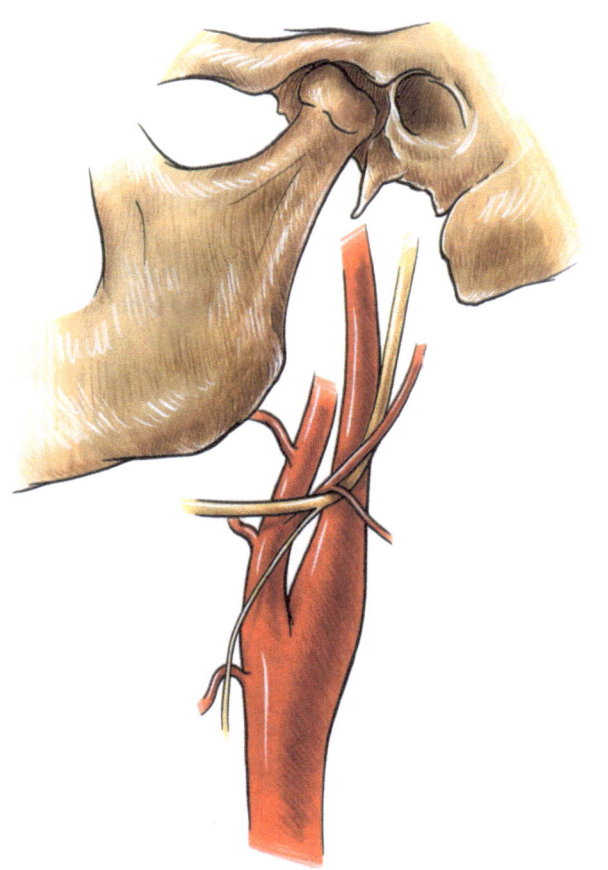

Figure 3.6 Occipital or sternomastoid artery may anchor and pull the hypoglossal nerve against the internal carotid artery.

may result in rare symptoms of hypoglossal nerve deficit.[56] The nerve itself may leave a visible indentation in the wall of the ICA and cause extrinsic compression of the artery during head rotation (Figure 3.7). Clinically, the pressure effects of the artery on the nerve (hypoglossal paresis) have been better documented than those of the nerve against the artery (symptomatic extrinsic compression of the ICA). A few cases of compression of the ICA by the styloid process and the muscles and ligaments that are attached to it have also been described (Eagle syndrome).

The VA may be compressed externally by the sympathetic chain, which anchors it to the spine, or by the tendon of the longus colli. However, the most common sites for external compression are in its intraspinal course, where it can be impinged by osteophytes that develop on the uncinate process or on the lip of the articular facet in patients with spondylosis.

Compression of the artery is often aggravated and may be seen only by rotating the neck. Extrinsic compression may also occur during hyperextension in children who have atlantooccipital instability, where exaggerated mobility of the atlantooccipital joint permits the posterior arch of the atlas to insinuate itself in the foramen magnum compressing both VAs.

With severe rheumatoid arthritis abnormal mobility and subluxation of intervertebral joints may also result in external compression of the VA. With the Klippel-Feil syndrome fusion of the cervical spine is partially compensated by exaggerated mobility of the atlantoaxial joint. Stretching of the vertebral artery at this level may cause intramural dissection and distal embolization (Figure 3.8).

The possibility that head rotation or extension/flexion may cause temporary occlusion of an ICA or VA must be borne in mind when positioning patients

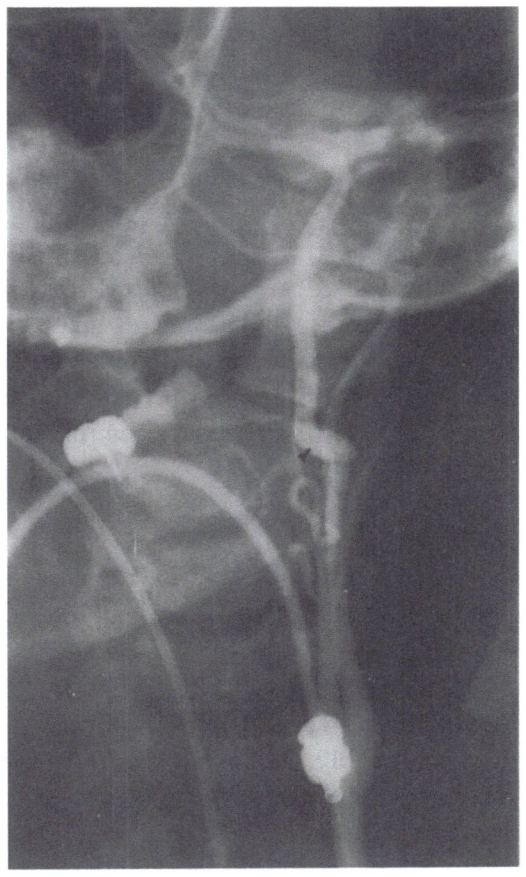

Figure 3.7 Compression of the internal carotid artery by the hypoglossal nerve.

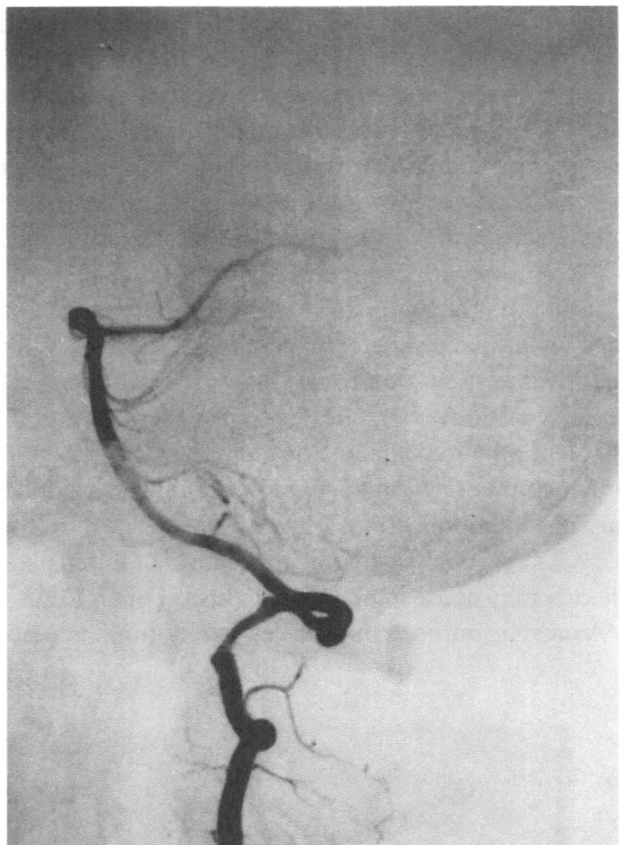

Figure 3.8 Dissection of the VA in its third segment in a woman with Klippel-Feil syndrome.

for an operation. The degree of rotation and extension that can be achieved may be underestimated in patients who are relaxed and asleep under anesthesia. The surgeon may inadvertently occlude the vertebral or carotid artery on which he is relying for collateral blood supply.

Dissection

Isolated dissections of the extracranial arteries usually involve the distal cervical VA (Figure 3.8) and ICA (Figure 3.9). These arteries have few or no important branches within their relatively long trajectories and presumably, therefore, fewer vasa vasorum. It has been postulated that these branchless segments with fewer vasa vasora in their media are more susceptible to damage by the normal stresses induced by the pulse wave or by external mechanical stresses.

Intramural dissection is slightly more prevalent in women and is thought to be facilitated by underlying fibromuscular dysplasia and female hormones. Acute or chronic trauma may also trigger a dissection (Figure 3.10). The role of bony trauma is suspected but not proved in dissection of the ICA where the transverse process of C1 has been considered a possible offending agent during hyperextension and rotation.

A common etiology of dissection of the VA is acute hyperextension trauma of its third segment following road accidents or chiropractic manipulations. Other causes of VA dissection are chronic trauma due to abnormally high entrance of the VA in the cervical spine (Figure 2.21), excursion of the VA around the transverse process of C1 because of the congenital absence of a transverse foramen (Figure 2.28), or the

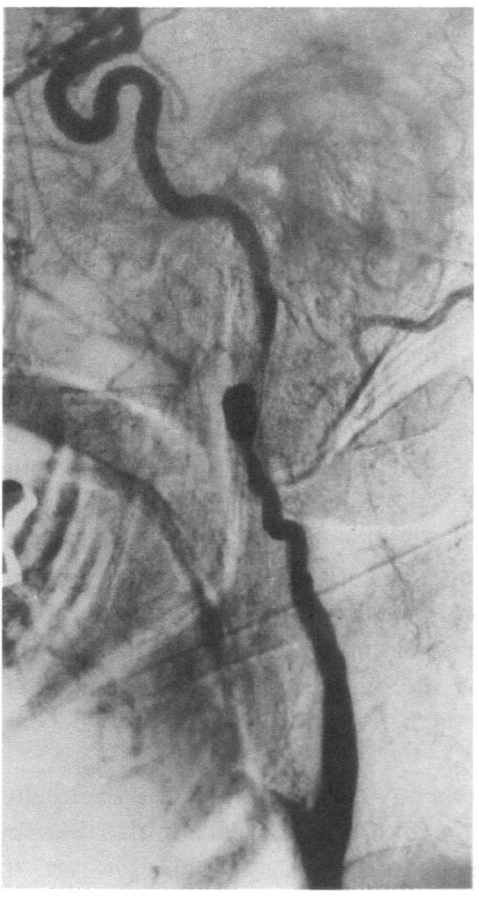

Figure 3.9 Intramural dissection of the ICA demonstrating two characteristic patterns; i.e., stenosis and aneurysm.

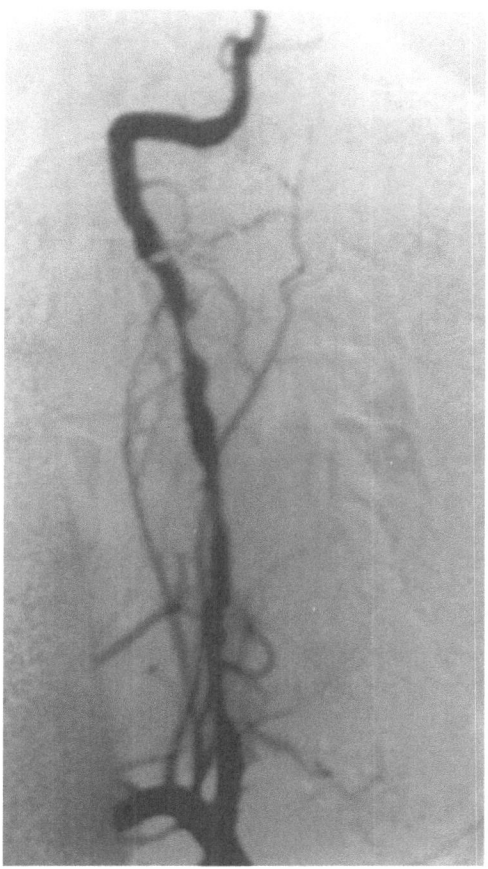

Figure 3.10 Intramural dissection of the second segment of the vertebral artery, presumed to be the cause of distal microembolization.

presence of abnormal neighboring bony elements in the second and third segments of the artery.

Dissection often appears macroscopically as an intramural hematoma, without intimal disruption. The presence of an intimal tear, as in aortic dissections, may be a primary or secondary event.

The intramural hematoma causes the usual "string" appearance of the dissected artery and may result in its early occlusion. Return to a normal appearance, however, is seen in a substantial number of cases within a period of weeks. "Complicated" dissections are associated with thromboembolic episodes due to superimposed intraluminal occlusive thrombus (Figure 3.10), an intimal tear communicating with the intramural hematoma within the arterial lumen, or the late development of an aneurysm.

Aortic dissections involving the aortic arch may disrupt the origin, or extend into, the SAT with or without superimposed thrombus formation. Although arterial damage may extend to the axillary artery, the VA and distal ICA are usually spared in the extension of an aortic arch dissection.

Arteritis

With *Takayasu's* arteritis involvement of the SAT is frequent but not constant. This disease of unknown etiology predominantly affects women in their second or third decades. Most patients have proximal involvement of the IA, left CCA or SA (Figure 3.11) often in continuity with aortic arch lesions (Figure 3.12). A few patients have isolated involvement of the CCA or distal SA. The ICA is usually spared by this disease.

The occlusive lesions of Takayasu's disease are characteristic in their extension and multiplicity (Figure 3.13). The hypertrophic intima usually has a smooth surface, accounting for the low embolic potential of these lesions. Thrombosis, however, may complicate tight stenoses and lead to extensive secondary occlusions, which may then include the ICA and the VA.

The histologic appearance of the lesions differs according to the phase of the disease. The lesions tend to be inflammatory during the acute phase and sclerotic during the chronic phase. They are located predominantly in the adventitial and intimal layers. The media may be partially destroyed, leading to aneurysmal formation in a few cases.

Giant cell arteritis rarely involves the proximal SAT. It may, however, affect the distal SA, often extending to the axillary artery or the ECA. It is usually seen in elderly patients. This feature helps to differentiate it from Takayasu's disease in the few cases where the topography and histology of the lesions are confusing.

Radiation arteritis is the result of a nonspecific arterial response that causes accelerated atherosclerosis in the irradiated arteries. It may take several years before the arterial damage becomes apparent, although the time frame depends on the radiation dose. Patients with radiation arteritis are often long-term survivors of head and neck cancer (Figure 3.14).

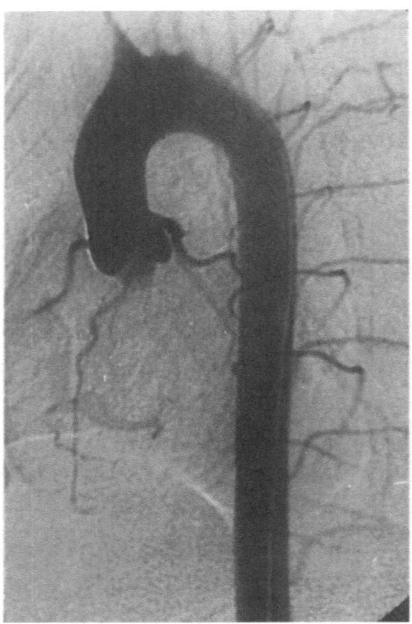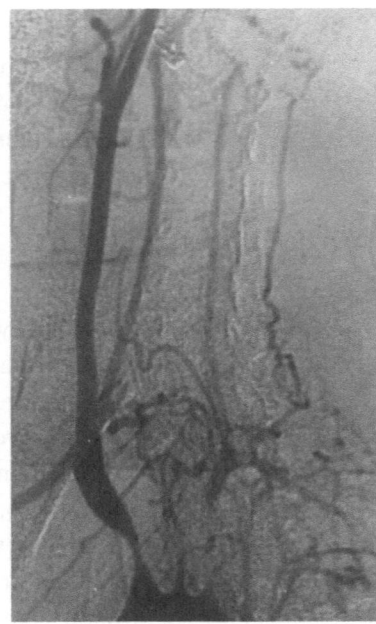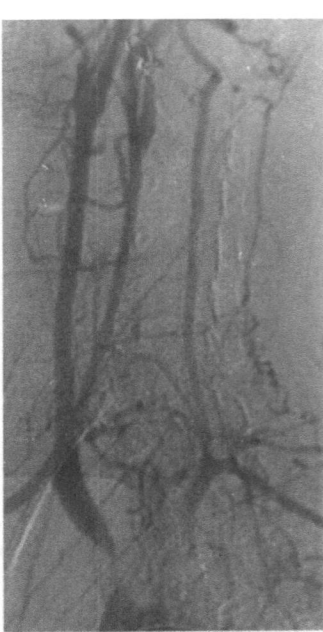

Figure 3.11 Takayasu's arteritis. The innominate, left common carotid, and left subclavian arteries are severely diseased. Both vertebral arteries and carotid bifurcations are patent. The left carotid bifurcation fills retrogradely from the external carotid and is superimposed over the right vertebral artery.

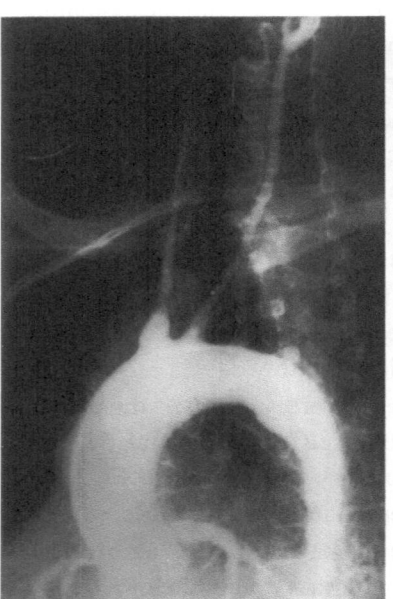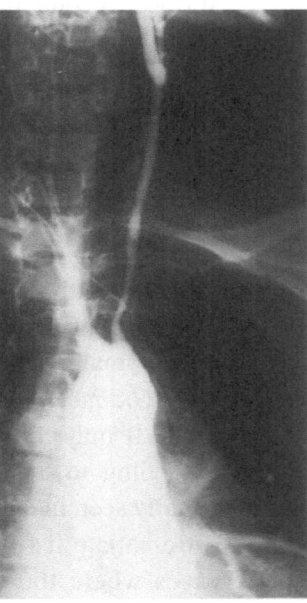

Figure 3.12 Extensive Takayasu's arteritis of all supraaortic trunks with involvement of the aortic arch. The left carotid bifurcation is patent.

In a few patients, however, radiation has been inappropriately prescribed for benign disease of the thyroid or tonsil.

The most common site of involvement for radiation arteritis is the cervical carotid artery (both CCA and ICA) following treatment of cancer of the head and neck. The SAT may be involved after radiotherapy for breast cancer, intrathoracic tumors or Hodgkin's disease (Figure 3.15). These patients often have associated involvement of the muscle, skeleton, and overlying skin as well as the accompanying veins. A tracheostomy is frequent in patients with previous head and neck cancer and may complicate their surgical management.

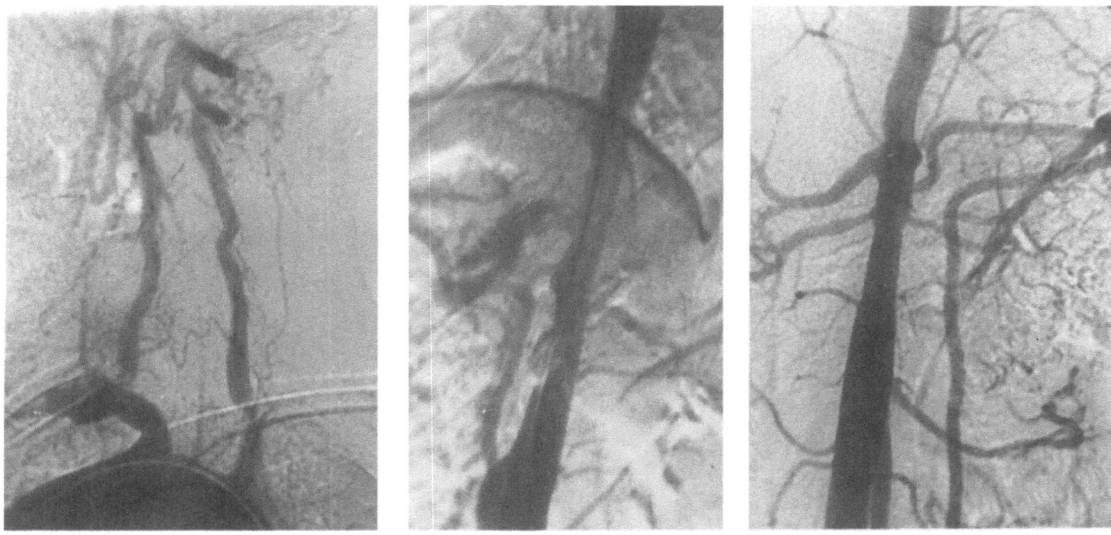

Figure 3.13 Takayasu's arteritis involving the supraaortic trunks and the thoracoabdominal aorta.

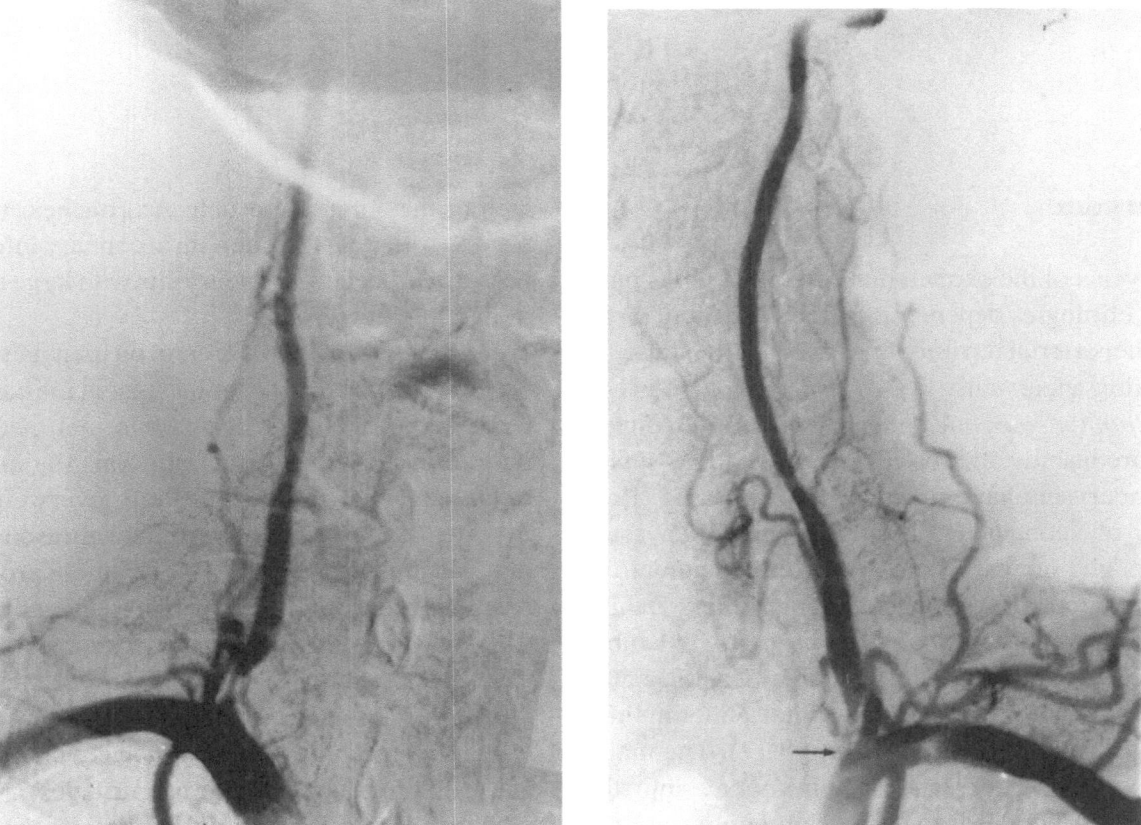

Figure 3.14 Severe symptomatic stenoses of both vertebral arteries following 8000 rads at the base of the neck for cancer treatment.

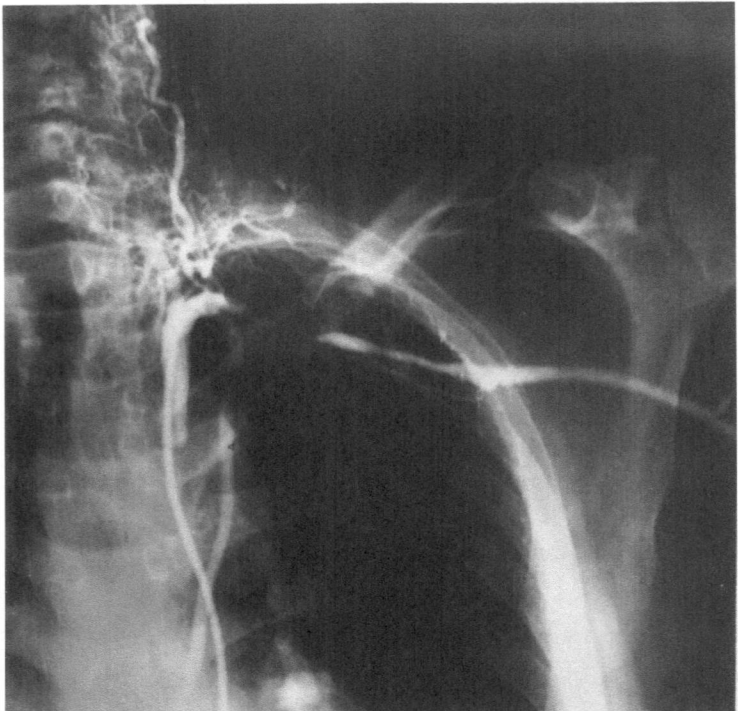

Figure 3.15 Radiation arteritis of the subclavian artery after radiotherapy for Hodgkin's disease.

Aneurysm

Aneurysms of the extracranial cerebral arteries have varied etiologies depending on their location. As in any other arterial territory they may be true, false, or dissecting aneurysms.

Spontaneous aneurysms of the SAT (Figure 3.16) are usually atherosclerotic in origin, as syphilitic aneurysms have practically disappeared. Rare causes of spontaneous aneurysms are Takayasu's arteritis and medial dystrophy (with or without the manifestations of Marfan syndrome, Ehlers-Danlos syndrome, or elastorrhexia). It is useful to remember that these aneurysms of the SAT are often associated with aortic aneurysms or congenital abnormalities such as aortic coarctation (Figure 3.17). The major risk of these aneurysms is their rupture into the mediastinum or pleura and, uncommonly, into the trachea, esophagus, and adjacent veins.

Thromboembolic complications from aneurysms are unusual, although they have been reported in the brain, eye, and upper extremities. Larger aneurysms may compress adjacent structures such as the arch of the aorta, the esophagus, trachea, veins, or nerves. Although uncommon, secondary infection is possible, especially in aneurysms with large amounts of intraluminal thrombus.

Redundancy of the IA and its branches (Figure 3.18) may result in a pulsating mass at the base of the right side of the neck or an abnormal mediastinal outline on chest roentgenogram. This finding seems to be seen more frequent in short, overweight, and hypertensive women. Palpation and ultrasonography may rule out an aneurysm. When single projections are used for arteriograms, such a redundancy (Figure 3.19) may give the impression of an aneurysm.

Spontaneous aneurysms of the ICA or VA have different characteristics. They are seen rarely in the carotid bifurcation (where occasionally they are difficult to differentiate from large carotid bulbs) and in the proximal segment of the VA. Dysplastic aneurysms may be multiple (see Figures 3.20 and 3.21) and associated with intracranial berry aneurysms. Their potential risk is mainly thromboembolic, as they usually do not become large enough to compress the neighboring structures or to rupture into them.

a
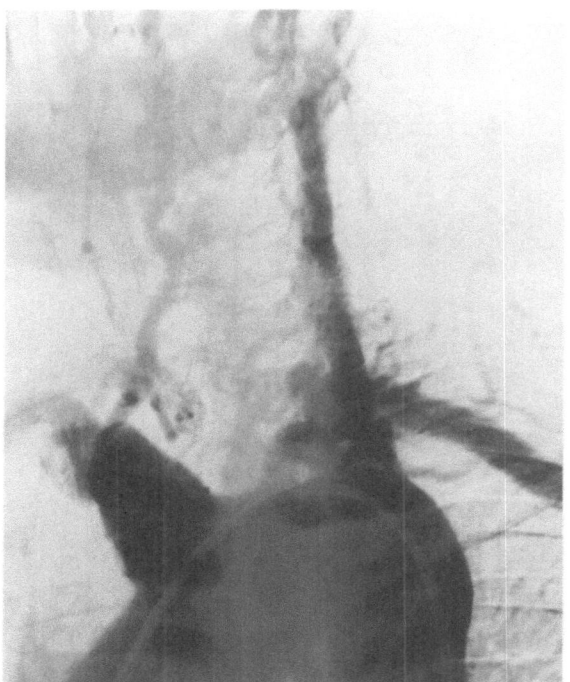

b
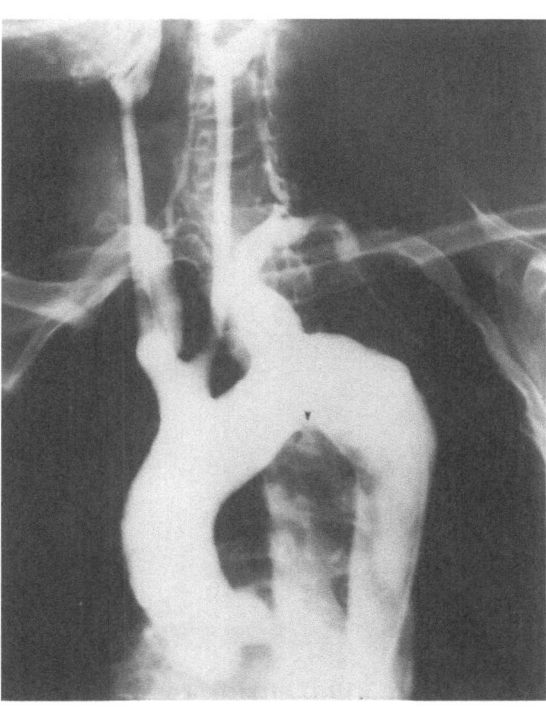

Figure 3.16 Aneurysmal disease of the supraaortic trunks may occur (**a**) isolated, as in this atherosclerotic aneurysm of an inominate artery or (**b**) associated with arch lesions as in this syphilitic aneurysm of the arch and left subclavian artery. The arrow points to a gumma in the concavity of the arch.

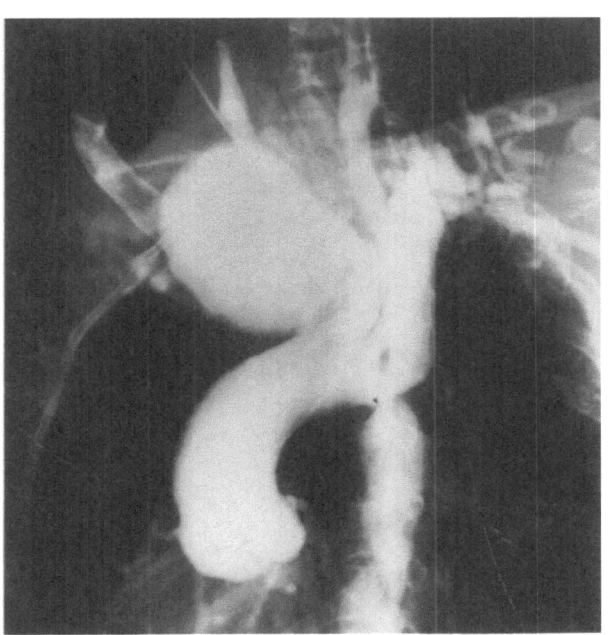

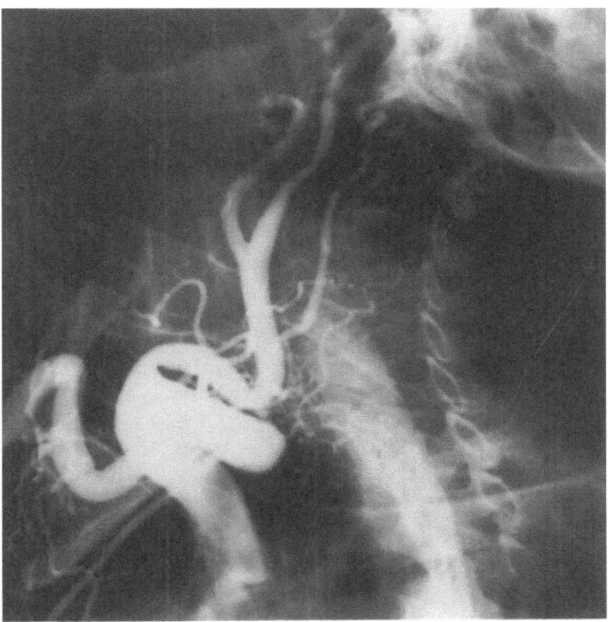

Figure 3.17 Coartation of the aorta associated with aneurysmal dilatation of both subclavian arteries.

Figure 3.18 Redundancy of the innominate, right subclavian, and common carotid arteries results in a pulsatile mass at the base of the right neck, which may raise the clinical suspicion of an aneurysm.

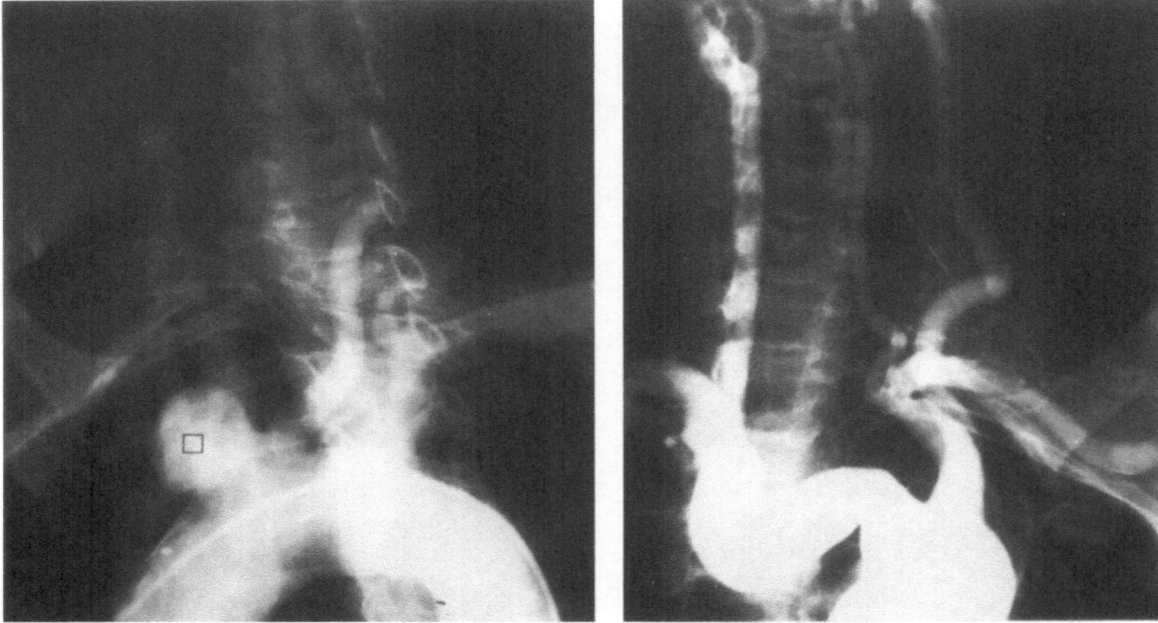

Figure 3.19 (**Left**) Right posterior oblique aortogram suggests an aneurysm of the innominate artery. (**Right**) Opposite oblique view shows what in fact is a redundant innominate artery.

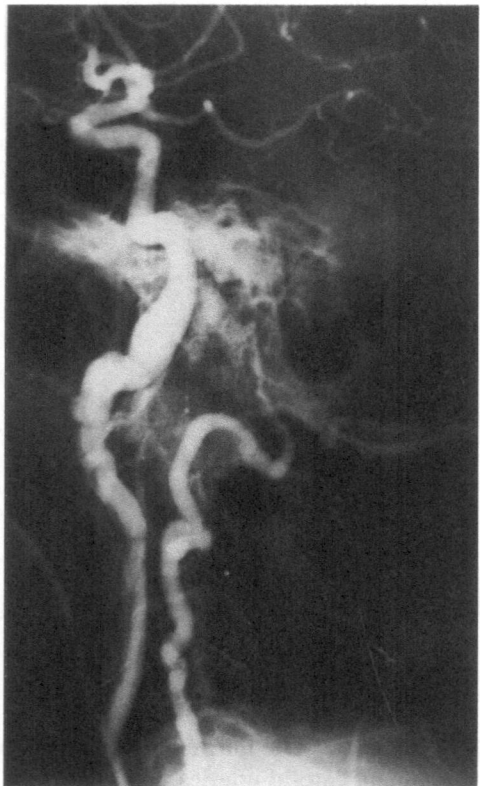

Figure 3.20 Fibrodysplasia of the internal carotid and vertebral arteries with aneurysm formation.

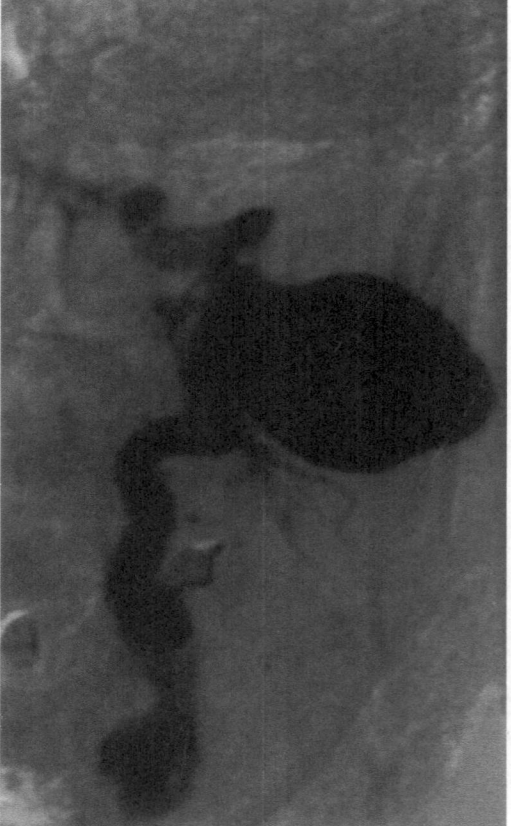

Figure 3.21 Large dysplastic aneurysm of the third segment of the vertebral artery.

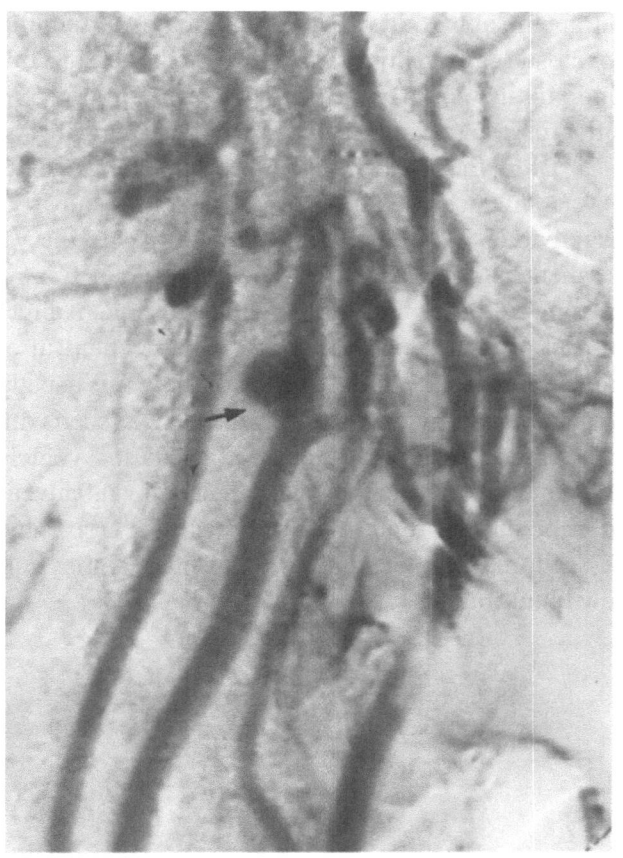

Figure 3.22 False aneurysm of the carotid bulb due to suture failure 10 years after a right carotid endarterectomy.

Noninfective postoperative aneurysms are rare. They usually occur years after the operation, and they may be true aneurysms (in grafts or patches made of vein) or false aneurysms due to the rupture of a suture line between a synthetic graft or patch and a native artery (Figure 3.22). Because operations on the carotid artery are common the most likely location for a postoperative aneurysm is the carotid bifurcation. These aneurysms may also be associated with restenosis of the ICA. Their major risk is thromboembolism.

The unusual late anastomotic aneurysm that develops in the proximal anastomosis of a bypass arising from the ascending aorta carries a major risk of intrathoracic rupture.

Infected aneurysms of the arteries to the brain are most unusual. Some patients have developed infected aneurysms on preexisting parietal lesions following bouts of systemic bacteremia. In drug addicts the mecha-

nism is mechanical trauma to the artery with a dirty needle and chemical injury by intramural injection of the various chemicals used to mix drugs.

Chronic traumatic aneurysms are the consequence of unrecognized or untreated trauma. Blunt trauma and subadventitial rupture result in aneurysms that involve either the intrathoracic SAT or the distal ICA. Penetrating trauma causes false aneurysms with or without associated arteriovenous fistulas. Traumatic aneurysms may cause embolism and rupture.

Trauma

Penetrating trauma may be secondary to a stab or bullet wound and is usually localized to the most vulnerable part of the carotid in the cervical portion. Injury to the wall of the CCA, ECA, or proximal ICA usually causes external hemorrhage or cervical hematoma. Injury to the wall of the proximal intrathoracic SAT (Figure 3.23) may cause bleeding into the pericardium, pleura, or mediastinum.

The incidence of *blunt* trauma, usually as a result of motor vehicle or industrial accidents, contin-

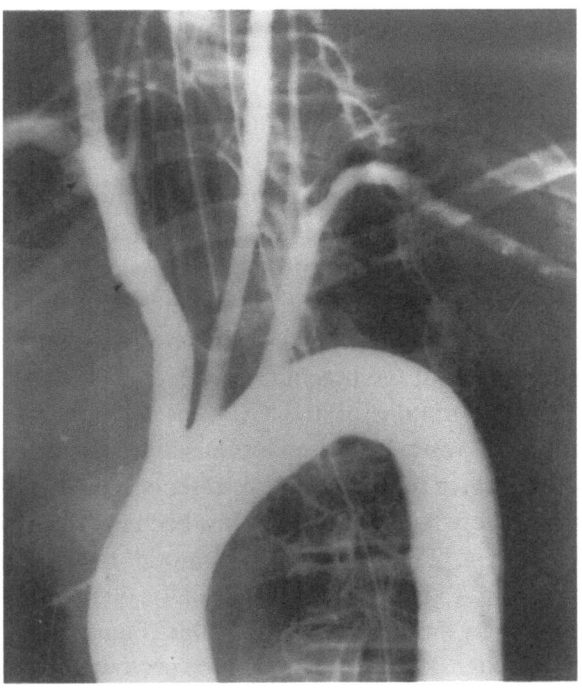

Figure 3.23 Blunt thoracic trauma resulting in subadventitial rupture of the innominate and right subclavian arteries.

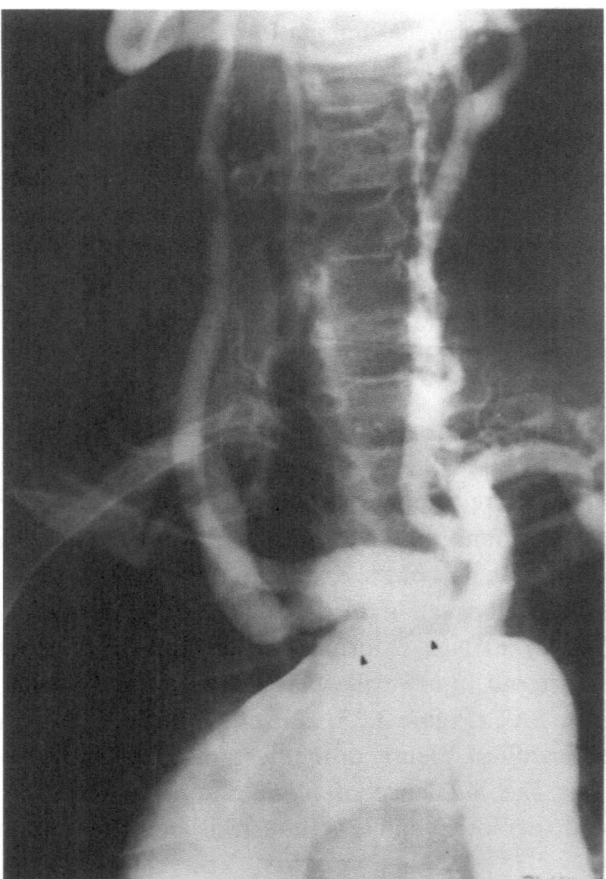

Figure 3.24 Disruption and hematoma of the origin of the innominate artery following blunt trauma.

ues to increase. The most common blunt deceleration injury to the SAT is avulsion of the IA from the aortic arch (Figure 3.24). Rupture of the intrathoracic portion of the left SA is seen less frequently. Impact trauma to the shoulder girdle and avulsion injury of the upper extremity are more frequent. Each may be associated with a fracture of the clavicle or compression/avulsion of the brachial plexus.

Blunt trauma of the CCA or its bifurcation usually follows a direct impact caused by sports (e.g., martial arts) or motor vehicle accidents. The shoulder loop of safety belt mechanisms has been involved in a few cases of blunt trauma to the carotid. In the distal cervical ICA, blunt trauma is usually due to direct contusion by the angle of the mandible (Figure 3.25) or to hyperextension and rotation of the neck with trauma to the ICA by the transverse process of C1 or by the styloid process. A fracture of the skull base may tear the

intrapetrosal carotid. In children another possibility for closed carotid injury is a fall with a pencil or a lollipop in the mouth, contusing the carotid in the tonsillar fossa and resulting in its secondary thrombosis.

Blunt trauma to the VA is seen at any level of its extracranial course. In the first segment injury is usually due to deceleration trauma. Injury to the V2 segment is seen in association with spinal trauma causing dislocation of the spine and subsequent direct impact or stretching of the VA. The mechanism of blunt trauma in the third segment of the VA is usually hyperextension and rotation of the neck, as seen with chiropractic manipulations or after motor vehicle accidents. Blunt trauma usually results in subadventitial or intimal rupture with or without associated dissection. Complete disruption of the VA may follow blunt trauma.

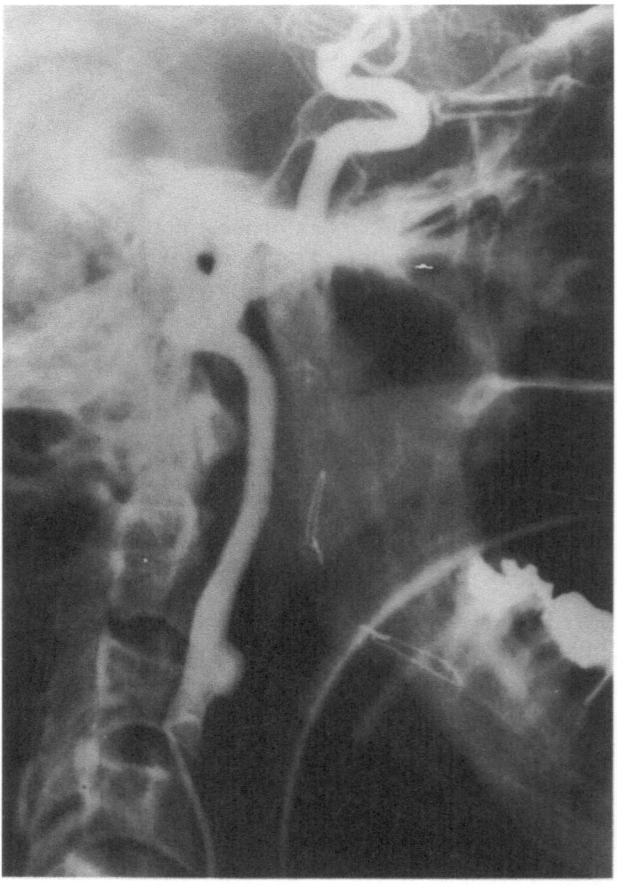

Figure 3.25 The now-wired fractured mandible was responsible for this false aneurysm of the internal carotid artery.

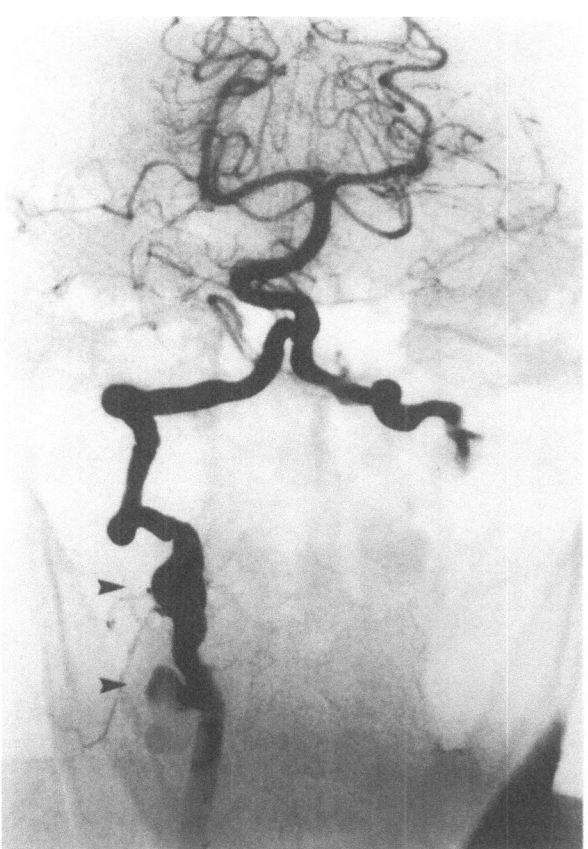

Figure 3.26 False aneurysms of the right vertebral artery after ill-advised balloon angioplasty of a stenosed segment. The latter was the result of dissection in a fibrodysplastic artery.

Iatrogenic trauma to the arterial wall is not unusual. Most of it occurs during attempted intravenous puncture (internal jugular or subclavian veins) for diagnostic or therapeutic purposes. After a needle injury to the CCA or SA, an arteriovenous fistula is as common as a false aneurysm. A few cases of iatrogenic trauma to the extracranial vessels have resulted from surgical procedures on the spine, balloon angioplasty of stenoses of the intraspinal VA (Figure 3.26), operations on the thoracic outlet and the sympathetic chain, or following mediastinoscopy or percutaneous thoracic drainage.

The arterial complications of prolonged endotracheal intubation, tracheostomy, or tracheal reconstruction (see Chapter 11) are more common in those patients when the IA exits from the arch in front or to the left of the trachea.

Arteriovenous Fistula

In the neck arteriovenous fistulas of *spontaneous* origin (either congenital or acquired) involve primarily the VA and the ECA. Congenital fistulas are not known in the IA or CCA and are exceedingly rare in the SA. Those found in the territories of the ECA usually have adjacent bone or skin components. Arteriovenous fistulas involving the mandible typically present in a young person who has a life-threatening hemorrhage following a tooth extraction. In the VA spontaneous fistulization is found in youngsters and young adults at the level of C2–C3. How many of these fistulas are congenital is debatable. Some are certainly due to fibromuscular dysplastic disease of the VA (more frequently in the third segment of the artery) (Figure 3.27). Acquired fistulas are probably a result of dissection or trauma of the VA related to spinal motion. Both trauma and dissection result in damage to the wall and rupture into the surrounding venous plexus with formation of a fistula. The fact that abnormal bone or skin components are not associated with arteriovenous fistulas of the extracranial VA supports the contention that they are probably acquired early in life rather than congenital.

Traumatic arteriovenous fistulas are common in the neck where the tightly packed arrangement of arteries and veins with little external protection makes them vulnerable to simultaneous injury. Traumatic fistulas are far less common in the retrosternal portion of the SAT owing to the protection provided by bone against low velocity injuries. The common causes of acquired arteriovenous fistulas are knife and bullet wounds (Figure 3.28), subluxation of the spine (VA), deceleration injuries with bone fracture, and accidental arterial puncture during catheterization procedures (Figure 3.29) or drug injection in addicts. Arteriovenous fistulas of the CCA or ICA are seen more often after knife injuries than after high velocity bullet injuries; the latter causes severe wall disintegration of arteries and severe hemorrhage, which usually necessitates an immediate operation to ligate the vessel or results in the thrombosis of the artery. With low velocity bullet and knife injuries the damage to the wall of the artery and accompanying vein may be limited. In these cases severe hemorrhage

Figure 3.27 Spontaneous arteriovenous fistula (arrows) of the second segment of the vertebral artery complicating fibromuscular dysplasia. A vertebrovertebral steal is present.

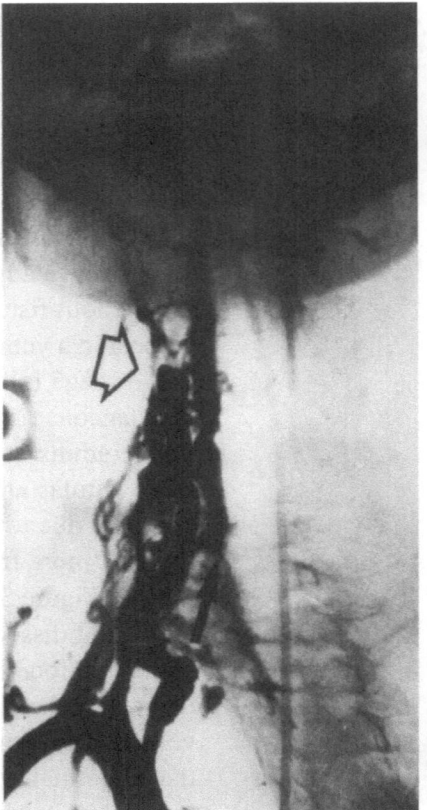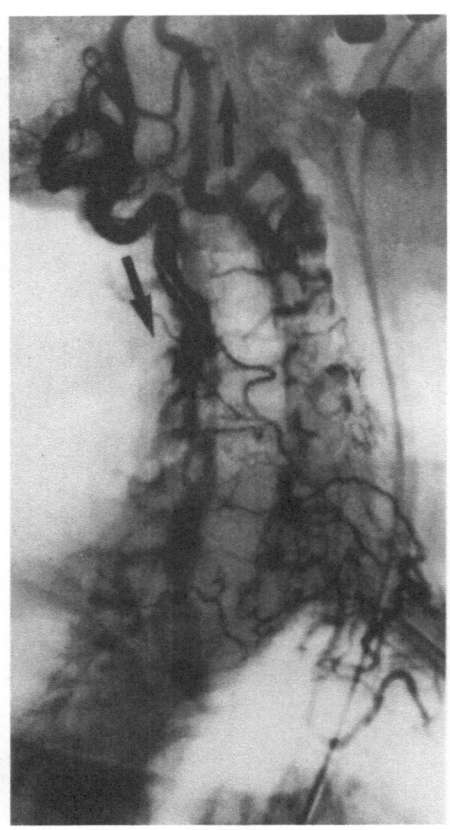

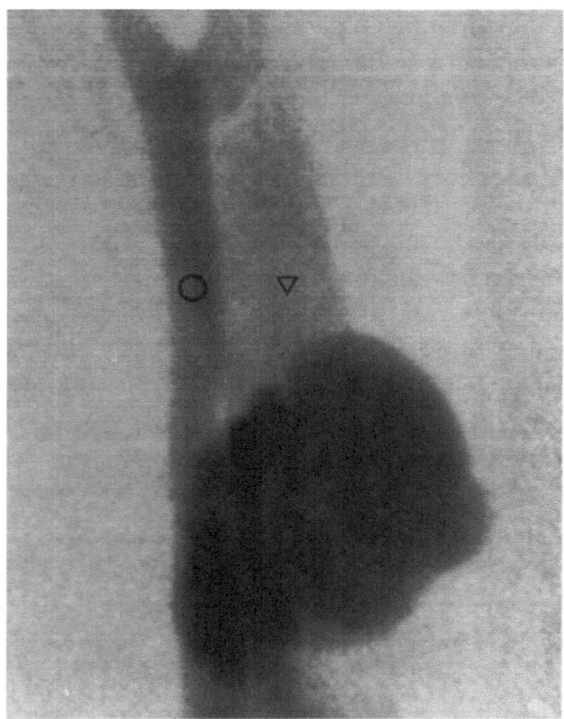

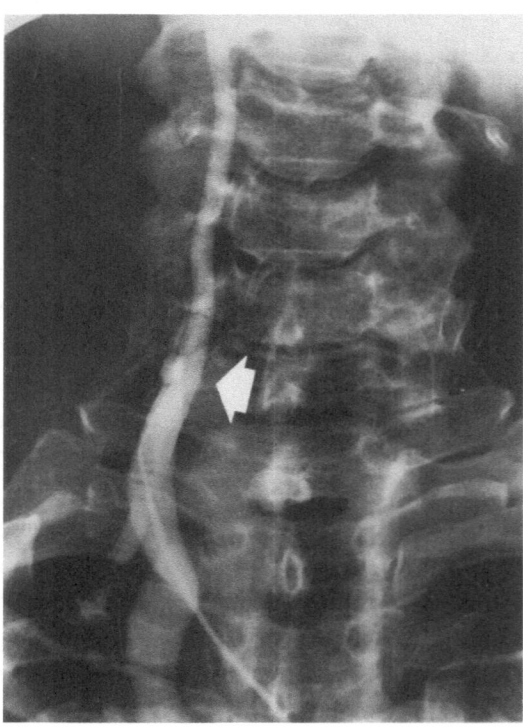

Figure 3.28 Arteriovenous fistula between the common carotid (circle) and jugular vein (triangle) following a knife injury.

Figure 3.29 Arteriovenous fistula between the proximal vertebral artery and vein following attempted catheterization of the jugular vein.

with external bleeding is rare, and the wound and the path of injury may not be explored, setting the stage for development of an arteriovenous fistula.

Patterns of Disease

Supraaortic Trunks

When involved by disease, the *innominate artery* develops a plaque, usually at its origin, that may show any of the degenerative features seen in plaques of the carotid bifurcation (Figure 3.30). This IA plaque may be continuous, extending over the entire dome of the aortic arch. When a stenosed IA has a common origin with the left CCA, the atheroma usually involves the origin of both vessels. The less common lesions of the middle or distal third of the IA usually extend into the right SA, right CCA, or both. The IA is often involved in patients with Takayasu's arteritis.

The most common lesion affecting the first segment of the *subclavian arteries* is atheroma. The left SA, which takes off at a right angle from the aortic arch, is frequently involved. Plaques involving the origin of the right SA may be part of a large distal IA plaque that often extends also into the origin of the right CCA.

The *common carotid arteries* are usually spared from atherosclerotic disease, except for their proximal and distal ends. The ostium of the left CCA at the dome of the aortic arch is involved more often than that of the right CCA. At their distal ends both common carotid arteries are often involved with the proximal extension of atheroma of the carotid bifurcation. CCAs may be involved throughout their length by Takayasu's arteritis or by a dissection originating in the aortic arch.

Internal Carotid Artery

The plaque characteristic of the carotid bifurcation is the most common of all lesions seen in the first and second order branches of the aortic arch. It most often develops at the origin of the ICA in the bulb and extends for some length proximally into the CCA and sideways into the orifice of the ECA. It has been our observation that plaques in the ICA appear to develop

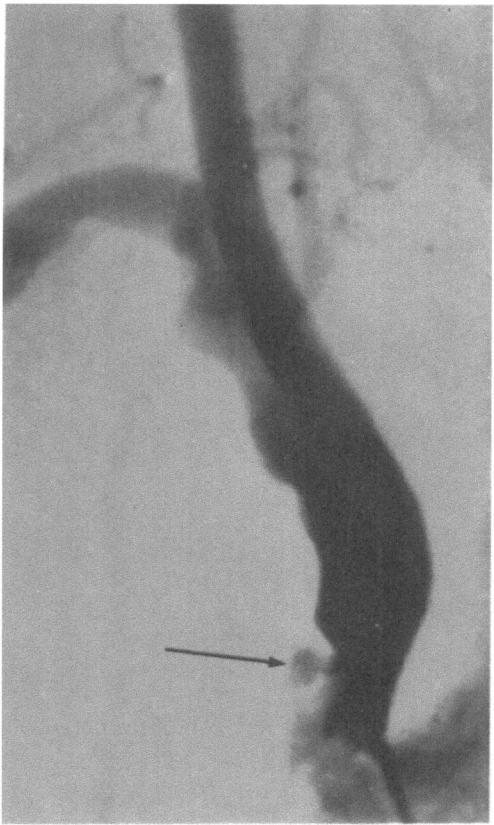

Figure 3.30 Ulcerated plaque at the origin of the innominate artery.

at about the same spinal level, regardless of where the carotid bifurcates, so that low carotid bifurcations present lesions that extend high in the ICA, whereas high bifurcations usually bear lesions confined to their bulbous portion.

The plaque of atheroma that forms in the carotid bulb is usually eccentric. Lusby et al.[57] have shown that there is substantial wall motion in the bulb with every heartbeat. In bulbs with atheromatous plaques, the thin areas of the wall distend more than other areas of the ICA wall, which cannot distend because they are splinted by the plaque they bear. These large differences in distensibility result in shearing forces acting on the plaque that may result in bleeding within its substance.

At the upper end of the carotid sinus its elastic wall changes abruptly into that of the musculoelastic cervical ICA. The intima becomes thinner, and lipid infiltration of the elastic media usually stops at this

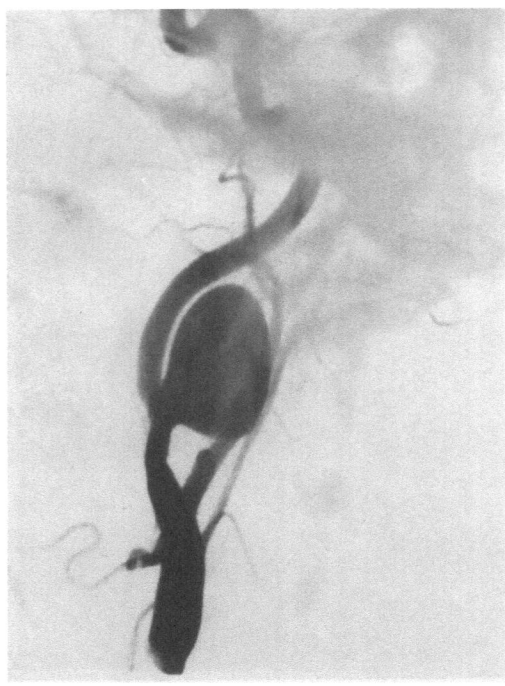

Figure 3.31 Dysplastic aneurysm of the cervical internal carotid artery.

Within these septa is a periarterial venous plexus communicating with the pterygoid and cavernous venous sinuses. It is likely that the changes that take place in the wall of the carotid as it enters the temporal bone result in termination of the intramural dissection or in its breaking through into the true lumen at this level.

The alternating series of curvatures formed by the petrous and cavernous segments of the ICA is called the carotid siphon (Figure 3.35). The radii of these series of curves become progressively smaller, with the pattern of flow generated by them probably determining their peculiar alternating histologic structure. In the young, the inner (convex) walls develop intimal cushions composed of collagenous material. The outer (concave) walls accumulate elastic elements in the subendothelial layer (Figure 3.36). Meyer

level. In the media of the cervical ICA, muscular fibers predominate over elastic elements; the latter are represented mostly by a prominent internal, and less prominent external, elastic lamina.

The cervical ICA above the bulb is usually free of atheromatous disease, although the lesions of fibromuscular dysplasia and dysplastic aneurysms (Figure 3.31) typically involve this segment. As it ascends in front of the lateral mass of the atlas, the ICA can be traumatized by this bony prominence (Figure 3.32), which moves forward when the head is turned to the opposite side. It is not known if this mechanism is the one that causes "spontaneous" intramural dissection.

Intramural dissection is typically seen in the cervical ICA (Figure 3.33). Whatever its mechanism, the dissection usually stops at the entrance of the artery into the temporal bone (Figure 3.34), where changes take place in and around the ICA. The architecture of its wall changes to that of a muscular artery, with most of its elastic fibers compacted into a single, internal elastic membrane and a media composed mostly of smooth muscle. The well-developed adventitia sends fibrous septa to the periosteum.

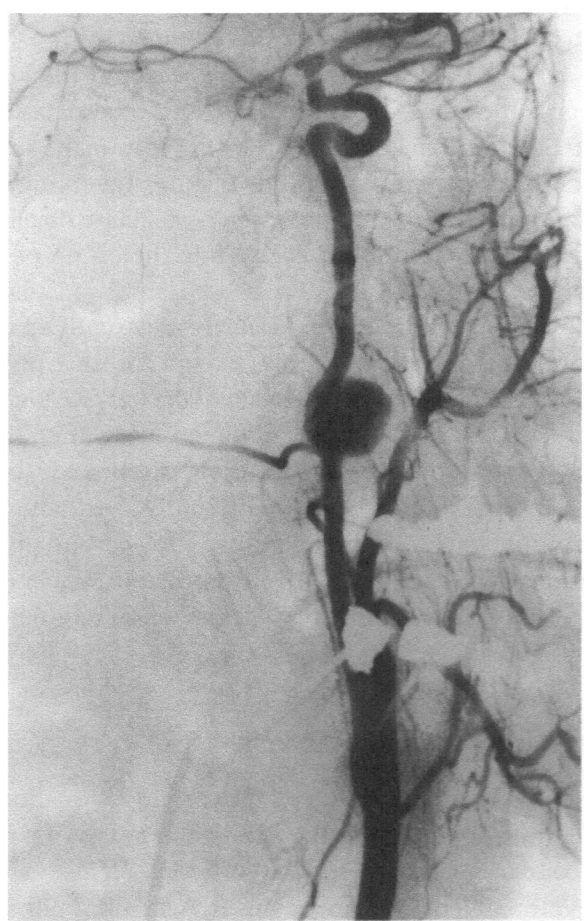

Figure 3.32 Traumatic aneurysm of the high cervical internal carotid artery.

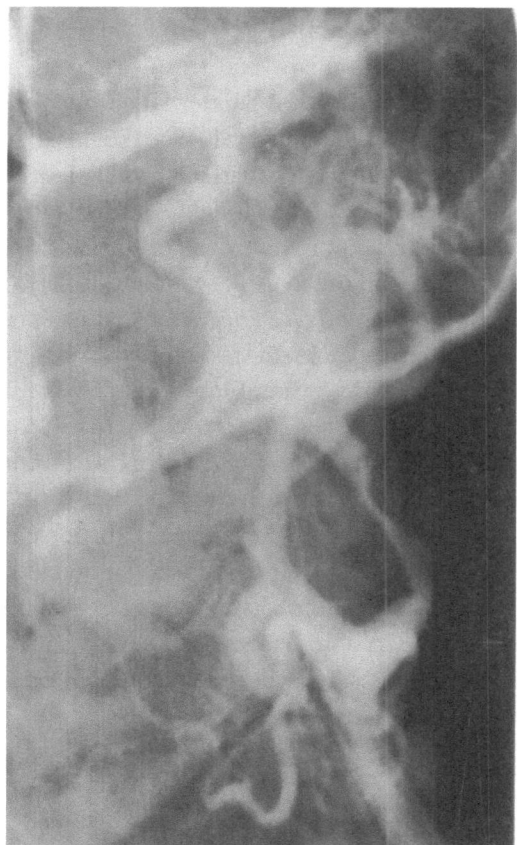

Figure 3.33 Localized intramural dissection of the cervical ICA.

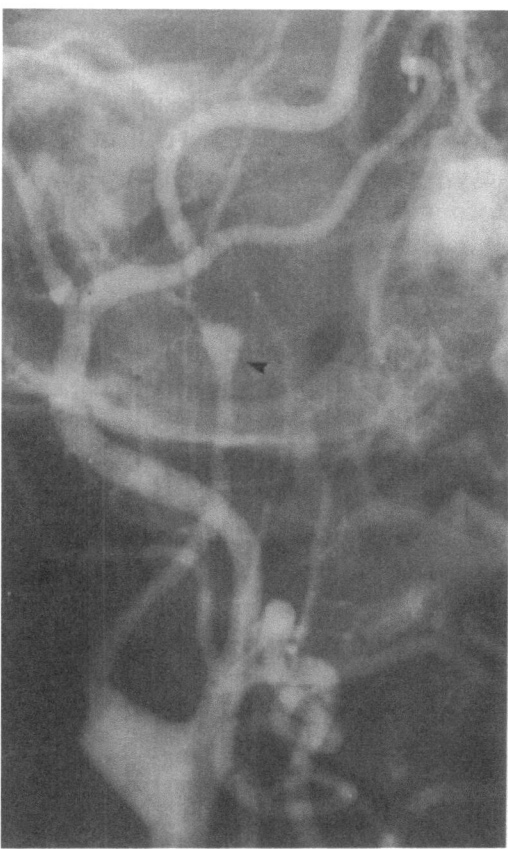

Figure 3.34 Long intramural dissection of the entire cervical ICA distal to the carotid bulb with an aneurysm (arrowhead) in its distal portion. The intrapetrosal carotid is normal.

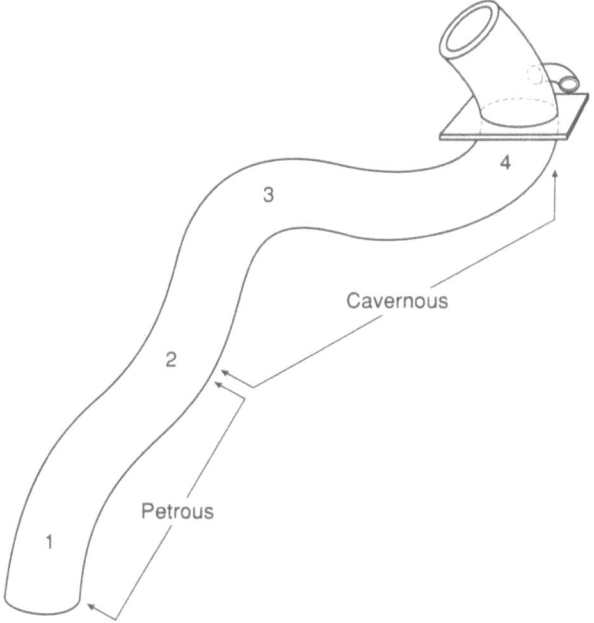

Figure 3.35 Four curvatures of the intracranial internal carotid artery. (Redrawn from Meyer et al.[58])

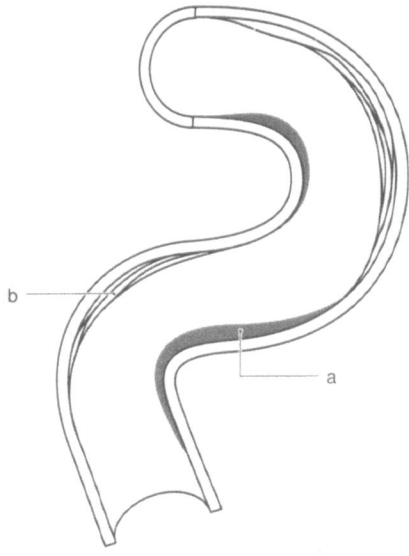

Figure 3.36 In the young, the inner convex walls (**a**) of the internal carotid develop intimal cushions. The outer concave walls (**b**) accumulate elastic elements in the subendothelial layer. (Redrawn from Meyer et al.[58])

et al.[58] have shown that lipid deposits, which already can be seen in adolescents, are preferentially associated with the hypertrophic elastic layers, whereas calcium deposits are associated with the collagenous intimal cushions. Later in life, when gross atheromatous formations develop, this preferential deposition of lipids in the concavities and calcium in the convexities becomes blurred.

Except for the unusual extensions of intramural dissection into it, the petrous segment of the ICA is usually spared from disease. Further up, the cavernous segment is the second most important site for stenosing and aneurysmal disease of the ICA (Figure 3.37).

The branches of the ICA may be involved by atheroma. Plaques in the anterior cerebral artery are best seen in the lateral view. In the middle cerebral artery the horizontal portion is the most common site of disease (Figure 3.38). These middle cerebral artery plaques are best seen in the anteroposterior view,

although this horizontal segment may be obscured by the bone density of the orbital rim.

Isolated stenosis of the external carotid artery is uncommon but often bilateral. The stenosis of the ostium of the ECA is usually part of a larger plaque at the carotid bifurcation. A few patients with advanced atherosclerosis have extensive lesions of the ECA involving the origin of all of its distal branches. Isolated ECA occlusion is uncommon. The artery is always patent above the occlusion, usually from the takeoff of the superior thyroid or facial arteries upward. Flow in the ECA may be maintained in these patients by a VA to ECA steal, wherein the occipital artery takes blood from the VA and feeds the ECA circuit by retrograde flow. In patients in whom this situation is present on both sides, a substantial amount of blood flow may be subtracted from the VA, causing vertebrobasilar ischemia. In this situation bilateral ECA thromboendarterectomy and angioplasty can reverse the steal and correct the symptoms.

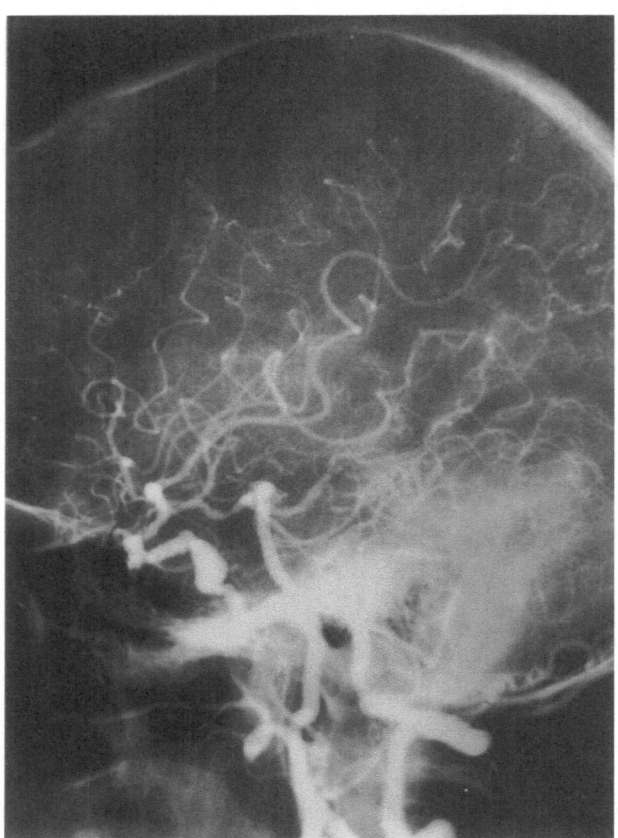

Figure 3.37 Aneurysmal disease of the cavernous internal carotid artery.

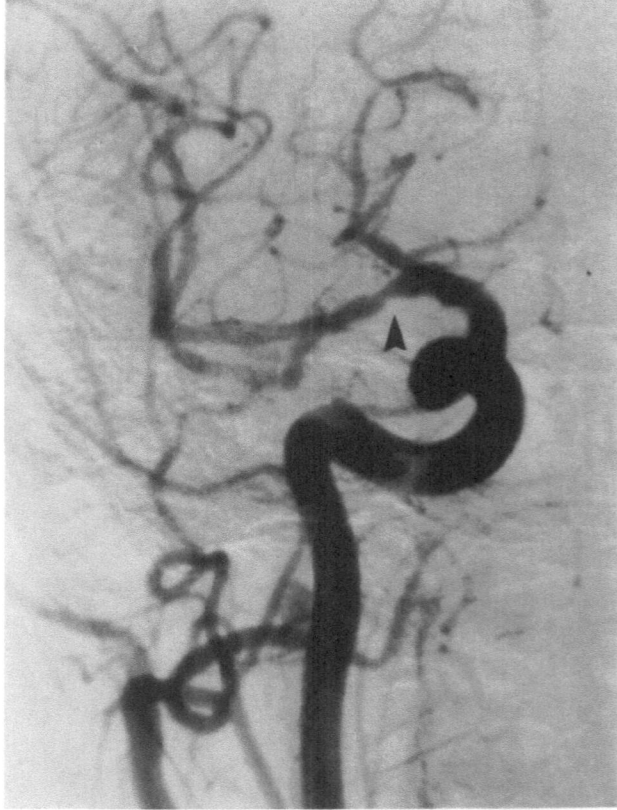

Figure 3.38 Stenosing disease (arrowhead) in the horizontal segment of the right middle cerebral artery.

Vertebral Artery

The VA also has specific sites for disease in its peculiar course. The most frequent site of narrowing occurs at its takeoff from the SA. This lesion is often missed in standard arteriograms because the curvature of the SA overlies and hides the origin of the VA (Figure 3.39). These orificial stenoses are usually short, measuring only a few millimeters in length. To demonstrate them, special oblique views may be needed to "throw" the SA aside (Figure 3.40) and show the VA takeoff from the posteromedial wall of the subclavian artery. Poststenotic dilatation is commonly seen with tight stenosis of the VA origin. A VA dilated immediately above its origin is commonly seen in patients with multiple and severe extracranial disease such as bilateral ICA occlusion. The artery undergoes hypertrophic dilatation in its extramural segment, whereas its orifice, splinted with plaque contiguous with that of the subclavian wall, does not dilate.

Shortly after its takeoff, the VA lies close to the upper pole of the lower cervical ganglion, which is usually posterior and inferior to the artery. There are sympathetic fibers in front of and behind the artery linking the lower and middle cervical ganglia. The fixation of the VA to these sympathetic structures may be the source of a kink, as with each breath a redundant VA moves up and down with the parent SA. Later in life when the aortic arch and the SA ascend in the neck in patients with long-standing hypertension, the VA may be permanently kinked by the stellate ganglion. Ipsilateral rotation of the neck (Figure 3.41) or hyperabduction of the arm may also cause temporary kinking of the VA owing to compression by the scalenus anticus muscle.

With arteritis of the Takayasu type, the VAs are often the only neck vessels spared from involvement by the disease and supplying most of the brain.

The close proximity of the VA to the single vertebral vein, both in their first segments, may result in the formation of an arteriovenous fistula following penetrating trauma at the base of the neck.

Higher up, the artery slips under the tendon of the longus colli muscle before entering the transverse foramen of C6. Although uncommon, this tendon can be stout and compress and occlude the artery against the transverse process of C7 when the muscle is pulled taut (Figure 3.42). Long-standing and critical

Figure 3.39 Severe stenosis at the origin of the right vertebral artery, which is seen only in the oblique projection (shown on the left).

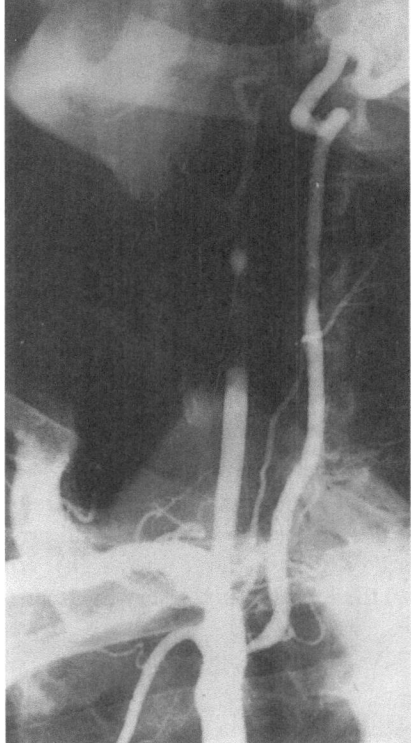
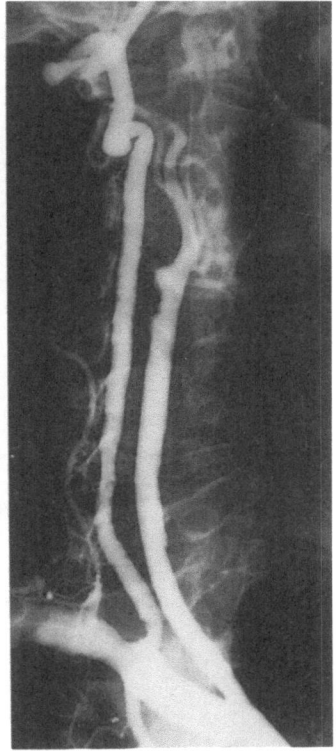

a, b

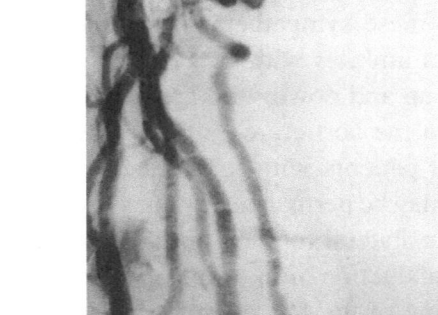
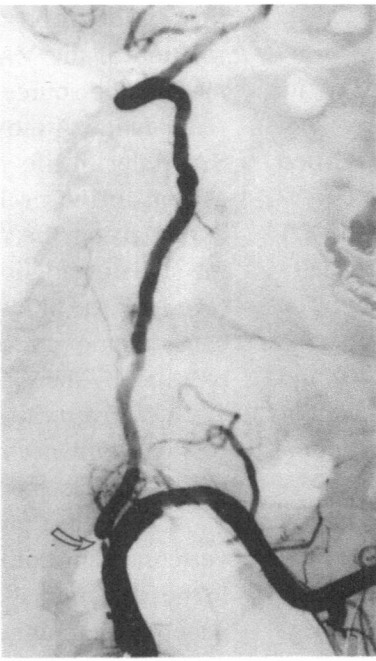

Figure 3.40 Origin of the left vertebral artery appears normal in the arch injection (**a**). An exaggerated oblique view (**b**) shows the stenosis of the vertebral artery (arrow).

a

b

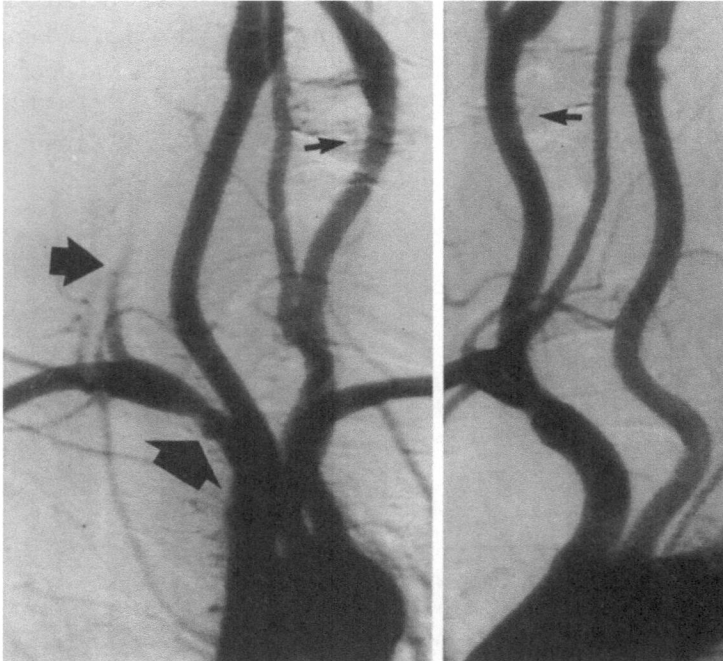

Figure 3.41 (a) In this patient the right vertebral artery occludes (large arrow) when the head is turned to the left (small arrow). There is an incidental right subclavian artery stenosis (large arrow). **(b)** When the head is turned to the right (small arrow) the left vertebral artery (large arrow) occludes.

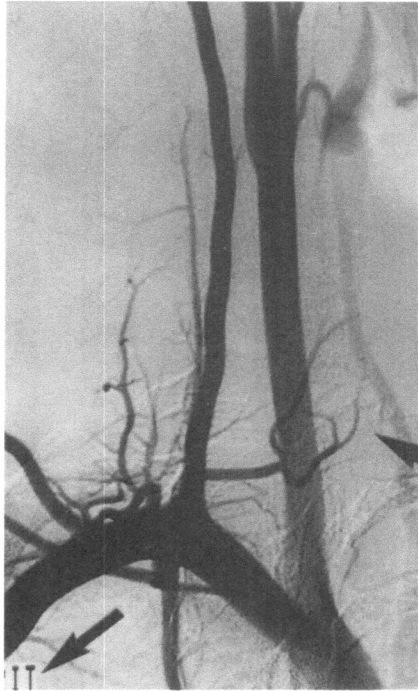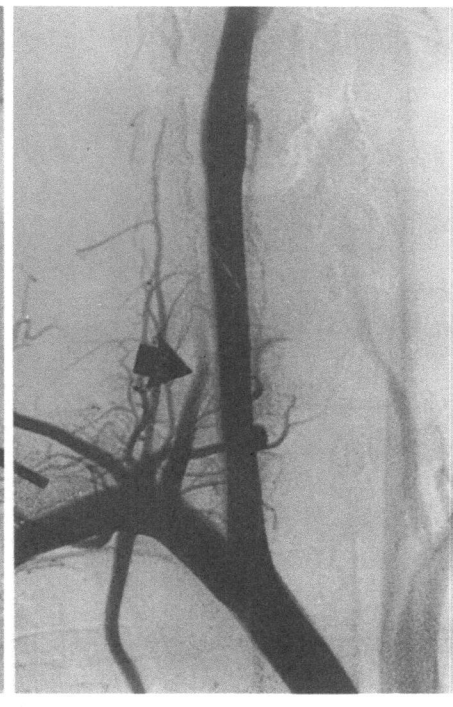

Figure 3.42 (a) Normal vertebral artery with the arm in adduction (small arrow). **(b)** With the arm in abduction (small arrow) the vertebral artery (large arrow) is compressed and occluded by the tendon of the longus colli.

compression can be inferred from an arteriogram when poststenotic dilatation is seen above an indentation of the artery at this level.

In its second segment the artery runs through the bony canals of the transverse processes of C6 through C2. There it may be deformed, impinged, or occluded by external pressure from osteophytes or torn by spinal trauma. The osteophytes may compress the artery only when the neck is rotated in a particular way, and this situation is mechanically aggravated when the patient sits up and bears the weight of the head. Unless the arteriogram is done with the neck in the position in which the patient has symptoms, the compression or occlusion of the artery may not be seen. It is noteworthy that the arteriographic appearance of the VA, particularly in its second segment, may be different with the patient lying down and standing up. Compression of the spine by the weight of the head and the splinting of the neck muscles in the upright position may reveal deformation and extramural compression, which are not seen on standard

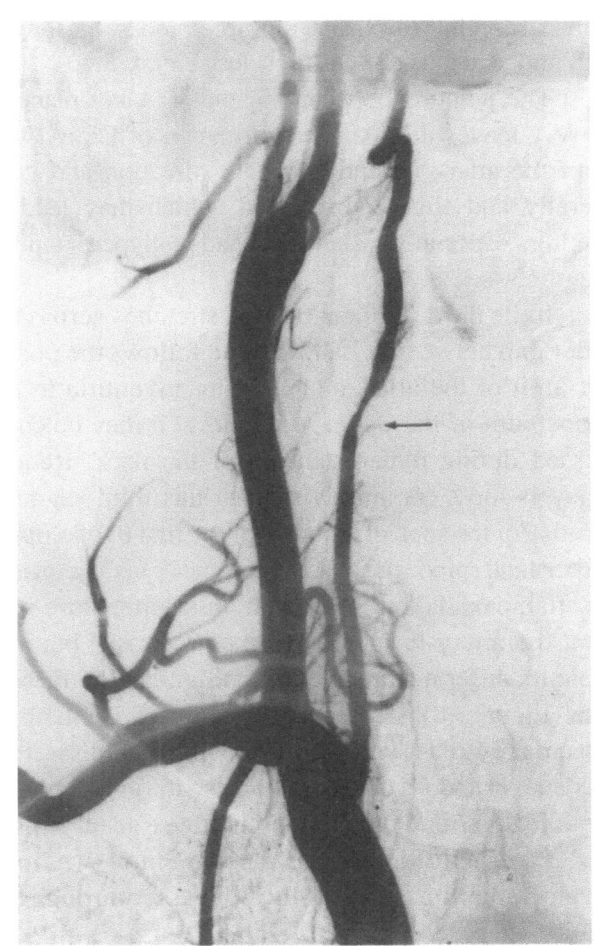

Figure 3.43 Compression of the vertebral artery by the longus colli and scalenus anticus muscles at an abnormally high point of entrance into the spine (arrow).

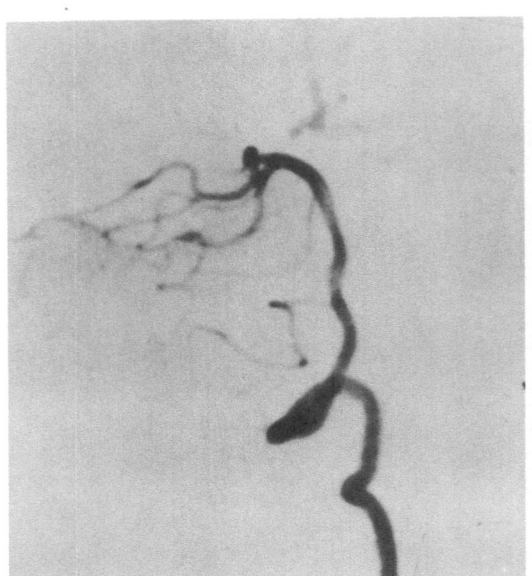 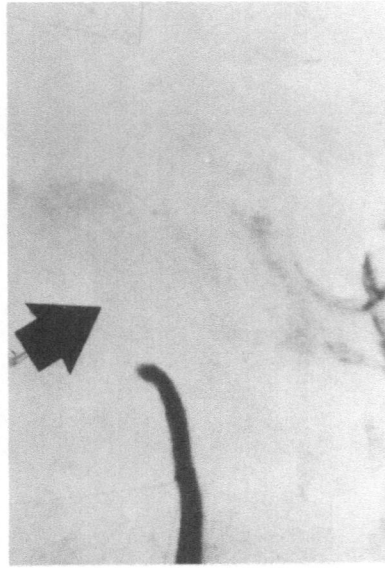

Figure 3.44 In its suboccipital course, as it exits C2, a normal vertebral artery (**a**) is compressed (**b**) by hyperextension of the neck.

arteriograms obtained with the patient lying down and the head resting on the arteriography table. When the VA enters the spine at an abnormally high level, it is more susceptible to extrinsic compression by the longus colli and scalenus anticus muscles (Figure 3.43).

The junction between V2 and V3 takes place as the VA leaves the transverse foramen of C2. At this point the artery abruptly changes direction and goes laterally and slightly backward, which may lead to kinking, especially when the head is hyperextended (Figure 3.44).

In its third segment the VA stretches across the wider gap between C1 and C2 and follows the posterior arch of the atlas, attaching its adventitia to the periosteum of the bone. At this level it may be compressed during hyperextension of the neck. Redundancy is most commonly seen in this third segment because of the special mobility of the first two joints of the cervical spine: the atlantooccipital ("yes") joint and the atlantoaxial ("no") joints. In this mobile third segment the artery is spared by atherosclerosis, but it is liable to suffer a stretch injury and intramural dissections (Figure 3.8). Vertebral arteries affected with fibromuscular dysplasia are particularly prone to dissection at this level and, as a consequence, to thromboembolic complications and the formation of false aneurysms.

In its fourth segment the intradural VA may develop atheromas, generally as it passes through the atlantooccipital membrane (Figure 3.45).

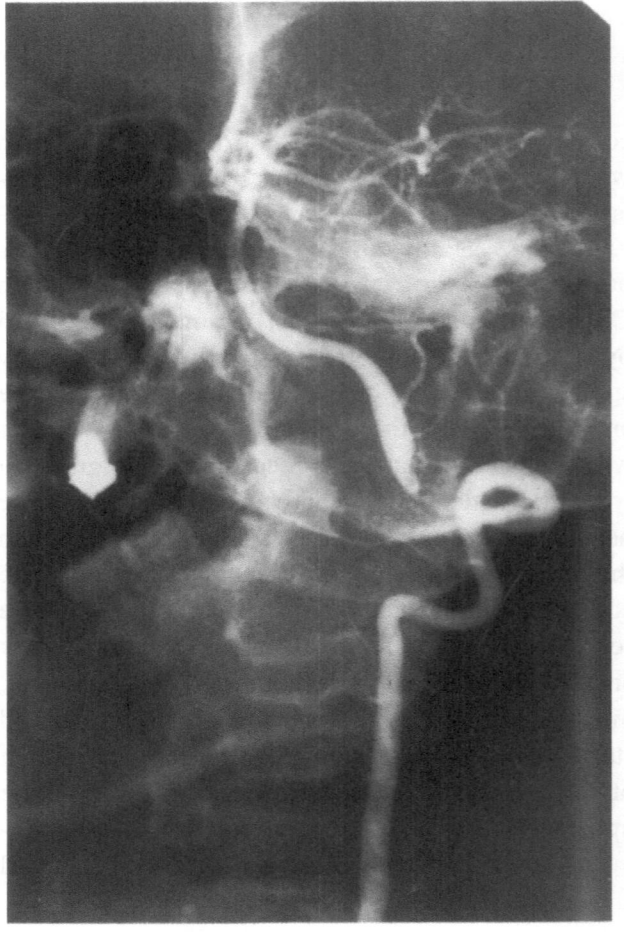

Figure 3.45 Severe atheroma of the vertebral artery at the junction of its third and fourth segments.

4 Mechanisms of Ischemia

Two mechanisms are involved in the production of symptoms in patients with lesions of the arteries that supply the brain: (1) The *hemodynamic mechanism* implies a regional drop in blood flow that is the result of either a restriction imposed by a proximal arterial blockage or failure of the heart pump mechanism to generate an adequate head of pressure (hypotension, arrhythmia). (2) The *embolic mechanism* is one in which particulate material—originating in the wall of the heart or of an artery—is carried by the flow stream eventually to lodge distally in some smaller vessel. This sequence usually results in occlusion of the vessel involved and damage to the tissue dependent on it if collateral flow cannot compensate for the arrest of blood flow. Some emboli may lodge in vessels but do not completely obliterate them, i.e., cholesterol crystals or emboli of irregular contour caught in a bifurcation. Other emboli fragment after lodging in a bifurcation and reembolize distally, as seen with fibrin-platelet plugs in the retinal arteries.

In the cerebral circulation both hemodynamic and embolic mechanisms can cause transient or permanent deficits. It is often difficult to determine whether a TIA or a stroke was due to severe restriction of blood flow or to an embolus. The flow restriction (hemodynamic) theory was prevalent at the time carotid surgery began to be performed and for years shaped the indications for it. There were, however, many inconsistencies between the hemodynamic theory of strokes and the clinical observations. For instance, it was difficult to explain the cure of TIA after thrombosis of the ICA, the tolerance of many patients to acute ligation of the CCA or ICA, and the intermittent nature of TIAs despite a stable narrowing of the ICA.

The embolic theory—that TIAs and strokes are primarily the result of embolization of the brain—is not new but has acquired clinical relevance primarily as a result of the work of Fisher and Adams,[59] Hollenhorst,[60] and Russell.[61] Today, the thromboembolic mechanism is ranked as the most important one in carotid artery disease. It is also increasingly recognized as a frequent mechanism in vertebrobasilar ischemia and of some TIAs or strokes secondary to disease of the supraaortic trunks (SAT). Both hemodynamic and thromboembolic mechanisms can lead to thrombosis of the distal arterial bed by a critical slowing of the blood flow, particularly if the distal arteries are severely diseased.

Hemodynamic Mechanism

The term *hemodynamic mechanism* implies that the tissue's requirements for blood flow are not being met because of a problem upstream. This perfusion deficit may be secondary to the proximal blockage of a large artery of supply or to a systemic cause. Stenosis or occlusion of a major artery supplying the territory may be due to intrinsic disease of the arterial wall or to its external compression. Systemic causes include failure of the heart pump, absolute loss of red blood cell mass (anemia), redistribution of blood (orthostatism), and increased peripheral resistance (tissue edema or hyperviscosity syndromes such as cryoglobulinemia or polycythemia).

Positional Changes in Blood Flow

Flow through the ICA and VA is affected by the movements of the neck. In their cervical course both of these arteries may be displaced, kinked, occluded, or injured by the bony cervical spine.

The most frequent point of compression of the ICA is at the level of the atlas. The large, wing-like transverse process of C1 projects forward when the neck is rotated to the opposite side and pushes the ICA, which rests on it (Figure 4.1). This mechanism was first described by Boldrey et al.[62] It is important to consider this possibility when positioning a patient for an operation in the carotid or vertebral artery. Excessive rotation of the neck to the opposite side, particularly if combined with some degree of extension, may in fact occlude the ICA that one plans to operate or rely upon during reconstruction of the VA. At a lower level, usually at C2, a severe kink of the cervical ICA may be aggravated with rotation of the neck and produce a drop in terminal ICA pressure (as shown by oculoplethysmography, symptoms, or both).

The VA is affected by neck movements to a greater degree than the ICA. In its second segment the artery traverses the foramina and is in close relation to the bone, making it likely that it could be compressed by osteophytes or by abnormally mobile intervertebral joints. In its third segment the artery has a redundancy—known in the French medical literature as the "safety loop"—that allows it to accommodate

the ample mobility of the atlantoaxial joint where one-half of the range of rotation of the neck takes place. It was DeKleyn and Nieuwenhuyse[63] who first showed that flow through the VA may cease with head turning. This finding is particularly relevant in individuals who have a dominant or single VA. In these patients vertebrobasilar ischemia may develop with head turning if compensatory flow from the ICA cannot be supplied by a good-sized posterior communicating artery.

Toole and Tucker[64] and more recently Koskas and Kieffer[65] quantified, in cadavers, the large variations in VA flow noted within the physiologic range of movement of the neck. These variations have also been demonstrated in healthy volunteers using radiographic techniques.

Positional changes in blood flow create a hemodynamic mechanism of ischemia by severely restricting flow through an artery. Position-induced extrinsic

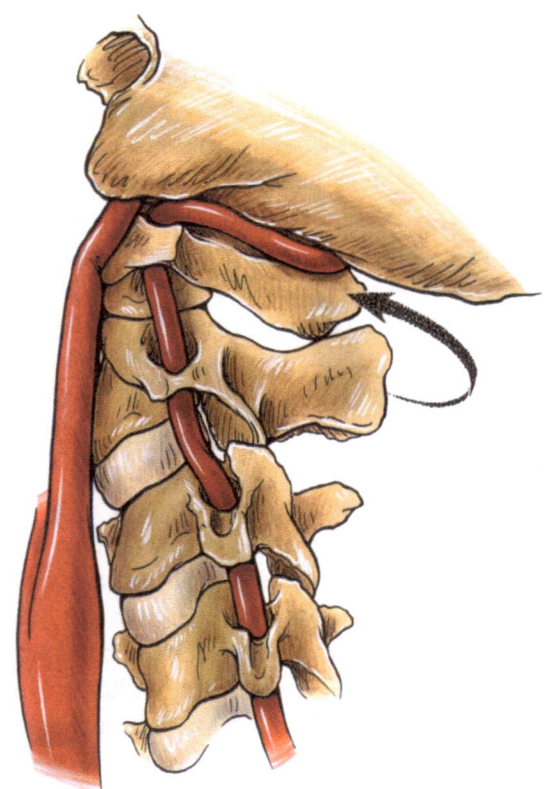

Figure 4.1 Compression of an internal carotid artery by the transverse process of the atlas during contralateral neck rotation.

Figure 4.2 Flow through a stenosis in a flow model. Flow streams are marked with dye. Note the orderly fast flow through the stenosed portion and the formation of vortices (turbulence) at the outlet. (Photograph obtained on a Hele-Shaw plate; fast flow depicted in red.)

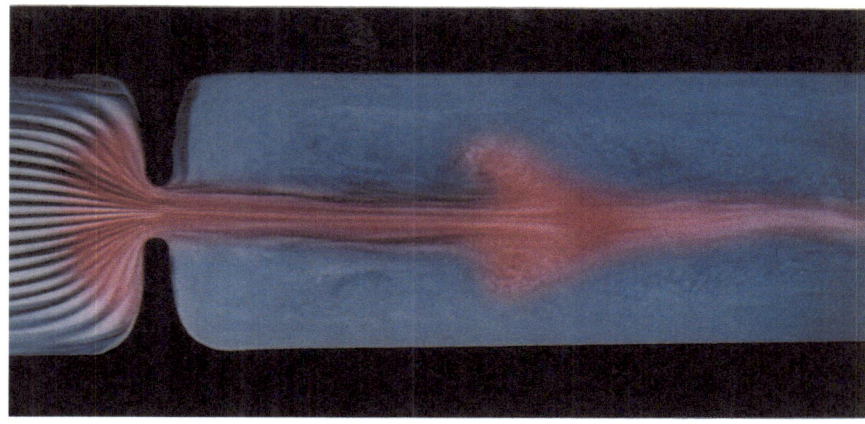

compression of an artery can also cause distal damage by embolization of thrombotic material formed in the traumatized wall. Moreover, the arterial wall traumatized by bone may become inflamed, develop an intramural dissection, or rupture its wall and develop a false aneurysm. All these pathologic variants of arterial trauma may result in partial or complete thrombosis of the ICA and VA as well as distal embolization.

Critical Stenosis

The most frequent hemodynamic mechanism of cerebral ischemia is the restriction of blood flow through a proximal artery of supply due to the presence of a critical stenosis. The mechanism by which a stenosis reduces flow is not straightforward. A vessel can be narrowed substantially without its flow rate being affected. When an artery is gradually constricted, however, there comes a point where there is a sudden drop in pressure beyond the constriction and in the flow rate through the artery. At this point the artery has reached a "critical" stenosis (commonly—and awkwardly—called a "hemodynamically significant stenosis"). This critical point is reached suddenly, without warning. Beyond this point, any further narrowing of the artery results in a precipitous drop in flow and distal pressure.

The term "subcritical stenosis" is sometimes used. A subcritical stenosis does not describe any specific flow pattern; it is mere anticipation. The term implies that a severe, but noncritical stenosis will became critical if a minimal change is added to the constricting lesion or to the velocity of the flow through it.

The appearance of the critical stenosis level with progressive narrowing is not a consequence of internal fluid friction as the flow squeezes through the narrowed segment. If that were so, it would be a gradual rather than a sudden occurrence. A critical stenosis is, rather, the consequence of the development of turbulence with massive dissipation of energy. The abrupt genesis of turbulence is a transition phenomenon that, to this day, has frustrated physicists and mathematicians attempting to explain it.

The mechanics involved, however, can be empirically understood[66] (Figure 4.2). As flow approaches the entrance of the stenotic segment, the constriction of the lumen imposes a sudden acceleration. The pressure energy in the artery (generated by the ventricular contraction) is converted to kinetic energy carried by the lumps of blood as they speed through the narrowed segment. The lateral arterial pressure energy drops by the same amount that the kinetic energy has increased (Bernoulli effect). Although flow across the stenosis is rapid, it continues to display an orderly, quasilaminar pattern. There is some increase in friction with the increase in velocity, but it accounts for only a negligible energy loss. At the outlet of the constriction, this accelerated fluid jet suddenly expands and enters the slow-moving flow in the poststenotic segment, like a fast mountain stream dissipating as it enters a lake.

The rapid, squeezed stream emerges into the poststenotic side where the flow channel abruptly recovers its normal size. As it hits the slower flow in

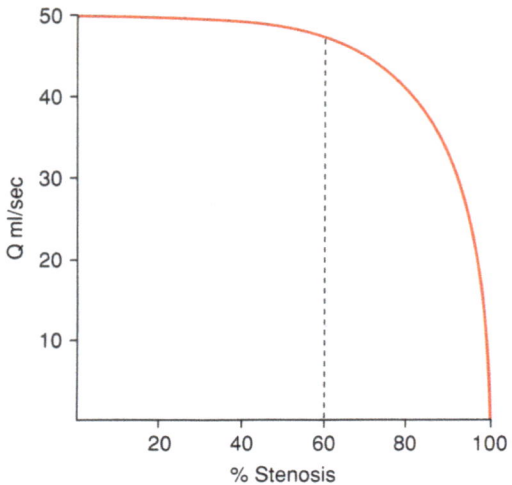

Figure 4.3 Concept of critical stenosis.

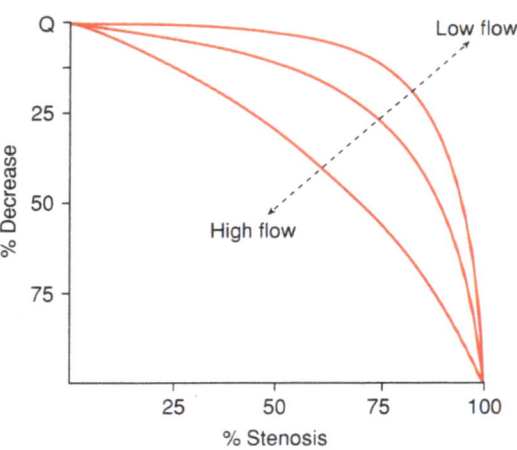

Figure 4.4 Percent stenosis at which the critical point appears varies depending on the initial flow rate.

the poststenotic segment, the emerging jet spends its high kinetic energy in the generation and maintenance of vortices (turbulence). These vortices are of different sizes and, as they hit the wall of the artery while they roll downstream, they make it vibrate, creating noise and heat. The frequency of the noise (vibration) produced is determined by the size of the vortices: Small ones produce high-pitched noise and large ones low-pitched vibrations. All the energy that had been transferred from the pressure (in the arterial wall) to the kinetic compartment (in the blood) for the fast trip across the stenosis is lost in the turbulence generated immediately beyond the narrowed segment. Consequently, the arterial pressure distal to the obstruction is lower and the distal perfusion decreases.

Mann et al.[67] in 1938 first studied the effects of a progressive stenosis on arterial flow (Figure 4.3). They noted that the critical point was not fixed at some specific degree of constriction, even for arteries that have the same diameter. Mann and associates noted that the critical point appeared at different percentages of stenoses for varying rates of flow (Figure 4.4). In vessels with high flow velocity (e.g., those supplying arteriovenous fistulas), a critical stenosis may develop with as little as a 20% cross-sectional constriction. On the other end, vessels with low flow velocities may have up to 90% of their lumen constricted without a drop in their flow rate.

There is nothing gradual about the effects of a progressive stenosis, just as there is nothing gradual about the start of turbulence in a pipe. The effects of a critical stenosis are caused by the sudden appearance of turbulence at the exit of the stenosis. To cause turbulence in an already narrowed artery we can either constrict the vessel further or increase the flow rate through it. Both result in higher velocity through the narrowed segment and early appearance of turbulence which spreads rapidly across the flow field. This explains the observation of Mann et al. that vessels with high flow rates (high flow velocity) develop critical stenoses early with a mild constriction, whereas arteries with low flow rates (low flow velocity) require a tighter stenosis before the onset of turbulence.

The length of the stenosis also affects the flow rate through it, although length ranks far below radius in determining the effects of a stenosis. The energy losses that take place as the length of a stenosis increases are primarily the result of fluid friction between the flow stream and the arterial wall. These losses are greater for fast and turbulent flows and for narrow and long segments.*

Finally, there is the question of what effect multiple stenoses have on the flow through an arterial

*For a steady flow system, whether laminar or turbulent, the loss due to length, is expressed by the Darcy-Weissbach formula

segment. From the point of view of flow mechanics, this proposition has as many variants as the infinite number of permutations that can be proposed for the severity of the various stenotic lesions and for the order in which they are placed. This matter is of such complexity it defies analysis. However, from an experimental point of view, a series of critical stenoses of the same severity has been shown to behave, if they are close enough to each other, as a continuous stenosis (over the segment containing the individual constrictions), with a uniform critical lumen.

If there is a critical lesion and another less severe stenosis in the same segment, the effects to be measured are largely those caused by the most severe constriction. In Weale's[68] words it is "analogous to a beam of light passing through diaphragms of different apertures. The smallest aperture controls the amount of light penetrating the combination."

Returning to the end-organ effects caused by a proximal critical stenosis, we should discuss a misconception occasionally cited in the interpretation of neurologic symptoms: that "focal" symptoms are derived from local disease, whereas "diffuse" symptoms arise from general systemic causes. Such a belief flies in the face of clinical evidence. Patients with smooth severe stenoses that have been proved at operation to be free of thrombus or ulceration may develop repetitive transient focal symptoms during episodes of transient hypotension that are cured by removing the carotid lesion. A simple conceptual model can explain the "focalization" of symptoms during transient systemic hypotension or a decrease in cardiac output (Figure 4.5). Let us assume that there is a stenosing plaque in a small arterial branch supplying the area that will eventually become symptomatic. This stenosis may decrease flow to its area of supply but not below the level where electrical or metabolic abnormalities will develop. A fall in central blood pressure causes an additional pressure drop in the stenotic branch territory beyond the tolerable level, and symptoms appear. The rest of the hemi-

$$Hl = f \ \frac{L}{D} \ \frac{V^2}{2g}$$

where Hl is the energy loss due to length, f is the resistance coefficient, L is the length of the stenosis, D is its diameter, and $V^2/2g$ is the kinetic energy per unit weight of the fluid flowing through the segment under consideration.

sphere, although hypotensive, is still within the perfusion level sufficient to function normally. In this situation a systemic problem (low cardiac output) causes a local lesion, e.g., a middle cerebral artery stenosis, to become symptomatic, which explains why some individuals with "fixed" stable carotid lesions suffer transient ischemic manifestations. A similarly localizing effect takes place when an area of the brain with a high metabolic activity has a marginal

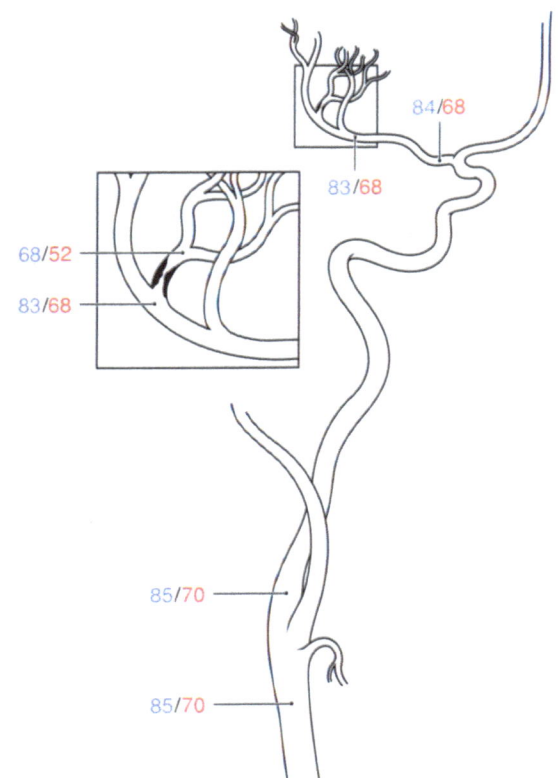

Figure 4.5 Intermittent, transient drops in systemic pressure may result in a discrete transient deficit, repetitively localized in the same area. Baseline pressures are shown in blue, and pressures after a transient drop in cardiac output in red. The critical stenosis at the origin of the branch of the middle cerebral artery causes a drop of 15 mm Hg in mean pressure (83 mm Hg → 68 mm Hg). The remaining pressure (68 mm Hg) is sufficient to perfuse its territory above the presumed level at which ischemic symptoms would appear (55 mm Hg). A drop in systemic pressure causes the intracerebral mean perfussion pressure to drop to 68 mmHg, still sufficient to provide adequate flow. However, the territory supplied by this stenotic branch now has a mean pressure of 52 mm Hg, which is insufficient to provide adequate perfusion; the area thus becomes ischemic, and symptoms appear.

flow situation, e.g., individuals with chronic poor retinal perfusion who are blinded by exposure to bright light.

Embolic Mechanism

Although it is sometimes difficult to determine whether TIAs and strokes are the result of hemodynamic or thromboembolic mechanisms, there is clinical and pathologic evidence suggesting that, at least in the carotid territory, thromboembolism is the more important of the two. More recent evidence is available showing that about one-third of VBI episodes are secondary to an embolus originating in the heart or in the subclavian, vertebral, or basilar arteries.

The thromboembolic mechanism is also strongly suspected to be the cause of symptoms in individuals with complex atheromatous plaques of the SAT. These lesions have the same degenerative features as plaques of the carotid bifurcation known to be associated with distal atheroembolization.

The source of embolization is either in the heart or somewhere in the arterial pathway from the heart to the site where the embolus lodges. Central embolization sources can be the pulmonary veins, left atrium (fibrillation, myxoma, thrombus), cardiac valves, or thrombus on the ventricular inner surface overlying a zone of infarction or within an aneurysm.

The ascending aorta is rarely a source of embolization to the brain. The arterial source of an embolus may be near the origin of the great vessels but more commonly is in the carotid bifurcation, in the first three segments of the VA, or in the basilar artery.

Within the arteries supplying the head a number of lesions may give rise to emboli. The most common sources are ulcerated plaques, aneurysms with layered clot, dissections of the arterial wall, intimal flaps, and arterial wall trauma causing mural thrombosis. From these sources emboli follow the current of flow to infarct the distal bed. Embolic material can be atheroma debris, platelet-fibrin aggregates, blood clots, or specks of calcium from the edges of an aortic valve. More exotic emboli are composed of the chemicals used to "cut" drugs, air from arteriographic catheters, or bullets entering the circulatory system.

The destination of an embolus carried by the blood flow stream is determined partly by its size and partly by the flow rate and flow currents in branches the particle encounters in its path. Obviously those arteries that carry the largest flow rates carry the largest amount of particulate material. It is not surprising that the ICA territory is a frequent site of infarction for many emboli. Within the ICA territory the middle cerebral artery, which carries 80% of the total ICA flow, is the one most likely to be entered by an embolus.

As an embolus travels downstream it may cause silent or overt complications. Like the proverbial tree falling in a deserted forest, an embolus may be entirely silent and be found incidentally at funduscopic examination, during arteriography, or at autopsy. We have seen silent embolic occlusions of the CCA, ICA, VA, and most of their branches where distal perfusion was maintained by collaterals from the time of occlusion. The patient has had neither symptoms nor findings of tissue damage distal to the occlusion. Some emboli partially block an artery, jammed between its walls but allowing flow around them, like a tree stuck in a stream. Emboli of this type are frequently composed of cholesterol crystals and can be seen in the branches of the retinal artery. Other emboli may cause a silent infarction, which in the brain is seen in about one-fifth of the patients with presumably asymptomatic carotid disease. These are infarcts that take place in areas of the brain with little or no somatic representation and in some of the peripheral areas of the retina. These silent infarcts are incidentally found on CT scans or at autopsy.

The location and shape of an infarction may give a clue as to whether its etiology is embolic or hemodynamic. Hemodynamic infarctions tend to occur in watershed areas, whereas embolic ones are usually in the core of the area supplied by a particular artery. Emboli may fragment and reembolize peripherally. This situation is occasionally seen when observing fibrin-platelet embolic material at the bifurcations of the branches of the retinal artery.

Embolic material from a lesion in the arterial wall may be dislodged when the soft core of a plaque bursts into the bloodstream. It is likely that this break is sometimes caused by the expansion and contraction of the arteries during the cardiac cycle. Lusby et al.[69] showed how an eccentric plaque may be noncompliant with respect to the rest of the more normal arterial circumference. As the artery expands and contracts, a break may occur at the interface between the distensible and nondistensible portions of the wall, with subsequent hemorrhage or intimal disruption. External trauma can also cause the release of embolic material as seen in the occasional reports of embolization of the hemispheres during carotid massage done for treatment of a cardiac arrhythmia. Probably some of the strokes observed after carotid endarterectomy are secondary to manipulation of the carotid bulb during dissection. When an osteophyte repeatedly traumatizes the VA, it may cause inflammation of the wall, deposition of thrombus, and eventually its release into the bloodstream.

Traditionally, the symptoms of ischemia in the vertebrobasilar territory have been considered to be of hemodynamic nature. There is, however, pathologic evidence[70] indicating that thromboembolism is common in the vertebrobasilar territory and can be incriminated in about one-third of the infarctions produced in it. This evidence comes from studies done in areas of infarction, primarily in the occipital lobes and cerebellum, showing that the thrombosed artery supplying the zone of infarction often has no evidence of atheroma in its walls. If the thrombus did not form on a previous atheroma, it must have come from a more proximal source. The site of this proximal source has been identified in many of the studies to have been in the VA, proximal SA, and heart.

Acute Cerebral Ischemia

The architecture of the arterial supply to the brain is such that the chance for collateral compensation decreases as the periphery is approached. This fact explains the apparent contradiction in the finding that extensive proximal occlusions (i.e., in the CCA) may cause few or no clinical consequences, whereas discrete and more distal blockages (i.e., in the middle cerebral artery) usually result in important neurologic deficits. As an artery supplying a small area of brain is occluded by an embolus or thrombus, the wedge shape of brain supplied by it becomes ischemic (Figure 4.6). Normal cerebral blood flow values are approximately 50 ml/100 gm/min. Brain tissue, however, can tolerate levels considerably lower than normal and remain functional until the blood flow rate drops below 18 ml/100 gm/minute. This level of perfusion is found at the outermost boundary of an acutely ischemic zone. Brain tissue perfused at this reduced blood flow level becomes electrically silent: the electroencephalogram is flat, the evoked poten-

Figure 4.6 Zones of ischemia in brain tissue following occlusion of the artery of supply: **(a)** normal brain; **(b)** edema and ischemic penumbra; **(c)** metabolic derangement and necrosis.

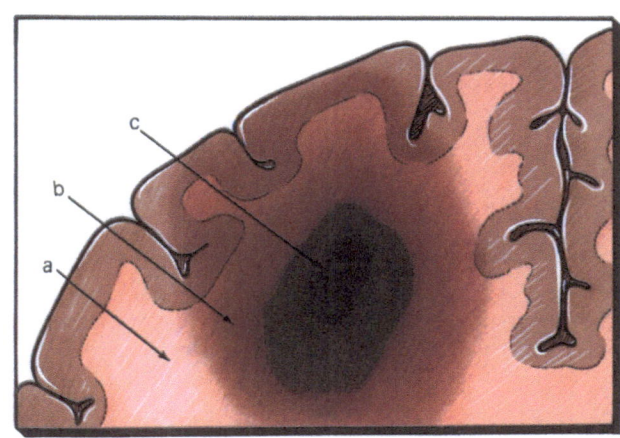

tials are abolished, and all electrical transmission ceases. Blood flow autoregulation is also absent. There are, however, no metabolic derangements. This is the zone that Astrup et al.[71] elegantly labeled the "ischemic penumbra." The cells are asleep, taking a siesta, and the reduced blood flow keeps their metabolic chains working at a basal rate. As in a Renaissance portrait this functional "chiaroscuro" is at the rim of the picture, at the boundary with normal functioning brain. If blood flow in the ischemic penumbra is restored to normal, the cells within resume their normal electrical activity. It is not known how long the penumbra cells remain viable and susceptible to being recruited back to normal function. As the acute changes induced by ischemia progress, the infarction may extend peripherally at the expense of the penumbra area, or it may recede as collateral supply of blood flow improves perfusion and tissue edema subsides.

Toward the core of the ischemic area, blood flow continues to decrease, and another important threshold is crossed. When cerebral blood flow decreases to 10 ml/100 mg/min, metabolic derange-

ments appear: among others, a massive egress of potassium to the extracellular compartment. The cells are damaged, and resumption of flow does not restore their normal function. At the core of the infarct, blood flow is zero and the cells are necrosed.

The outcome of an infarction in the brain is partly determined by the extent of the edema that surrounds it. Edematous brain tissue has increased pressure and may not allow flow through the tenuous collaterals with low intravascular pressure that traverse it. The rigid cranium does not allow room for further tissue swelling, and extensive damage to the rest of the brain may be caused by increasing edema and the anatomic dislocation that follows it.

Abnormal values of cerebral blood flow and abnormal function are also noted in areas remote to the infarct. This phenomenon is termed *diaschisis*. The remote effects are a consequence of the cessation of facilitating impulses previously generated in the now infarcted area, redistribution (steal) of local blood flow, abnormal production of neurotransmitters, and the mechanical effects of edema.

5 Presentation and Selection of Patients

Clinical Syndromes

The clinical manifestations of ischemia of the brain caused by disease of its supplying arteries are traditionally classified as transient (TIAs) or permanent (stroke) neurologic deficits. Conventionally, a deficit lasting less than 24 hours is called a TIA and one lasting longer than that is called a stroke. For a while it was popular to insert a third category between these two known by its acronym, RIND, a reversible ischemic neurologic deficit. To qualify as a RIND, such a deficit was arbitrarily said to be present for longer than 24 hours but less than 3 weeks. The sequestration of deficits into this third clinical category has no discernible practical use or specific pathologic correlation. Most of the so-called RINDs have been shown by modern imaging techniques to be strokes. Therefore the use of RIND as a category in clinical description is no longer justified.

With postmortem studies of the brain being the exception rather than the rule, there was for many years a dearth of clinicopathologic correlation in the study of cerebrovascular disease. The advent of computed tomographic (CT) scanning of the brain and more recently of magnetic resonance imaging (MRI) has provided important information from which correlations between specific symptoms and specific brain lesions have been derived, at least within the limits of resolution of which these instruments are capable.

The term TIA, like stroke, is merely the description of a clinical event and should not be associated with a transient disturbance that, after compensation, leaves behind an intact brain. In fact, brain infarction is frequently the anatomic lesion responsible for a clinical TIA. Many patients with TIAs sustain substantial loss of brain tissue but manage to compensate rapidly for the physiologic deficit.

The routine scanning of patients who have anatomically demonstrated ICA disease has shown that approximately 17% of those presumed asymptomatic already have zones of infarction in the brain ("silent infarctions") seen as hypodense areas in the CT scan.[72] Of those with a history of TIAs, approximately 20% show an infarct in the brain by CT scan. If the TIA is referable to a hemisphere, rather than to the brainstem or cerebellum, the incidence of silent infarction is even higher. On the contrary, only 64% of those with a fixed neurologic deficit show a CT lesion suggestive of an infarct. We know, however, that the CT scan cannot resolve small infarcts, which may cause serious neurologic deficits.

It is not within our competence to discuss in detail the lengthy list of ischemic brain syndromes associated with occlusion of one or another of the branches of the carotid or vertebrobasilar systems. For a brief general description, the symptoms caused by occlusive or embolic disease of the arteries supplying the brain may be grouped into two large categories: carotid (or anterior) and vertebrobasilar (or posterior) syndromes.

There is not always a precise correspondence between the territory that produces the symptom and the main artery of supply involved. For instance, patients with severe and bilateral narrowing of both ICAs may present exclusively with VBI. The posterior communicating arteries permit supply of the posterior circulation from the ICA in patients with small or occluded VAs and vice versa. If most of the supply of the vertebrobasilar territory depends on the ICA, a decrease in perfusion pressure in the latter causes the first symptoms to appear in the territory that is the farthest away and has the highest peripheral resistance—hence the symptoms of VBI.

Even allowing for this occasional crossover of arterial lesions and symptoms, most patients with ICA disease manifest anterior (or ocular/hemispheric) symptoms, whereas those with VA or basilar artery disease present posterior circulation symptoms.

The location of the watershed between the anterior and posterior circulations depends on the source of supply of the posterior cerebral arteries. In 80% of patients the posterior cerebral arteries arise from the terminal basilar artery, and therefore the occipital lobe is generally considered posterior circulation territory. In this circumstance the boundary between the two circulations in these patients is drawn roughly across the posterior tip of the temporal lobe. In the 20% of patients in whom the posterior cerebral artery arises from the ICA, the entire hemisphere is in the territory of the latter.

The ICA syndrome encompasses manifestations arising from the frontal, parietal, temporal, and occasionally occipital lobes supplied by it. In addition to the cortical involvement in these lobes, ischemia of the ICA also involves the internal capsule (which has tightly packed and therefore vulnerable bundles of sensory and motor fibers originating in the cortex), optic radiations, globus pallidus, and nucleus caudatus. In the dominant (usually left) hemisphere, Broca's or Wernicke's aphasias may be present. Involvement of the optic tracts as they travel through the parietal and temporal lobes results in more or less complete hemianopsias.

Unilateral eye symptoms are an important feature of the ICA syndrome. Transient loss of vision (amaurosis fugax) is more frequent than the more serious ischemic injuries such as infarction of the retina, occlusion of the central retinal artery or one of its branches, or infarction of the optic nerve due to thrombosis of the posterior ciliary arteries.

The ophthalmoscopic findings in patients with amaurosis fugax are usually negative. The mechanism of these symptoms can be either an embolus that eventually fragments and lodges in a more peripheral location or hypotension of the central retinal artery with subsequent transient ischemia of the retina it supplies. Patients with severe occlusive disease of the ICA or of the ophthalmic artery and branches may have a hypotensive retinal artery and experience a form of retinal claudication when, after exposure to bright light, they are briefly blinded.

The symptoms caused by disease of the VA or basilar artery are less well defined than those arising in the hemispheres from carotid artery disease. The mechanisms of vertebrobasilar ischemia are the same as those of carotid artery disease: either thromboembolic or hemodynamic. The thromboembolic source may be in the VA (occluded or diseased), the basilar artery, the proximal SA, or the heart chambers. It is estimated that at least one-third of the ischemic infarctions of the vertebrobasilar territory are of thromboembolic origin.[70] Low perfusion pressure in the basilar artery is more often due to systemic causes, e.g., low cardiac output, shock, or orthostatism. However, severe occlusive disease of the VA (or basilar artery) is also a frequent cause of symptoms due to hypoperfusion. A systemic cause (e.g., orthostatism) and segmental occlusion or stenosis of the VA may be present, compounding each other's effects.

The manifestations of VBI are dizziness, vertigo, tinnitus, ataxia, blurring of vision, diplopia, perioral numbness, and drop attacks. Intrinsic disease of the inner ear can cause vertigo, tinnitus, and deafness. Patients with vertebrobasilar symptoms of hemodynamic origin tend to have diffuse symptoms that are brief, transitory, and repetitive and seldom result in brain infarcts. Patients suffering from thromboembolic VBI have more discrete, more persistent symptoms and a high incidence of brain infarction. Infarction of the vertebrobasilar territory is often missed by the CT scan but can be seen on MRI scans.

Patient Selection

Disease of the Supraaortic Trunks

Patients with disease of the branches of the aortic arch may present with symptoms of the carotid or vertebrobasilar distribution or both and, occasionally, symptoms of upper limb ischemia. Restriction of blood flow is the most common mechanism, although embolization from ulcerated plaques or aneurysms is also seen.

An arteriogram is indispensable for evaluating these patients. The definition of an arterial lesion by arteriography is best achieved when the lumen of the vessel is outlined in two projections, usually perpendicular to each other, e.g., anteroposterior and lateral views. Right and left oblique projections are traditionally obtained to evaluate the supraaortic trunks (SAT). The branches of the aortic arch may be visualized without superimposition in the right posterior oblique projection. The left posterior oblique view shows the trunks as they emerge from the top of the arch superimposed on each other, raising the possibility that the only view that separates the trunks (right oblique projection) may miss an eccentric plaque that faces the viewer in this projection.

In addition to the SAT, the arteriogram should also display both carotid bifurcations, the cervical course of both VAs and the intracranial arteries. When the carotid bifurcations are involved and there is no intracranial disease contraindicating the procedure, arterial repair of the SAT is carried up to the carotid bifurcation. Before repairing any trunk it must be established that its outflow tract is open. For instance, a bypass of the CCA carried onto the bifurcation requires demonstrating the patency of the carotid bifurcation branches beforehand. In extreme cases where the occlusion of the SAT does not allow proper visualization of the branches of the CCA, a direct exploration of the bifurcation may be required

before opening the chest. Radiologic evidence of subclavian steal does not constitute a surgical indication by itself. A CT scan of the brain is also part of the workup for these patients because silent hemispheric infarction may result from atheromas of the IA or the CCA.

In patients who have not had coronary revascularization and are candidates for transthoracic reconstruction of the branches of the aortic arch, we advise coronary arteriography. It is worth considering simultaneous SAT and coronary repair given the high incidence of coronary artery disease in this group and the difficulty of coronary revascularization in patients who have had a previous transternal repair of the SAT. Once the indication for a transthoracic approach has been met we advocate complete revascularization of all critical lesions including those lesions of the SA, even if the latter are not symptomatic. This technique allows secondary cervical repair should the IA or left CCA reconstruction occlude at a later time.

Our indications for repair of the SAT are as follows.

1. Symptomatic lesions of the SAT causing ischemic symptoms of carotid, vertebrobasilar, or upper limb distribution. Symptoms often involve the carotid and vertebrobasilar territories simultaneously and occasionally the upper extremities. The mechanism for production of symptoms is either severe restriction of flow due to critical lesions, usually at the origin of the SAT, or embolization from irregular or ulcerated atheromatous plaque.

2. Asymptomatic patients with complex plaques in the SAT and no evidence of intracranial arterial disease who present with ipsilateral silent brain infarctions.

3. Asymptomatic but severe (> 75% of diameter) lesions of the IA and CCA because we believe that these lesions have the same potential risks as those found in the carotid bifurcation.

4. Severe asymptomatic lesions of the SA (> 75% of diameter) in patients who are candidates for coronary artery revascularization to ensure adequate internal mammary artery inflow. Revascularization of the SA is also indicated in patients who have had a previous myocardial revascularization using the in-

ternal mammary artery and have recurrence of angina due to progression of disease in the ipsilateral SA. Finally, asymptomatic occlusions of the SA are also revascularized to allow blood pressure measurement in patients with bilateral subclavian occlusions and to provide inflow in those patients who require hemodialysis or axillofemoral bypass grafting.

The choice between the transsternal and supraclavicular approaches is discussed in Chapter 8. If there is associated disease of the carotid bifurcation, the latter should be treated at the same operation either as a separate procedure or by performance of a distal anastomosis of the bypass to an endarterectomized carotid bifurcation.

When SAT reconstructions are done in patients who have suffered silent infarctions or clinical strokes, the timing for the operation is a bit different than what is used for isolated carotid disease because the incidence and extent of revascularization hyperemia appears to be greater after reconstruction of multiple proximal trunks. We do not advise reconstruction of the SAT following an infarction until 1 month has elapsed. This general rule is particularly important in patients who have lost their autoregulatory blood flow mechanisms in the brain (as can be seen on contrast CT scans or in studies of regional cerebral blood flow) because of large infarctions or extensive disease of all three trunks.

It is worth adding that no operation should be done during the active phase of Takayasu's disease when the patient has an elevated erythrocyte sedimentation rate. Steroid therapy for a few weeks can cool the inflammatory phase and allow a safer reconstruction.

Carotid Artery Disease

Arteriography remains the keystone to defining the extent of disease and the possible contraindications to an operation. The arteriogram must outline the entire circulation from the aortic arch to the intracranial branches. Proper visualization of the branches of the arch shows if there is a proximal lesion. The cervical and intracranial ICA is best defined by selective injections for anteroposterior and lateral views. The intraarterial digital techniques today permit a com-

prehensive arterial survey using reasonable amounts of contrast material.

The presence of severe or diffuse intracranial disease is generally a contraindication to an extracranial arterial operation. In the carotid territory severe disease of the siphon or of the middle cerebral artery, usually in its horizontal portion, generally precludes an operation on the ipsilateral carotid system.

In disease of the carotid bifurcation the arteriogram permits a rough rating of the degree of stenosis and of any gross surface irregularity, e.g., a deep ulceration, that may be present. If the carotid lesion does not appear "threatening" on the arteriogram and there is no evidence of an intracranial or cardiac etiology for the symptoms, the carotid duplex may outline additional plaque features, e.g., ulceration and intraplaque hemorrhage, that may not be evident on the arteriogram and that, if present, suggest that the carotid lesion is the source of the symptoms.

Computed tomography is an important part of the evaluation of patients presenting with symptoms of carotid distribution, as it may reveal the nature of the lesion that causes the symptom or provide evidence of previous silent infarctions. The localization (central or watershed territory) and the shape of the infarction may suggest whether the etiology is thromboembolic or due to low perfusion. During the acute phase of an infarction the brain CT scan is usually obtained without and with contrast. The former method is best for detecting the presence of hyperdense blood, the latter for defining the intracerebral architecture. The CT scan, however, is a poor tool for detecting the hypodense area that corresponds to a brain infarction during the first 48 hours after the event. Small but clinically important infarctions in the internal capsule may never be seen by CT scanning. For utilization reasons MRI is not yet routinely used for evaluating the consequences of carotid artery disease, though it may be utilized in the future.

Our indications for operation on carotid artery disease are as follows.

1. Symptomatic patients with TIAs or minor residual symptoms from a previous stroke who have evidence of carotid artery disease. Although atheromatous carotid disease frequently coexists with hemispheric symptoms or findings of brain infarction

by CT scan, one cannot always presume a cause-and-effect relation. The elements of judgment that allow the presumption of causality and eventually the indications for surgical reconstruction are the clinical course and the findings on the CT scan of the brain. The clinical course of a neurologic deficit suggests its etiology. Vascular events have a rapid onset and usually improve rapidly as collateral flow or fragmentation or distal migration of the embolus improves perfusion. Massive infarctions, however, may progress and worsen as the original damage is compounded by edema and, eventually, dislocation of the brain anatomy. Patients in whom the arteriogram or the duplex scan has shown a carotid lesion and who have had a TIA or who have minor residual deficits from a previous stroke are candidates for repair of the carotid lesion. Most symptomatic patients should undergo a cardiac workup to rule out a cardiac source for their symptoms. A carotid operation is also indicated in a second group of symptomatic patients, those presenting with manifestations of vertebrobasilar ischemia who have intact hemispheres on the brain CT scan but are bearers of critical carotid lesions.

Another group of patients, those having silent brain infarctions, are considered with this group, even though they are asymptomatic, as their carotid lesions have already proved their potential morbidity by causing an infarct. Whether an infarct is silent or not depends mostly on the size of the embolus and the part of the brain involved.

2. Asymptomatic patients with a severe (> 75% diameter) stenosis of the ICA or complex plaques with a large ulceration or thrombus on the surface of a plaque that is not critically reducing flow. If the patient is a good surgical risk, such potentially threatening lesions should probably be removed.

The main contraindications for a carotid operation are severe intracranial disease and a massive ipsilateral brain infarction. Age is not a contraindication, as carotid endarterectomy is a reasonably atraumatic cervical operation. Finally, cardiovascular disease, particularly severe coronary artery disease and hypertension, may contraindicate a carotid operation. On occasion, the coronary artery and carotid corrections are done at the same operative session. Hyper-

tension, if present, should be controlled with drugs before subjecting the patient to surgery.

The only emergency primary operation on the carotid bifurcation takes place in those patients who have an acute occlusion of the ICA. The diagnosis of an acute ICA occlusion is usually suspected when the patient undergoes a duplex scan of the carotid bifurcation following a stroke. If a patient is alert, we proceed with immediate arteriography and CT scanning of the brain (without contrast) to determine if there is an indication for an emergency thromboendarterectomy. Assuming that (1) there is no evidence of bleeding in the CT scan, (2) the distal siphon is patent and filling by collaterals, (3) the blood pressure is under control, and (4) mentation is normal, the patient is operated on an emergency basis to avoid additional brain damage.

In patients who have sustained an acute stroke and are found to have a severe carotid lesion, the timing of the operation is a source of controversy. Tradition has it that these patients should wait 6 to 8 weeks before an operation is done for fear of reperfusing an altered blood-brain barrier and thus transforming an ischemic into a hemorrhagic infarction. Practice has shown that during this period of waiting a larger deficit may develop because of repeated embolization or when a tight preocclusive ICA lesion progresses to thrombosis. The evidence supporting this 8-week delay is traceable to work done 25 years ago when the surgical management of patients with carotid disease was in its infancy and CT scans were not available. It has been our practice for the last 15 years to wait, at most, a week after a stroke before repairing the carotid lesions suspected of being the source of an infarction. We do, however, delay the operation if the patient has any degree of obfuscation or stupor or if the brain CT scan shows evidence of edema, dislocation, or uptake of dye within the area of infarction. Operations are delayed in the patients until disappearance of the contraindications just mentioned.

The natural history of fibromuscular dysplasia, kinks, and radiation arteritic lesions in the carotid is not sufficiently well known to allow prediction of stroke rates in asymptomatic patients. For this reason observation is advised in asymptomatic patients who do not have a severe plaque associated with the fibrodysplastic lesion. However, we advocate intervention on one side in asymptomatic patients who have severe bilateral fibromuscular dysplasia and who have evidence of critical restriction of flow bilaterally, demonstrated by oculoplethysmography, as well as in patients who have secondary pulsatile tinnitus that interferes with their well-being.

Vertebral Artery Disease

The selection of patients with VBI is more difficult, as a number of medical conditions may cause these symptoms. Their workup tends to be more fragmented than that of those presenting with carotid symptoms. Patients may first be seen by different specialists, each placing emphasis on causes related to their respective field of expertise. Patients seen by otolaryngologists, for example, are likely to undergo a full workup of the territory of the eighth cervical nerve, including brainstem-evoked potentials, and electronystagmography, whereas primary consideration is rarely given to arteriography or to the monitoring of cardiac arrhythmias. Vascular surgeons, on the other hand, may request an arteriogram before ruling out the nonsurgical causes of VBI.

The mode of presentation of VBI symptoms sometimes suggests the cause. Palpitation associated with dizziness suggests the possibility of a supraventricular arrhythmia. Concomitant deafness, tinnitus, or vertigo requires investigating the possibility of inner ear disease as the etiology. A clear and repetitive association between a specific head position and drop attacks or syncope suggests mechanical compression of the VA. The symptoms can usually be reproduced after a few seconds by slowly and deliberately rotating the head to the trigger position. In contrast, the immediate appearance of symptoms with brisk rotation, flexion, or extension of the head speaks of an inertial mechanism more suggestive of a labyrinthine disorder.

Computed tomography is of limited usefulness in the diagnosis of ischemic lesions in the VB territory because small infarctions are seldom seen. MRI is a far better tool to detect brainstem infarctions and is part of our workup of patients with symptomatic VBI.

The decision to obtain an arteriogram in a patient with VBI is controversial. Some specialists never order them because they have not traditionally been aware of the importance of hemodynamic and thromboembolic mechanisms in the production of VBI. Our indications for arteriography are (1) any VBI event suspected of being thromboembolic (e.g., with a posterior circulation infarction, shown by MRI); (2) concomitant carotid disease demonstrated by duplex scanning and requiring arteriography (VA visualization should be part of the arteriogram); and (3) patients with hemodynamic VBI who continue to have symptoms after correction of associated diseases such as anemia, arrhythmia, or postural hypertension or after adjustment of their antihypertensive therapy (including suppression of beta-blockers) and a 2- to 3-month trial with alpha-blockers.

Arteriography in patients with posterior circulation symptoms requires special views to demonstrate some important features of the pathology of the VA (these views are discussed in Chapter 3). The vertebrobasilar system needs to be fully displayed by the arteriogram, and when indicated special views are obtained. Failure to obtain these special views often results in missed significant VA lesions.

The dominant VA should be noted on the arteriogram. It is the larger one and is on the side to which the concavity of the basilar artery opens when seen in anteroposterior projection. In approximately 40% of individuals the two VAs are of comparable size. The determination of both the dominant VA and the completeness (or otherwise) of the opposite VA is necessary during the selection of surgical candidates. When the stenoses of both VAs are comparable, the lesion on the dominant VA should be the one that is corrected. If one VA is incomplete, the lesion on the opposite VA has greater relevance. Finally, it can be said generally that if a VA is normal (including evidence that it is not externally compressed during neck rotation and extension) there is no reason to presume that repairing a stenosis in the opposite VA will result in increased flow in the basilar artery. This consideration does *not* apply to individuals who have thromboembolic VBI and who constitute about one-third of the patients with symptoms of VBI. In these patients, if they have appropriate symptoms, the demonstration of a possibly embologenic lesion justifies VA repair regardless of the status of the opposite VA.

The ubiquitous stenosis at the origin of the VA should be studied by special oblique projections. The possibility of extrinsic compression in the intraspinal segment can only be excluded on views taken with the neck in rotation, extension, flexion, or compression. In some cases the demonstration of extrinsic compression cannot be shown with the patient in a supine position. The head's natural weight in the standing position influences the mechanics of the cervical spine and contributes to the degree of compression or deformation seen in the VA. To demonstrate this mechanism[73] the arteriography may have to be performed with the patient sitting up (transtrachial route) or, alternatively, (transfemoral route) with the arteriography table tilted head down and the head supported by blocks so the weight of the body compresses the neck (see Chapter 3).

Delayed subtraction views may show a patent VA beyond its thrombosed first and second segments. This information is essential for planning a reconstruction of the third segment of the VA. The integrity of the basilar artery should be ascertained in lateral projections. Finally, the caliber of the posterior communicating artery needs to be noted, although failure to visualize this artery does not imply that it is occluded or absent.

Patients presenting with systemic problems (e.g., anemia, arrhythmia) that may cause vertebrobasilar insufficiency ought to have these corrected before the need for an operation is considered. The presence of intracranial disease, usually in the basilar artery, is a contraindication for operating in the VA.

Our indications for a VA reconstruction are as follows.

1. In symptomatic patients with hemodynamic VBI, and (1) stenosis of a dominant or single VA that is more than 75% of its diameter; (2) the same degree of stenosis involving both VAs; or (3) segmental occlusion of the second portion of the VA with a small hypoplastic VA remaining on the opposite side.

2. In patients with thromboembolic VBI or MRI evidence of infarction who have a demonstrated embologenic source in any VA.

3. In patients who need an ipsilateral carotid operation if they satisfy the anatomic conditions described under item 1.

6   Surgical Maneuvers

Ligature was, for many years, the only operation done on arteries. Many of the approaches to the vessels of the neck used in reconstructive surgery today were worked out decades ago in order to ligate injured or aneurysmal arteries. The advent of balloon occlusion and distal embolization have made surgical ligature uncommon; it is now done almost exclusively for trauma. For surgical reconstruction of the arteries of the neck the classic techniques of endarterectomy and bypass are still the ones most frequently used, although transposition techniques are becoming commonplace.

Ligation/Intravascular Occlusion

Supraaortic Trunks

Ligation of the IA is part of the treatment of tracheoinnominate fistula. However, the situation created by ligation of the IA may result in massive flow reversal in the right carotid and vertebral arteries (see Chapter 2). The proximal SA is used by pediatric cardiac surgeons as a patch for the treatment of aortic coarctation or in systemic-pulmonary shunts for the palliative management of cyanotic congenital heart disease. Ligation of the IA or SA may also be needed to treat the rare patient with mycotic aneurysm or with infection of a previously placed prosthetic graft. In these cases the surgeon is faced with the dilemma of whether to preserve the IA bifurcation or the most important branching of the SA, usually the VA. Although saving these bifurcations creates the possibility of a steal, it is still preferable to sacrificing their branches with the attendant risks of extensive occlusion and ischemia. In addition, if the bifurcations of the IA or the vertebral-subclavian junction have been preserved, a secondary reconstruction at a later date is made much easier (see Chapter 11).

Carotid Artery

Ligature is frequently done in the CCA or ICA for trauma. Ligations are double, above and below the wound to the vessel, with the surgeon relying on other arteries to supply the distal bed.

With trauma a common dilemma is when to reconstruct a carotid artery versus when to ligate it. The expediency of ligature is favored when there is loss of a substantial amount of arterial wall after an injury to the distal cervical ICA or when there are other serious problems that need to be taken care of in a patient who is comatose or in shock and whose neurologic condition cannot be properly evaluated. Reconstruction is favored when the wound in the vessel wall is small and partial (as with a knife wound) and the patient is stable and alert without evidence of brain damage.

Ligation of the CCA or ICA for bleeding is also favored when contamination or infection is suspected, as with associated pharyngoesophageal tears, fistulas following radical neck dissection, or the rare postoperative infection following carotid endarterectomy where a prosthetic patch was used to close the arteriotomy and a more distal autogenous vein repair is not feasible. Rarely, ligation of the ICA may be offered as an alternative to reconstructive surgery in a patient with an embologenic lesion of the distal cervical ICA, such as an aneurysm or a dissection.

For many years, ligation of the CCA was part of the treatment of intracranial aneurysms. The aim of ligation was to find the difficult balance between decreasing pressure in the distal ICA feeding the aneurysm and maintaining enough blood flow to avoid a stroke. Because of the vagaries of the anastomotic pathways between the basilar and the two carotid arteries, the surgeon ligating a CCA had no reliable way to predict the resulting pressure head in the ICA feeding the aneurysm and therefore the outcome of the procedure.

Blood flow studies performed in the operating room during ligation of the CCA for aneurysm or malignancy have shown that immediately after ligation the ICA or ECA may display retrograde flow with forward flow into the other branch. More recent studies have shown that most patients perfuse the ICA at the expense of retrograde flow in the ECA. In patients who at the time of ligation had shown reversal of ICA flow, anterograde flow was noted to have returned usually within hours, sometimes minutes. This pattern is the expected consequence of an ICA territory that offers less resistance to flow than does that of the ECA.

The extensive experience with ligation of the carotid system has taught us other facts about the arterial supply to the head. Neurosurgical reports reviewing ligations of the CCA for intracranial aneurysm give a stroke incidence of approximately 10%; which probably represents the general inci-

dence of stroke following CCA ligation. It is important to note that some of these strokes do not become evident when the patient awakens from the ligation procedure but, rather, 2 to 4 days later. This delay suggests that the mechanism of stroke in these patients is not the sudden decrease in perfusion caused by the ligature but, rather, thrombosis of the ICA propagated to the intracranial vessels. Following ligation of the CCA, the ICA may thrombose, often up to the ophthalmic artery because the minute branches exiting the petrosal and cavernous ICA carry an inadequate amount of flow to maintain patency of these segments. As the thrombus reaches the distal ICA, it may grow a tail that can float into or embolize the anterior and middle cerebral arteries. Because of this mechanism it is suggested that following ligation of the ICA patients should be maintained on intravenous heparin for 5 to 7 days, so that growth of the thrombus tail may be curtailed until its thrombogenicity decreases and a delayed stroke may be avoided. Obviously, in some situations heparin cannot be used.

There are therefore two mechanisms for cerebral infarction that may follow ICA (and CCA) ligation. The first is the immediate consequence of decreased cerebral perfusion in the corresponding hemisphere. Measurements of cerebral blood flow at the time of occlusion show that most patients recover to near-normal within 30 minutes of clamping. The second mechanism is propagation of thrombus into the distal ICA and its branches. This mechanism is usually delayed for hours or days.

The immediate effects of ICA ligation may be anticipated by preoperative testing, such as compression of the ipsilateral CCA with clinical, electro-encephalographic, ocular plethysmographic, or transcranial Doppler monitoring or by temporary balloon occlusion of the ICA with or without monitoring of the distal stump pressure. However, most patients in whom a carotid ligation is indicated are seen in emergency situations, which precludes the possibility of such testing. For these cases we have been satisfied with the reliability of measuring the distal stump pressure intraoperatively and have considered 45 mm Hg of mean arterial pressure a safe level at which to ligate the ICA. For cancer resections where the tumor is attached to the distal CCA and where the

ICA back-pressure is marginal, we have occasionally used the expedient measure of a direct anastomosis of the ECA and ICA to preserve flow through the latter.

Operative ligation of the ECA has been done mostly to control bleeding from tumors or arteriovenous malformations supplied by this artery. It usually provides only temporary relief, as the ligation is generally done at the trunk of origin or, at best, at the origin of its primary branches. The extensive anastomoses between the two ECAs and between the ECA and branches of the VA and the SA take little time to resupply blood to the previous tumor or malformation with resumption of bleeding or continued growth of the malformation. Once bleeding recurs, the previously ligated ECA no longer permits passage of the catheters used today to embolize the distal lesion.

In these circumstances one may need access to the distal portion of an ECA that had previously been ligated to control bleeding. This measure can seldom be done by direct puncture of the ECA distal to the ligation point but may be resolved by its reconstruction using a vein graft from the CCA so the percutaneous catheter can be passed through it to a more distal destination.

Under elective conditions most proximal (truncal) occlusions are achieved today by detachable intravascular balloons rather than by ligature. In the internal carotid artery, balloon occlusion is used in rare cases to obliterate the outflow of an ICA aneurysm inaccessible at the base of the skull. It may be done in conjunction with a superficial temporal to middle cerebral artery anastomosis.

Vertebral Artery

False anerysms of the VA are often located in its second or third segment and can be difficult to expose surgically. The technique for treating such a false aneurysm by balloon occlusion is to occlude the artery above and below the aneurysm. If only a proximal occluding ballon is used, retrograde flow from the distal VA may continue to expand the false aneurysm. Sometimes, however, it is impossible to pass the balloon through the false aneurysm and into the distal vessel. In that case only a proximal balloon is inserted; if it fails to cause thrombosis of the false aneurysm, the removal of the aneurysm and distal ligature may have to be done surgically as a second step.

Surgical ligation of the VA has been done mostly to treat bleeding or false aneurysms secondary to trauma. A bizarre use of the ligature of this vessel was reported a century ago by Alexander[74] who, claiming to treat epilepsy, performed 27 such operations in Liverpool. The fact that he got away with these ligatures, in some cases done bilaterally, is not surprising. Generally, the ligature of one VA does not result in ischemia, provided the contralateral VA is open and reaches the basilar artery. However, brain infarction has been reported following ligation of the VA done to stop reversal of flow. In these instances it is likely that the thrombus distal to the ligature propagated beyond the junction of both VAs and into the basilar artery.

Classic Reconstructive Techniques

Endarterectomy

Endarterectomy is the most frequent technique used in the arteries of the neck, mostly to remove atheromatous plaque at the carotid bulb. It is also used in the ECA, usually in combination with some patching procedure. Although endarterectomy was the technique originally used to correct stenoses of the ostium of the VA and of the first segment of the SA, it has been superseded by better technical solutions and is used now only in special circumstances (see Chapters 7 and 9). Endarterectomy of the IA remains a valid technique to clear obstructions of the distal two-thirds of this vessel (see Chapter 7)

In general, the endarterectomy plane follows the external elastic membrane. In the SA and IA the wall remaining after following this plane is too thin. Primary closure of a thin-walled vessel requires small bites and may result in serious bleeding from tears. On the other hand, reports of false aneurysms following endarterectomy of the supraaortic trunks are rare. An endarterectomy of a large artery (IA, SA, CCA, and the ICA bulb) can be closed primarily without a patch, but an arteriotomy with ragged edges is best closed by patching it.

After opening the artery, the plane of endarterectomy is entered in the middle third of the length of the plaque. Toward the distal end, in order to achieve a smooth end, the plane of endarterectomy needs to become more superficial, at the level of the internal elastic membrane. This point is particularly important when removing a plaque from the ICA. The media that remains in this transition zone is composed of smooth muscle fibers arranged circularly like the hoops of a barrel. They can be easily pulled across the artery using loop magnification and fine grasping forceps (Figure 6.1). However, this "pull" debridement should not reach the edge where the intima broke off. If it does, it undermines the intimal edge and creates a flap.

Three maneuvers can be used to free the distal end of a plaque (Figure 6.2). The first is torsion and gentle traction of the plaque along its axis, usually with gentle counterpressure on the remaining wall, which results in a tapered detachment of its distal end. The second is to cause a pressure fracture with the spatula on the distal tapered end while pulling the plaque axially. The third is the technique of eversion endarterectomy. If the end of a plaque does not feather and needs to be cut, it may be done with sharp, fine scissors at a slanted angle to create a "ramp" rather than a "step." The sharp cut end of a plaque can also be smoothed by imbricating adjacent wall of endarterectomized artery (Figure 6.3).

Patching

A patch is meant to compensate for the inevitable loss of wall circumference taken up by the suture that closes an artery and, less commonly, to "splint" an endarterectomized segment. After removing a large circumferential plaque, the remaining arterial tube, when distended with normal pressure, is a bit larger than the original artery. Radial dilatation of an artery is coupled with its elongation, and so an artery that has been endarterectomized for a substantial length is longer when pressure is reestablished in it. This predicament follows endarterectomy of the carotid

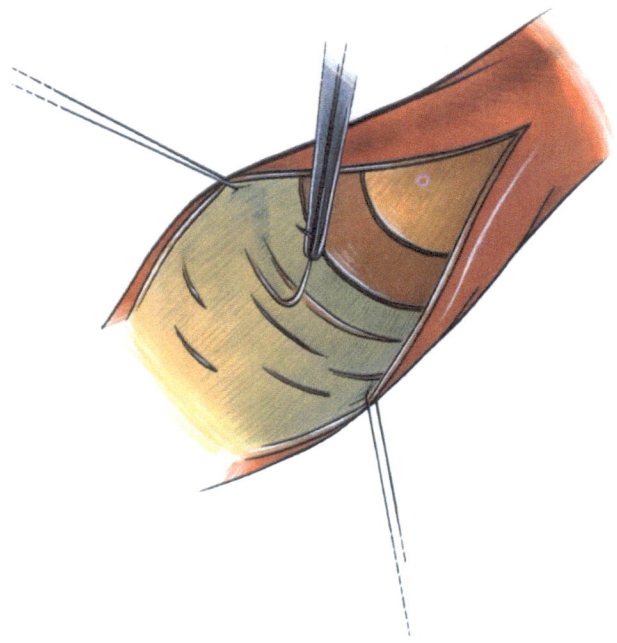

Figure 6.1 Removal of small circular debris of smooth muscle fibers of the media from the distal end of an endarterectomy site.

bulb and may result in kinking, usually at the point where the endarterectomy ends. If a patch is placed so that it extends slightly beyond the endarterectomized wall, it may splint the artery and avoid a kink.

Three types of material are available for patching: autogenous vein, prosthetic, and autogenous artery. The latter is used occasionally when closing an endarterectomy of the ECA after excising the occluded ICA. In this case, the thrombosed artery is opened along its length and, after endarterectomy, provides a convenient autogenous patch. Autogenous vein (usually saphenous) makes an ideal patch for vessels of medium and small diameter, but a valuable saphenous vein should not be spent in such a maneuver. Internal jugular vein patches can also be used. Although thin and a bit awkward to handle, the wall of the jugular vein withstands pressure well; and, contrary to traditional reservations, it does not become aneurysmal. In cases where a prosthetic patch is not advisable and the opposite jugular vein is suspected to be occluded (evidence provided by ultrasonography or the venous phase of the arteriogram), we have removed a patch from the ipsilateral jugular

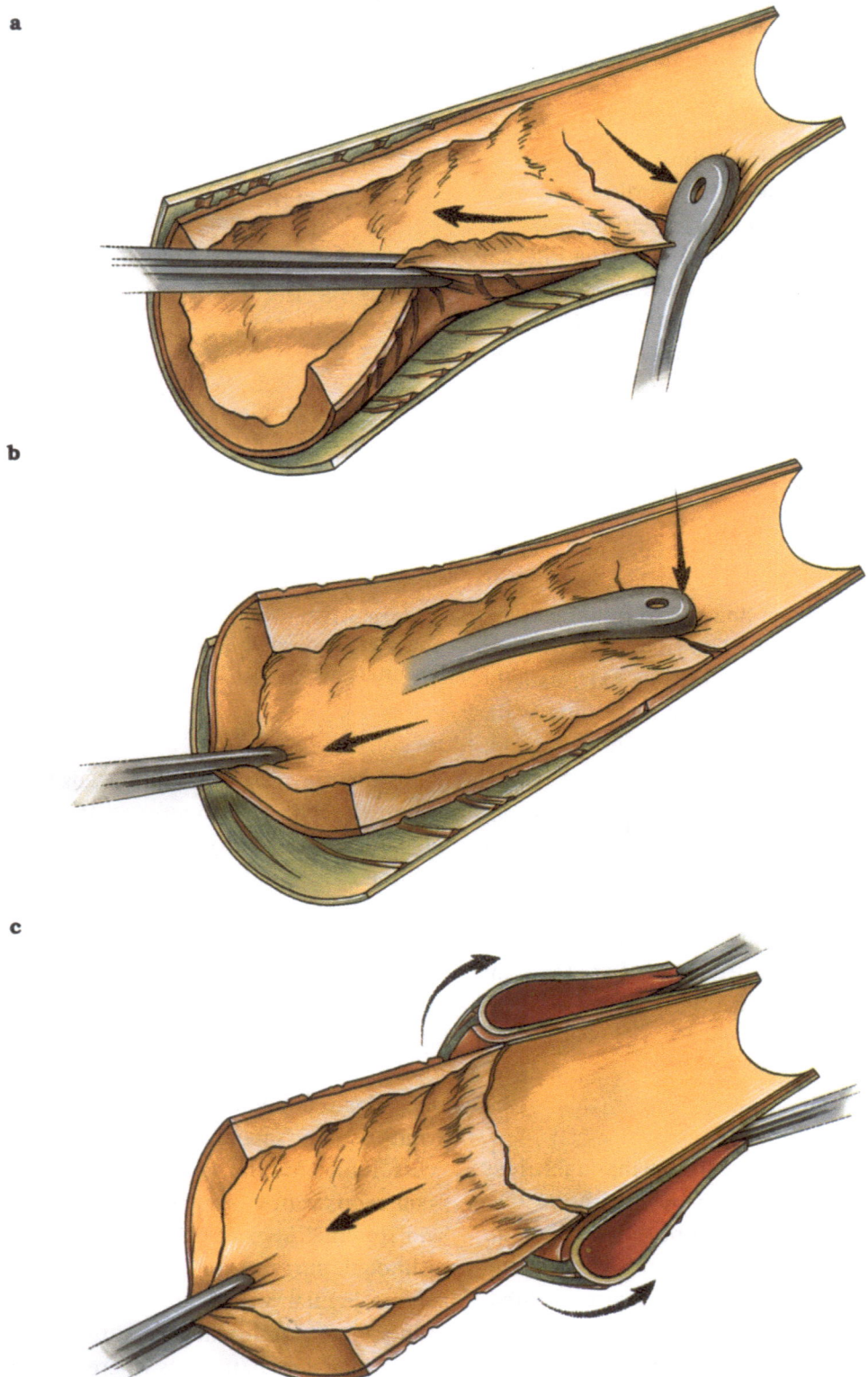

Figure 6.2 Three maneuvers used for the termination of endarterectomy. (**a**) Torsion and gentle traction of the plaque along its axis with gentle counterpressure on the remaining wall. (**b**) Pressure fracture of the plaque with the spatula while pulling the plaque axially. (**c**) Eversion endarterectomy.

a

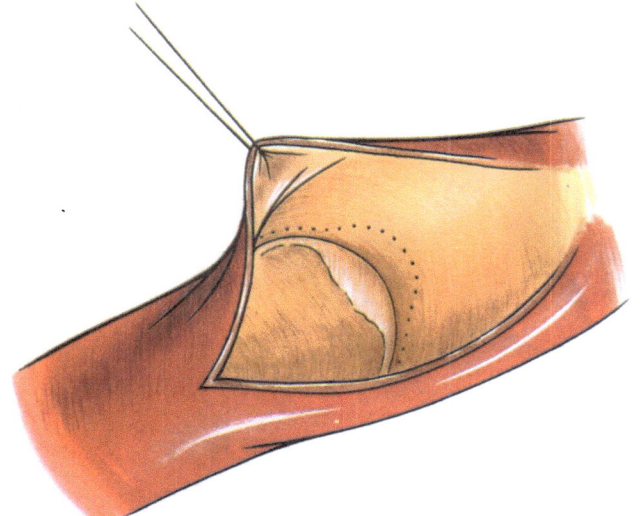

Figure 6.3 Smoothing the sharp, cut end of a plaque (a) by imbricating adjacent wall from the endarterectomized artery (b).

b

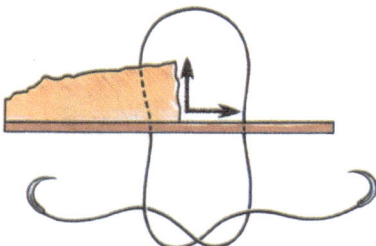

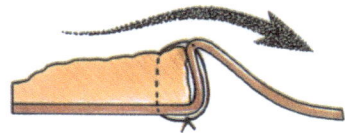

It may be done using either interrupted or continuous (c) sutures.

c

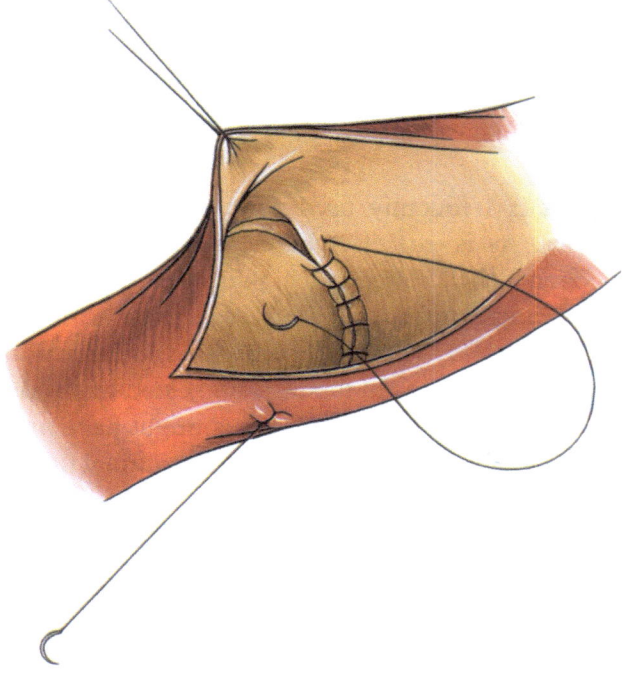

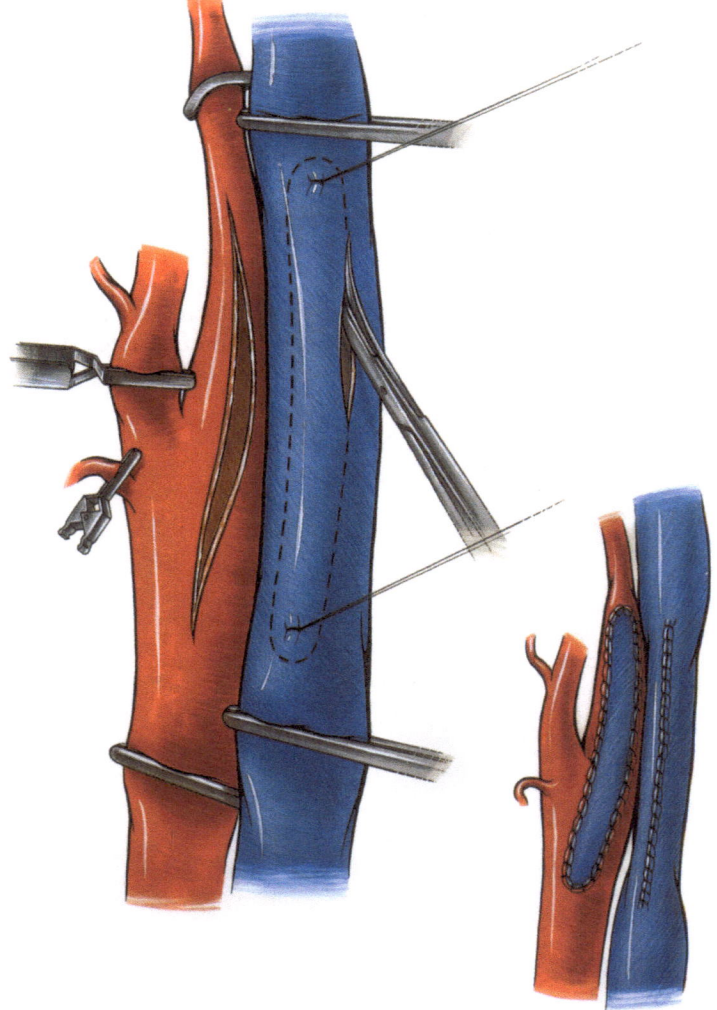

Figure 6.4 Internal carotid artery patch made of jugular vein, with preservation of the latter.

vein, closing the venotomy so as to preserve venous flow in the jugular (Figure 6.4). Plastic patches fare well in the neck, and they are our choice for arteries the size of the ICA and larger. A preclotted Dacron patch bleeds less through the suture holes than one made of polytetrafluorethylene (PTFE); the latter however, does not require preclotting.

The most common error made when cutting a patch is to make it too wide. A too wide patch results in an aneurysmal dilatation in the carotid bulb with thrombus deposition in its wall and intimal hyperplasia at the tip of the dilatation where the ICA recovers its normal size.

Bypass

Bypass is frequently used for the repair of neck arteries. As is true elsewhere, prosthetic bypasses function well if they carry a high flow rate, if they are a good caliber match to vessels larger than 6 mm, and if they are short. Years ago, surgical experience with prosthetic bypasses in the legs suggested that when implanted in the neck these tubes might have poor patency rates or might embolize their intimal lining. This inference was wrong. Prosthetic bypasses are the material of choice for replacement of the branches of the aortic arch and can be extended up to the carotid bifurcation with good long-term results, no doubt due to their high flow rates. They are also less likely to kink and twist than saphenous vein bypasses, and they do not dilate the way vein grafts, carrying high flow rates, often do. Saphenous vein, however, is still the material of choice to replace the ICA and the VA.

A bypass used in an artery supplying the brain must be placed excluding the offending atheroma from the pathway of blood. Not doing so may result in embolization from the complex plaque for which the bypass was constructed or in the formation of a thrombus in the native artery (which now has a sluggish flow), insinuation of the tail of the thrombus into the distal anastomosis, and distal embolization.

Usually, the proximal anastomosis of a bypass is made end-to-side to a good donor vessel (ascending aorta, SA, CCA). The distal anastomosis, if made to the carotid or vertebral arteries, should function as an end-to-end construction. It may be constructed as such or may be done end-to-side and then converted to an end-to-end anastomosis by precise ligation or clipping of the recipient vessel below the distal anastomosis. The latter method makes it easier to construct and vent an anastomosis of proper dimensions and avoids the problems of axial rotation and mismatch that may occur in an end-to-end anastomosis. Axial rotation is sometimes a nuisance when anastomosing a vein graft to a divided distal cervical ICA or distal VA. These arterial ends, once dissected free of attachments, twist and move about during the performance of the end-to-end anastomosis to the vein graft. Bypass with autogenous vein is reserved for the distal ICA and VA; their delicate wall and small size advise against the choice of a synthetic tube.

Resection and Anastomosis

A tortuous neck artery may present a kink at the site of a plaque. If this combination becomes symptomatic, it may be resolved by simple segmental resection and reanastomosis. This technique is used sometimes for the correction of ICA kinks.

Intraluminal Dilatation

Intraluminal dilatation may be used to relieve stenoses secondary to fibromuscular dysplasia. It may be done by the surgeon through an arteriotomy or percutaneously by the arteriographer. Although the intima appears shaggy immediately following the dilatation, the surface becomes smooth after a few months. A good long-term outcome after this crude tearing of diaphragm-like lesions is predicated on the existence of an intact endothelium covering the intimal surface and the absence of concomitant atherosclerotic disease. Intraluminal angioplasty is rarely used to dilate an intimal hyperplastic lesion at the site of a previous operation.

Percutaneous angioplasty has been used by some to compact atheromatous plaques in the ICA and VA. In the ICA this procedure is not safe unless coupled with an effective trapping device to collect all the particulate material that may be fragmented and float into the bloodstream during angioplasty. Transluminal angioplasty has also been used to dilate lesions of the origin of the VA. The assumption here has been that plaques at the origin of the VA are fibrous and unlikely to embolize. As we have noted before (see Chapter 4) this conclusion is presumptive, not factual. The limited experience reported with balloon angioplasty of proximal VA stenoses indicates that it carries a higher morbidity than correction by operation. Balloon dilatation of stenotic lesions of the second segment of the VA should not be undertaken, as its thin wall may easily rupture. Furthermore, stenosing lesions in the intraspinal course of the VA are frequently associated with external compression by bony abnormalities that cannot be modified by balloon dilatation.

Stenosis of the first segment of the SA may be corrected by balloon angioplasty. The problem here is the possibility of embolization of the vertebrobasilar territory. Digital compression maneuvers that attempt to temporarily arrest VA flow during angioplasty are unreliable. An absent VA on the side of the SA to be dilated appears to be the only situation where this technique can be used safely, although under this

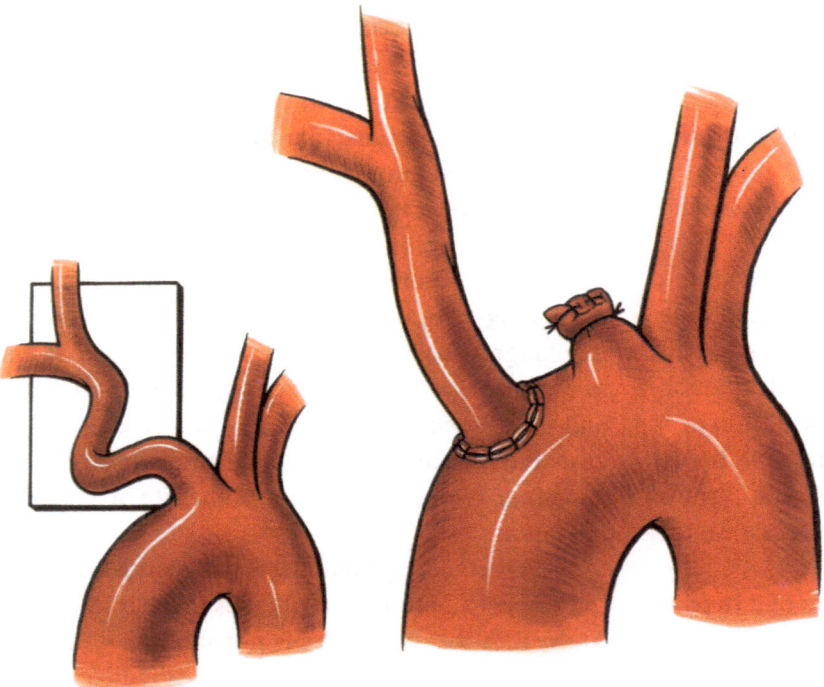

Figure 6.5 Redundancy of the innominate artery may allow its transposition to the adjacent aorta.

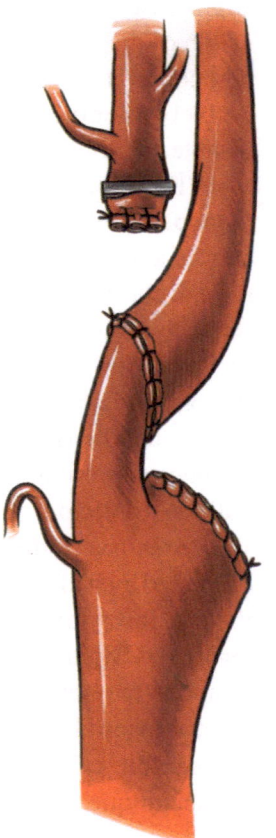

Figure 6.6 Transposition of the external carotid artery to the internal carotid artery distal to its diseased segment.

circumstance a proximal SA lesion falls outside our subject because it is no longer in an artery supplying the head.

Transposition Techniques

Transposition techniques are suited to the anatomy of the neck because the neck arteries run close to each other and some degree of tortuosity provides extra length. There are two types of transposition. With the first, an artery is divided distal to a stenosis and then transposed by anastomosing it to another vessel in its proximity. The proximal stump containing the lesion is tied off and excluded from the circulation. With the second type of transposition, a nonessential artery is used as a source of blood by switching its distal end to the artery that needs to be revascularized.

The *proximal* type of transposition is the most common in the neck arteries because most lesions occur at arterial origins. Rarely, a redundant IA originating to the left of the trachea and bearing a proximal stenosis can be transposed directly to a more proximal site in the ascending aorta (Figure

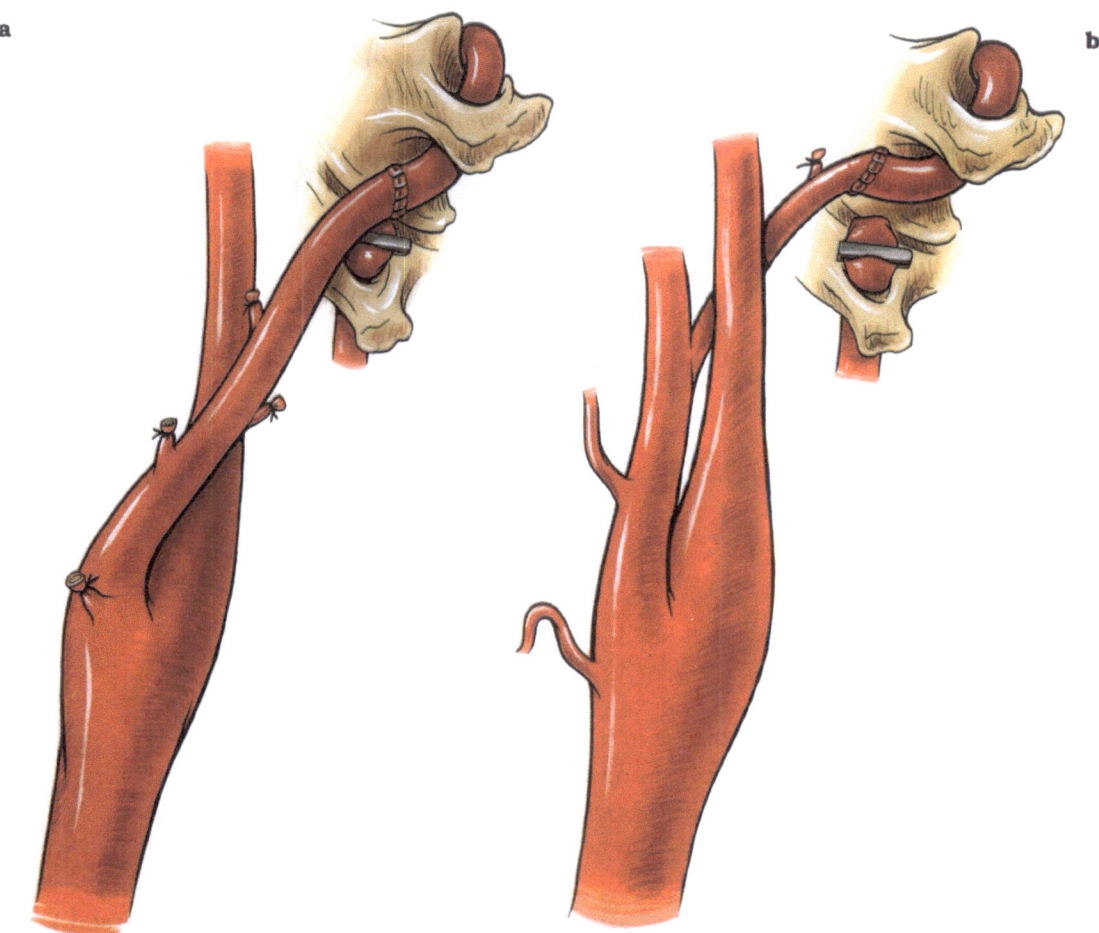

Figure 6.7 Transposition of the external carotid artery (**a**) or occipital artery (**b**) to the distal vertebral artery.

6.5). The CCAs can be transposed to one another. Either SA can be transposed to the neighboring CCA and vice versa (see Chapter 7), and the left CCA may be transposed to the IA. A redundant and diseased ICA may be endarterectomized and reimplanted further down in the CCA to correct a concomitant redundancy or kink (see Chapter 8). The VA can be transposed to the CCA or to another site in the SA, and the distal VA can be transposed in the ICA (see Chapter 9). A retroesophageal SA may also be transposed to the right CCA or to the ascending aorta (see Chapter 11).

It is not as common to switch the *distal end* of an arterial site in the neck as it is during coronary revascularization using the internal mammary artery. The ECA may be transposed to the cervical ICA, as was done at the first carotid operation performed to relieve ischemic attacks from a carotid plaque (Figure 6.6). Either the ECA or the occipital artery may be anastomosed to the distal VA to provide flow (Figure 6.7).

Transpositions are increasingly preferred in situations where a bypass was heretofore the standard technique. The appeal of a transposition is that it requires a single autogenous artery-to-artery anastomosis and eliminates the problem of procuring a suitable vein or the drawbacks of a synthetic graft. On the down side, a transposition entails simultaneous clamping of the recipient and donor vessel. There are individuals with advanced arterial disease who have only one carotid supplying directly the brain. In these cases the risk imposed by clamping this remaining vessel of supply for a transposition procedure may be lessened by the temporary use of a carotid shunt.

7 Repair of the Supraaortic Trunks

The SAT as described here begin at the aortic arch and extend up to the bifurcation of the carotid and the takeoff of the vertebral arteries. Within these boundaries are included all the arteries supplying the head and upper extremities.

Three types of operation are done on these arteries: *axial or transthoracic repairs*, where the reconstruction takes place along the axis of the vessel, reestablishing a semblance of normal anatomy; *cervical bypasses* that run transversely in the neck, sometimes crossing from one side to the other ("crossover"); and *transpositions*, where an artery is divided distal to an obstruction and reimplanted into a neighboring source.

From a clinical point of view, when reconstruction of these arteries is contemplated, one must decide first whether the approach will be made through the neck or the chest. Generally, *transthoracic repairs* are riskier but more durable. They are the best choice when the repair involves the IA or more than one trunk. Transthoracic techniques are preferable in young individuals. They may be difficult and risky after a coronary bypass operation has scarred the anterior mediastinum and crowded the space available for clamping of the ascending aorta.

Cervical reconstructions, whether by bypass or transposition, are usually advisable for single trunk disease (except of the IA) and carry a lower risk than transthoracic repairs, although the long term follow-up of cervical bypasses indicates a lower patency rate. Cervical reconstructions are the preferred approach in older individuals and occasionally in patients in whom a previous median sternotomy has been done.

There are rare indications for remote bypasses to the supraaortic trunks originating from the descending and supraceliac aorta or iliac or femoral arteries. These techniques are used in patients in whom the ascending aorta is not accessible and no form of cervical bypass is feasible (see Chapter 10).

Transthoracic Repairs

We discuss first repair of the left CCA and the IA and its branches through a median sternotomy. Repair of the left SA through a left thoracotomy is described under a separate heading.

Although not often performed, endarterectomy of the IA was for years the preferred technique for treating lesions of this vessel. Today the most common transthoracic technique for repair of the branches of the aortic arch is bypass grafting.

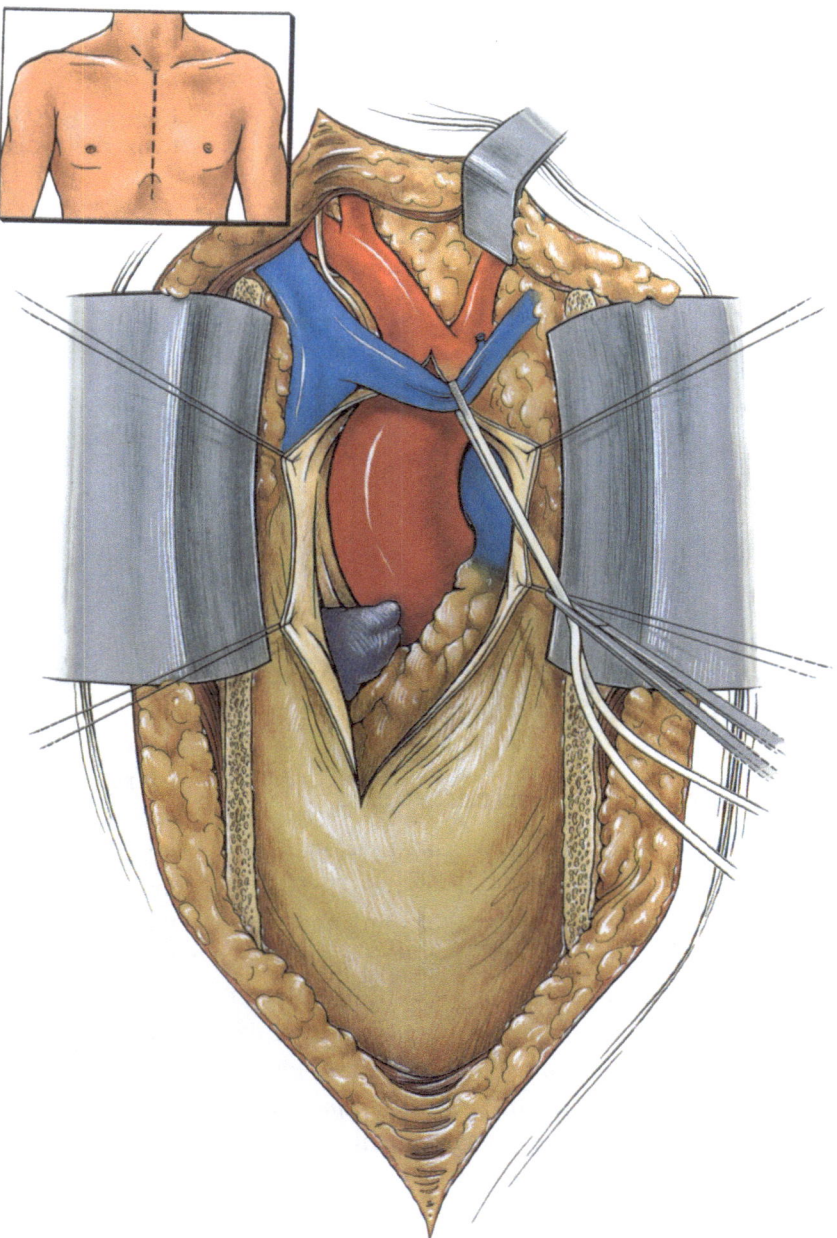

Figure 7.1 Approach to the anterior trunks through a median sternotomy.

Preoperative Care

The left jugular and left subclavian vein cannot be used to insert a Swan-Ganz catheter if we anticipate the need to revascularize the left SA, which requires division of the brachiocephalic vein. The right jugular approach cannot be used for insertion of a Swan-Ganz catheter when simultaneous exposure of the right carotid bifurcation is anticipated. Alternatively, in this case the Swan-Ganz catheter may be placed through the right femoral vein and may later be rotated to a right subclavian venous site if monitoring is needed beyond 24 hours. An arterial line is placed on the left radial artery, provided the arterial supply to the left arm is normal. If not, a femoral arterial line is used. Antibiotics are started on the eve of the operation. Once the patient is on the operating table, a pneumatic cuff is placed on the right arm. (It will be

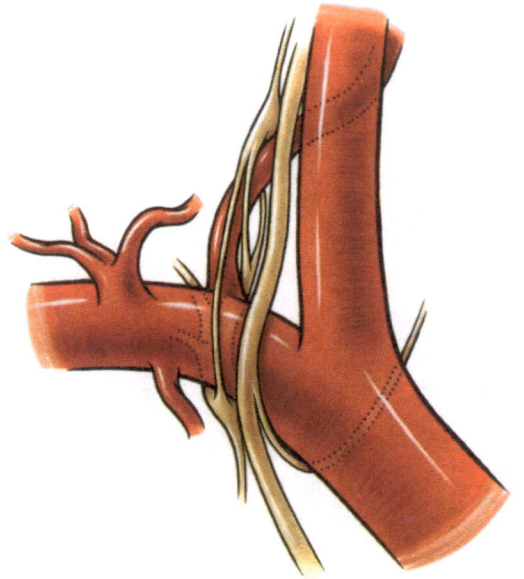

Figure 7.2 Relation of the innominate artery bifurcation to the right vagus and recurrent laryngeal nerves.

helpful later to decrease the reversal of VA flow while the origin of the right SA is clamped.)

Approach to the Anterior Trunks

A median sternotomy extended slightly to the right (Figure 7.1) along the anterior edge of the sternomastoid provides easy access to the ascending aorta and the IA and its branches. The two lobes of the thymus are separated in the midline; they will be useful later to isolate the arterial repair from the sternum at the time of closure. The strap muscles on the right side are cut. At closure, they and the thymus will be part of the soft tissue coverage of the arterial repair. The brachiocephalic vein is isolated and its small branches divided so the vein may be retracted upward or downward provided the sternal retractor is not too widely open, making the vein taut across the incision. The origin of the IA lies behind the brachiocephalic vein. The pericardium is opened, exposing the ascending aorta and the right side of the heart. Dissection of the IA should be done with care to avoid distal embolization. The IA exposure is extended over the origins of the right CCA and SA, avoiding injury to the right recurrent laryngeal nerve as it curves behind both branches of the IA (Figure 7.2). The steps that follow are different for endarterectomy and for bypass originating from the ascending aorta.

Endarterectomy

Although endarterectomy is not our primary choice for repair of IA lesions, there are situations where it should be considered: (1) in the presence of a lesion involving the distal two-thirds of the IA with a grossly uninvolved proximal portion; (2) in a small woman with a narrow thorax and a small thoracic inlet; and (3) when there has been a previous aortocoronary bypass graft, and a cervical reconstruction is not feasible. A generous portion of the wall of the aortic arch surrounding the IA should be dissected, clearing the origin of the left CCA in order to avoid interference later when placing the proximal aortic clamp. The proximity of the origin of the left CCA may present a problem here because its origin and that of the IA are shared or separated only by a flow divider in 16% of individuals. In another 8% of persons, the left CCA is actually a branch of the IA. Therefore in about 25% of cases one can anticipate difficulty avoiding the left CCA while placing an exclusion clamp around the origin of the IA. The plaque at the orifice of the IA may be continuous with plaque at the orifice of the left CCA, and the clamp may frac-ture the intima of the left CCA resulting in embo-lization, dissection, or occlusion of this artery. Endarterectomy of the IA should not be attempted when the proximity of the left CCA origin presents a problem or in cases where the IA plaques blend with extensive atheromatous disease of the dome of the arch.

If the endarterectomy appears feasible, systemic heparin is given, usually 5000 to 7000 U. Systemic arterial pressure is lowered to 100 to 110 mm Hg systolic. The cuff in the right arm is inflated. The distal vessels are clamped first to avoid embolization. The proximal clamp excludes a generous bite on the arch of the aorta. The systemic arterial pressure is monitored. If a drop is noted, it is caused by too large a bite of the partial exclusion clamp creating left ventricular outflow obstruction; the clamp should be replaced in a manner that avoids this problem.

The longitudinal arteriotomy of the IA should extend into the wall of the arch already excluded by the clamp. Distally, it extends to its bifurcation or into the SA or CCA, depending on findings. For the endarterectomy, an effort should be made to develop a more superficial endarterectomy plane than the one usually obtained (Figure 7.3). If one follows the usual plane of the external elastic lamina, the remaining IA wall may be too thin and friable to perform a safe closure. This predicament may require abandoning this technique and turning to a bypass based on the ascending aorta. Proximally, the IA plaque seldom has a clean break-off point, and the intima/media complex needs to be cut and affixed to the aortic wall by suture. A thin IA wall with a jagged edge usually requires a prosthetic patch for closure. Before completing the closure, which is done with a running 5-0 or 6-0 polypropylene suture, the distal vessels and the aorta must be sequentially and gently released, bled, and reclamped. When the suturing is finished, the right brachial cuff is released and flow is reestablished by opening first the right SA clamp, then the aortic clamp, and finally the right CCA clamp.

Endarterectomy is appealing because it is simple, provides a normal blood flow pathway, and avoids the need for prosthetic material. Its disadvantage is its limited application. If the left CCA shares either the ostium or a common trunk with the IA, the IA cannot be exclusion-clamped without interrupting flow to both arteries, which poses a great risk to the brain.

Endarterectomy may still be indicated in a small woman with a narrow thorax (in whom a prosthesis may occupy too much space) who has a common trunk bifurcating into an IA and a left CCA. In such cases an endarterectomy of the common trunk can be done, provided one maintains perfusion of one of the branches of the trunk by a shunt originating from the ascending aorta (Figure 7.4). An alternative solution is to transpose the left CCA into the left SA and then proceed with the IA endarterectomy. This situation is, however, a rare occurrence because the left SA is seldom free of disease when there is severe involvement of the remaining SATs.

Single lesions involving the distal two-thirds of the IA are a good indication for endarterectomy. In this case the IA may be clamped at its origin allowing a smaller operation where the exposure may be obtained by a partial upper midsternotomy without opening the pericardium.

a

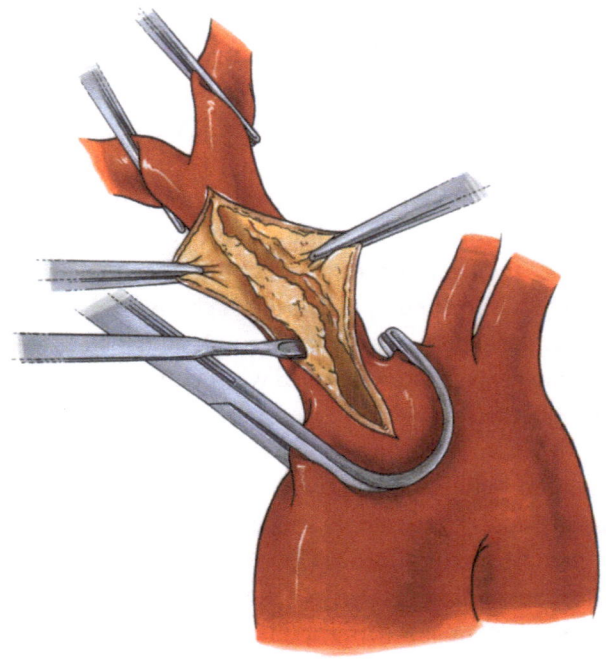

b

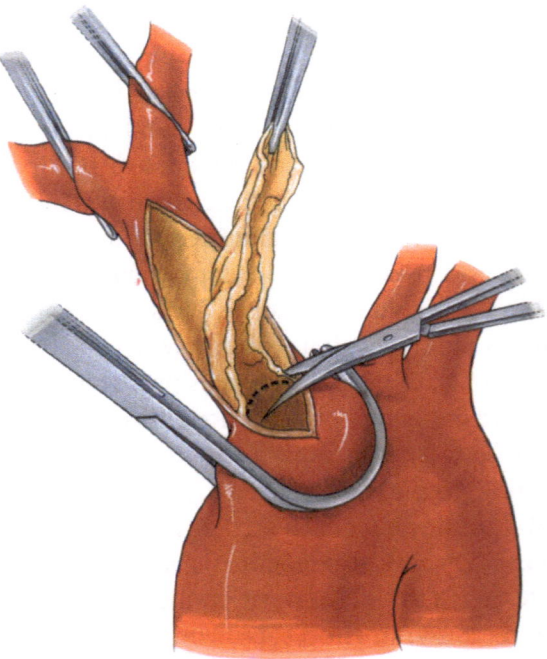

c

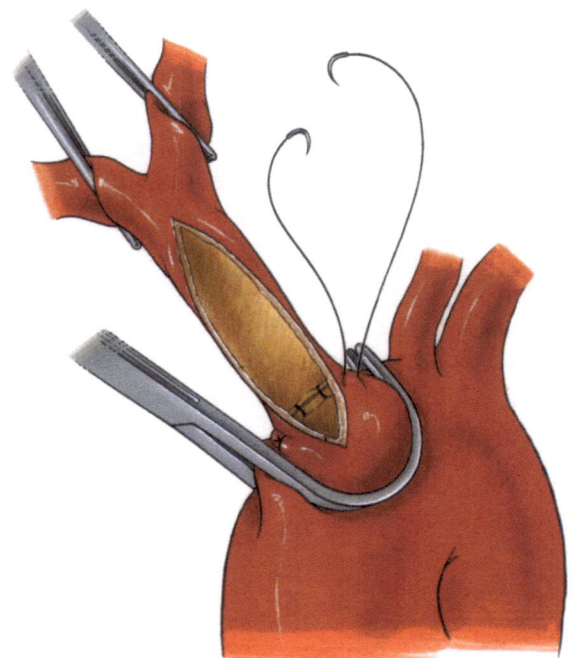

Figure 7.3 Innominate artery endarterectomy. (a) After clamping the arch about the orifice of the innominate artery, endarterectomy is performed in a superficial plane. (b) Transection of the proximal part of the plaque. (c) Tacking the intima of the aortic wall around the orifice of the innominate artery.

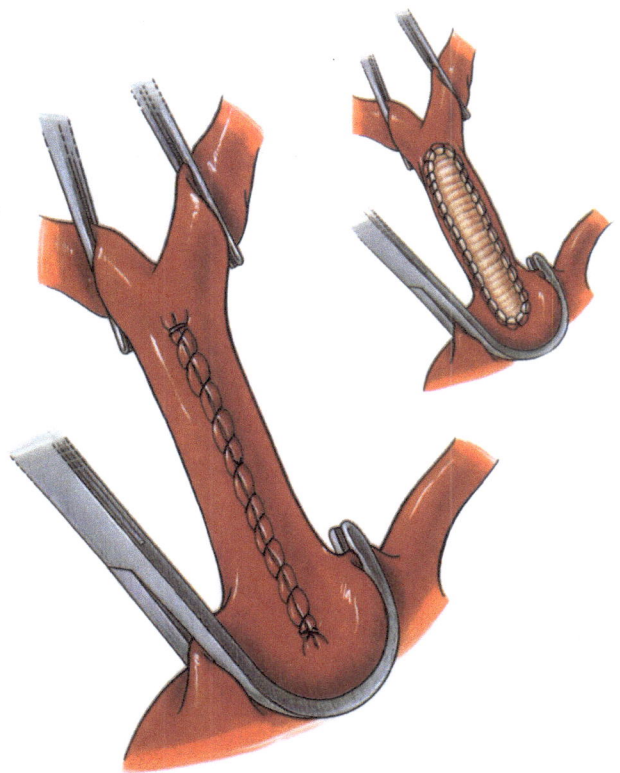

(**d**) Primary and patch (**inset**) closure of the innominate arteriotomy. (**e** & **f**) Sequence of declamping at the completion of the procedure.

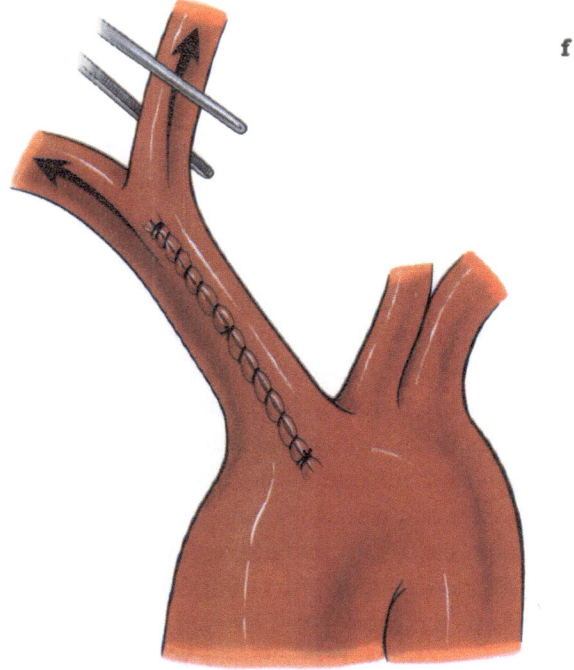

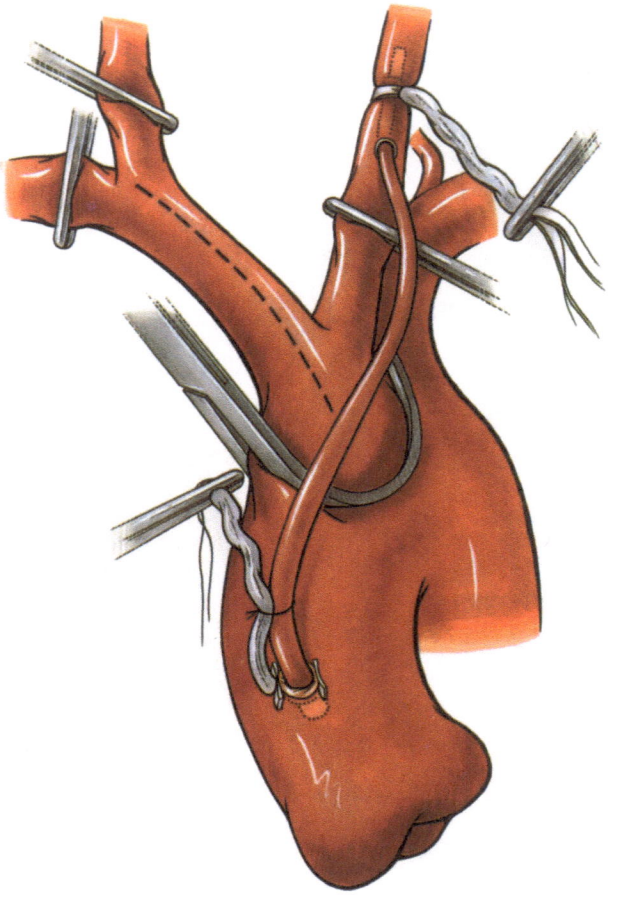

Figure 7.4 Preparing for an innominate endarterectomy with the help of an ascending aorta to left common carotid shunt in a patient with a common trunk for the innominate and left common carotid arteries.

Bypass from the Ascending Aorta

Our preferred technique for reconstructing the IA and multiple branches of the aortic arch is a bypass originating from the ascending aorta. The proximal portion of the ascending aorta is chosen because this segment is generally spared from the calcification and atheroma that may involve the dome of the arch. The proximal anastomosis is made easier if heparin is not used during this part of the procedure. By adding one or more branches to the main prosthesis, the other neck vessels can be revascularized in sequence without simultaneous or lengthy cross-clamping of the involved arterial trunks (see Chapter 10).

The pericardium is opened and tented outward with stay sutures (Figure 7.1). (Note of caution: Excess tension in the pericardial stays of the right side may obstruct the superior vena cava.) The IA and origins of the right SA and right CCA are dissected, avoiding injury to the right recurrent laryngeal nerve (Figure 7.2). If the left CCA is to be revascularized, it is exposed at the desired level. On the left side there is no need to cut the strap muscles because the anastomosis to the left CCA is planned either proximal or distal to these muscles. In the latter case, the left carotid bifurcation is exposed through a standard separate high presternomastoid incision. Exposure of the left SA origin in the posterior mediastinum requires division of the brachiocephalic vein and of the left-sided strap muscles.

Once all the vessels that are to be anastomosed are exposed, the ascending aorta is cleared for placement of a partial exclusion clamp (Figure 7.5). The aortic systolic pressure is lowered with nitroglycerin or isoflurane to 100 to 110 mm Hg. A Lemole-Strong clamp is placed on the anterior wall of the aorta, excluding enough wall so the anastomosis can be done with ease. Arterial pressure is monitored during clamping to ensure that there is no drop in pressure or change in the arterial pressure waveform. The excluded aorta is then aspirated with a needle, ensuring that the excluded aortic wall collapses and does not refill. The aortotomy is made in the anterior wall, and a small sliver is excised from both edges. The anastomosis is done with 3-0 monofilament suture, taking large bites on the aorta. If the aortic wall is friable or the sutures cut through, the anastomosis is made by "sandwiching" the aorta between the graft and a strip of Teflon felt applied outside.

Before testing the anastomosis, the table is tilted head-down 15 degrees to avoid embolization from air bubbles trapped around the proximal anastomosis. The proximal clamp is released gently, allowing short bursts of controlled bleeding from the distal end of the graft while applying pressure to the anastomosis. The proximal end of the graft is then clamped, and the table is returned to horizontal. Bleeding from any small tear that might occur at the anastomotic edge is controlled with a pledgeted suture. Once the anastomosis is sealed, the patient is given heparin.

The necessary side branches are then sewn to the main graft. The sequence of the distal anastomoses is determined by the severity and location of the existing lesions. The most severely stenotic trunk is repaired first to take advantage of the collateral support provided by the less diseased trunk(s). If the IA is the first to be bypassed, the cuff on the right arm is inflated above systolic pressure to decrease the vertebral steal, and the right SA and CCA are occluded. The IA is then clamped in its middle third and cut. The distal IA is trimmed back to near its bifurcation, and the prosthesis is cut to appropriate length. If the IA is cut perpendicular to its axis, the opening to which the prosthesis is to be anastomosed faces medially and downward. The prosthesis is beveled to face the distal opening of the IA (facing right side, 90 degrees clockwise from the plane of the proximal anastomosis). Like the SA, the IA has a thin wall and requires thin sutures (5-0) and noncutting needles. When the plaque in the IA extends into the first portion of the right CCA

or right SA, a number of solutions can be used including eversion endarterectomy or beveled or sequential anastomoses (Figure 7.6).

Once the anastomosis is completed, its two ends are bled into the wound or through the sidebranch if one has been sewn. The pressure cuff on the right brachial artery is released, and flow is resumed first into the subclavian and then into the carotid artery. The distal anastomosis of the branch or branches to the left carotid, the left SA, or both are then completed. The proximal stump of the IA is oversewn; and if the condition of the vessel permits, it is also ligated proximally not closer than 1 cm from its origin in the aortic arch. The reason to avoid a ligature at the takeoff of the IA is fear of a tear of its origin, retrograde dissection into the dome of the arch due to intimal fracture, or embolization of debris from the ostium of the IA into the distal aorta or left CCA. If ligation is difficult because of calcified atheroma or because the wall is too frail, the artery is closed over a Teflon felt strip.

The anastomosis of the prosthesis to a carotid may be done to the CCA below the strap muscles or to the bifurcation if the CCA is extensively diseased. Anastomosis to a carotid bifurcation is done in a manner that allows endarterectomy of the carotid bifurcation, a concomitant step that is frequently needed. There are two techniques for it. With the first, the CCA is transected 1 cm below the bifurcation, and the ICA and ECA are dissected (Figure 7.7). Care is taken to not injure the superior laryngeal nerve when dissecting behind the carotid bulb to mobilize it. The posterolateral wall of the bifurcation is opened. Eversion of the plaque may facilitate the endarterectomy. After endarterectomy the edges are trimmed, and the prosthesis is cut to reach snugly to the top of the opened carotid bulb. When the CCA is cut and the ICA and ECA are dissected free from their posterior attachments, the bifurcation retracts upward. If this retraction is not taken into consideration when measuring the length of the prosthesis, the limb will be too long and the anastomosis will buckle when flow is resumed. The prosthesis is then spatulated to match the large opening. The generous patching achieved

a

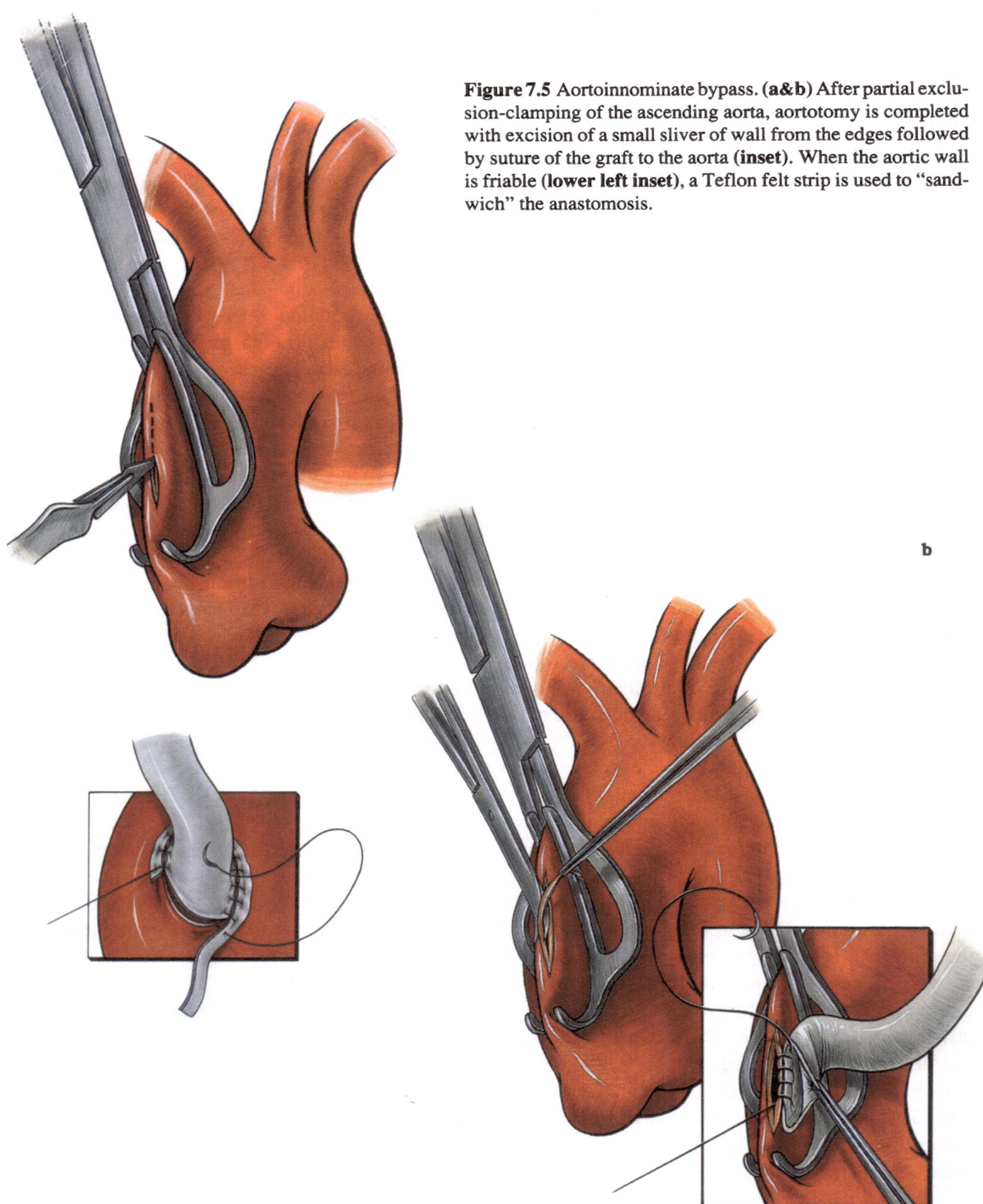

Figure 7.5 Aortoinnominate bypass. **(a&b)** After partial exclusion-clamping of the ascending aorta, aortotomy is completed with excision of a small sliver of wall from the edges followed by suture of the graft to the aorta **(inset)**. When the aortic wall is friable **(lower left inset)**, a Teflon felt strip is used to "sandwich" the anastomosis.

b

c

d

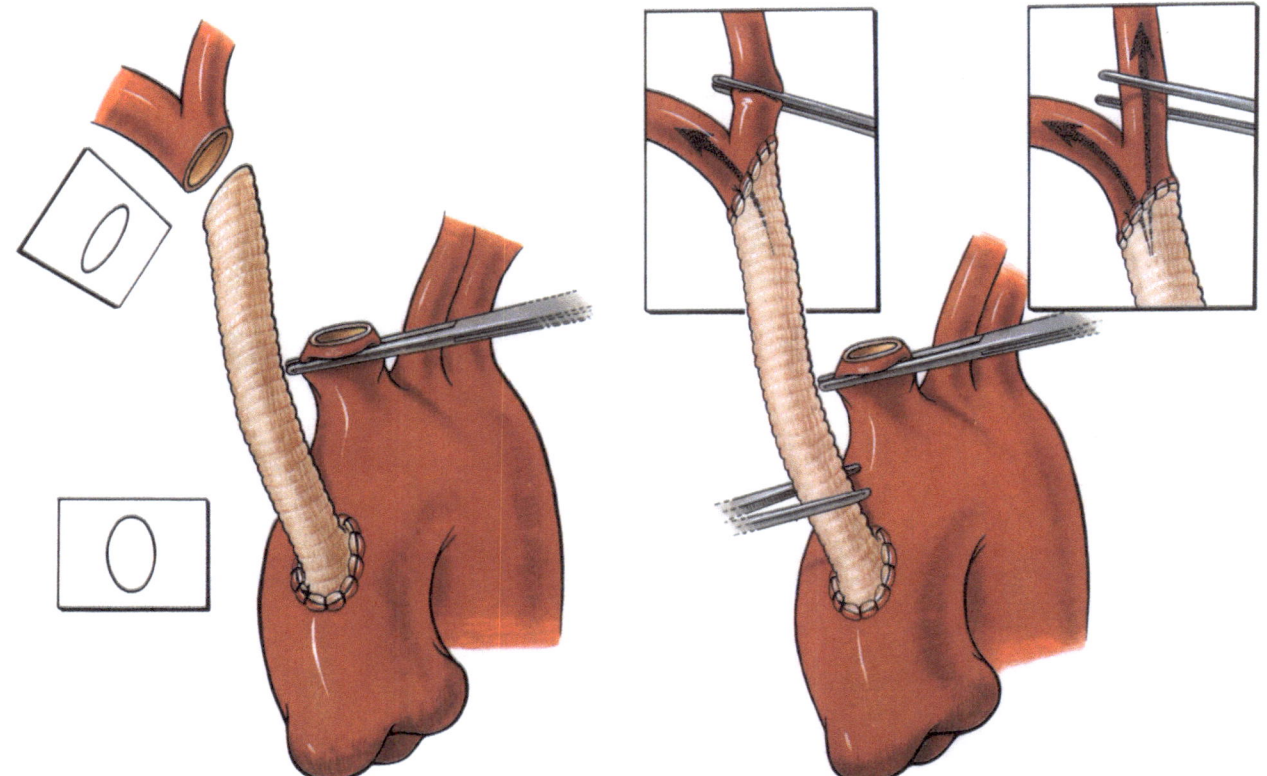

(c) Planes of the proximal and distal anastomoses are at 90 degree angles to each other. (d) Sequence of declamping at the completion of the procedure.

e

f

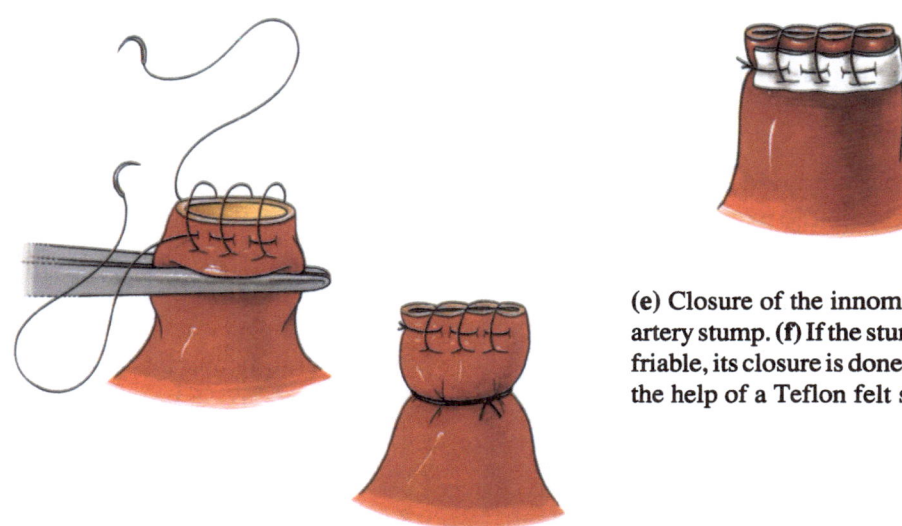

(e) Closure of the innominate artery stump. (f) If the stump is friable, its closure is done with the help of a Teflon felt strip.

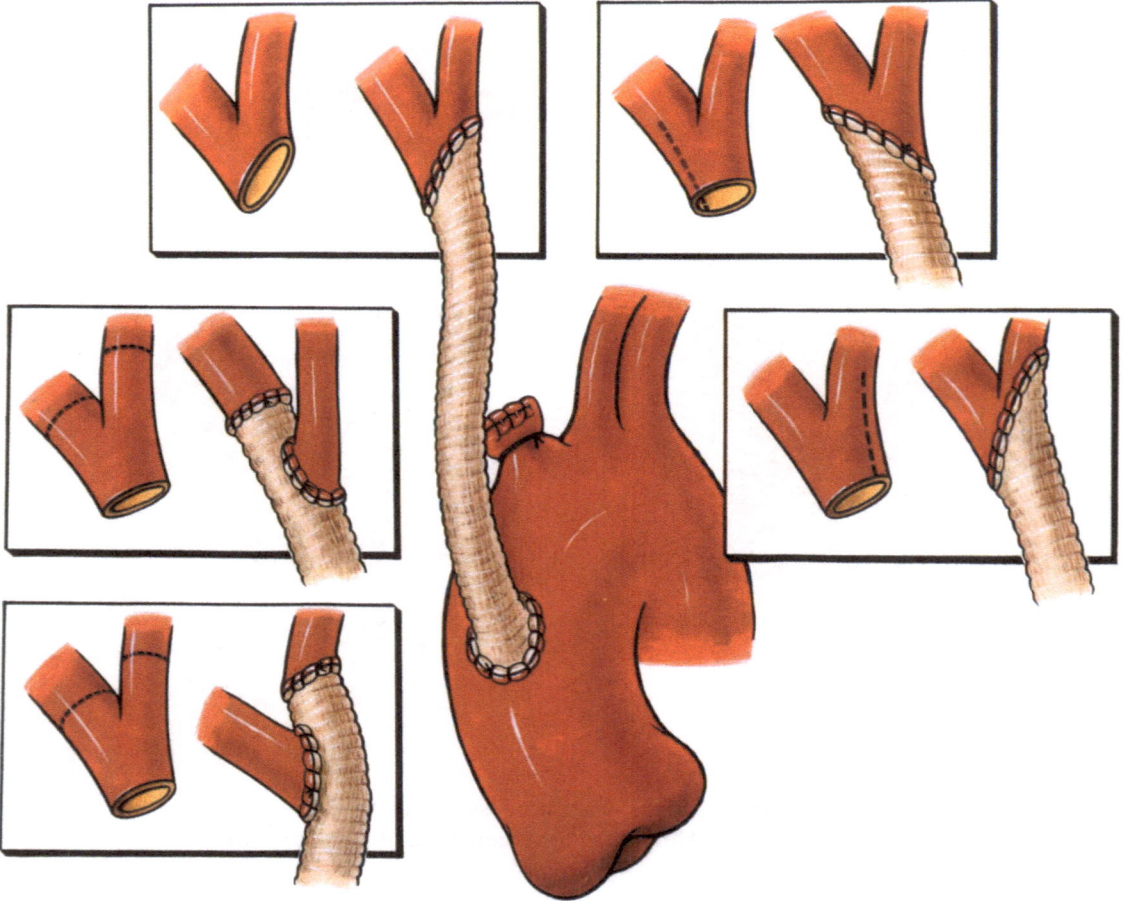

Figure 7.6 Various solutions for the distal anastomosis of a bypass between the ascending aorta and the bifurcation of the innominate artery.

with this geometry permits good-sized bites throughout the anastomosis with the exception of its apex.

The alternative for this distal anastomosis is to open the carotid bifurcation, after clamping its components, in the same manner as is done for a carotid endarterectomy. After completing the endarterectomy of the bulb and of the distal segment of the CCA in the usual fashion (see Chapter 8), the distal end of the prosthesis is anastomosed end-to-side as an onlay patch (Figure 7.7). Flow is resumed first in the ECA and then into the ICA. The distal CCA, which now has a soft wall after its endarterectomy, is closed with two large hemoclips placed obliquely and secured with transfixion ligatures of 4-0 polypropylene.

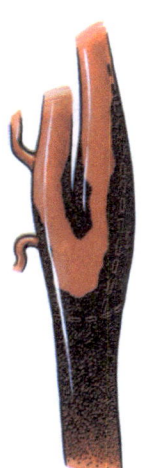

Figure 7.7 Techniques for distal anastomosis of a bypass to the carotid bifurcation. (**a**) A spatulated end-to-end anastomosis follows the eversion endarterectomy of the internal carotid artery.

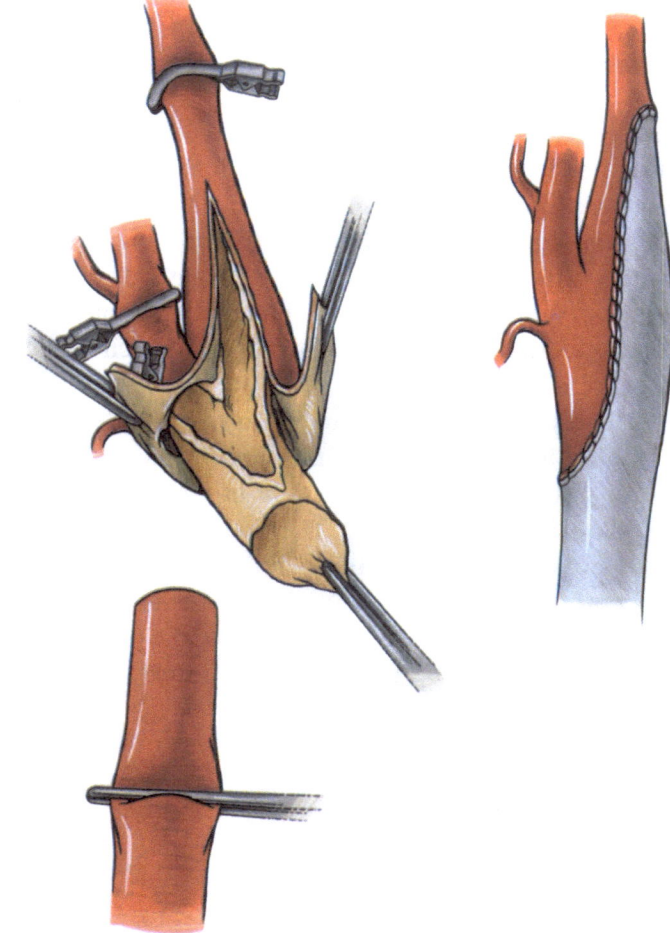

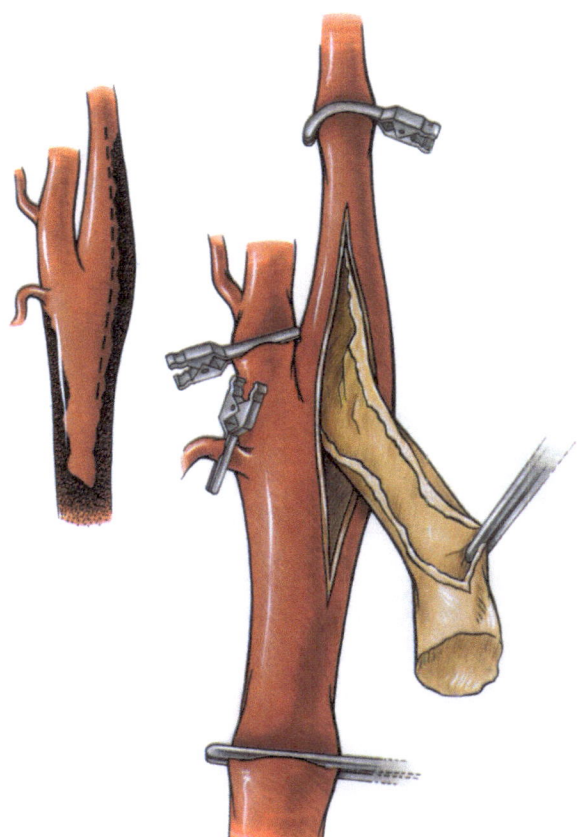

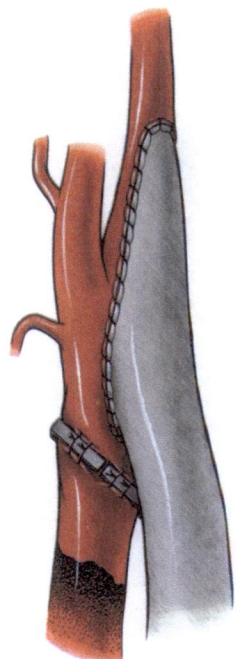

(**b**) End-to-side anastomosis of the limb of the graft to the carotid bifurcation after a conventional endarterectomy using a longitudinal incision, followed by exclusion of the proximal common carotid artery by two large hemoclips affixed with sutures.

Transthoracic Approach to the Left Subclavian Artery

Correction of isolated lesions of the left SA is nearly always accomplished through a cervical approach. There are, however, specific indications for the transthoracic repair of such lesions provided they are limited to the first portion of the SA: In patients who have inoperable occlusions of the left CCA and in those undergoing a concomitant operation on the descending thoracic aorta.

The transthoracic approach to the left SA is through a left posterolateral incision (in the fourth intercostal space) with the patient in the full right lateral position (Figure 7.8). The first portion of the SA is covered by the pleura and can be dissected easily after dividing the superior intercostal vein that runs in front of the vagus and behind the phrenic nerves. Care must be taken to avoid injury to the nerves, which run nearly vertically and in close proximity to the artery. The SA is dissected from its origin up to the takeoff of the VA; a short portion of the latter can be seen before it disappears into the supraclavicular space. The extent of SA disease may be assessed by palpation. Atherosclerotic lesions usually involve the first segment of the SA but occasionally extend into the origin of the VA.

The usual technique for transthoracic reconstruction of the left SA is a bypass graft originating from the descending aorta (Figure 7.9). The aorta is partially excluded with a Satinsky clamp below the isthmus. A preclotted 7 or 8 mm Dacron or 8 mm polytetrafluorethylene (PTFE) graft is anastomosed end-to-side to an aortotomy long enough to fit the beveled end of the graft. If the wall of the aorta is thick, the anastomosis of a 7 or 8 mm Dacron graft is facilitated by obtaining it from the limb of a bifurcation graft. This flared edge provides a wide implan-

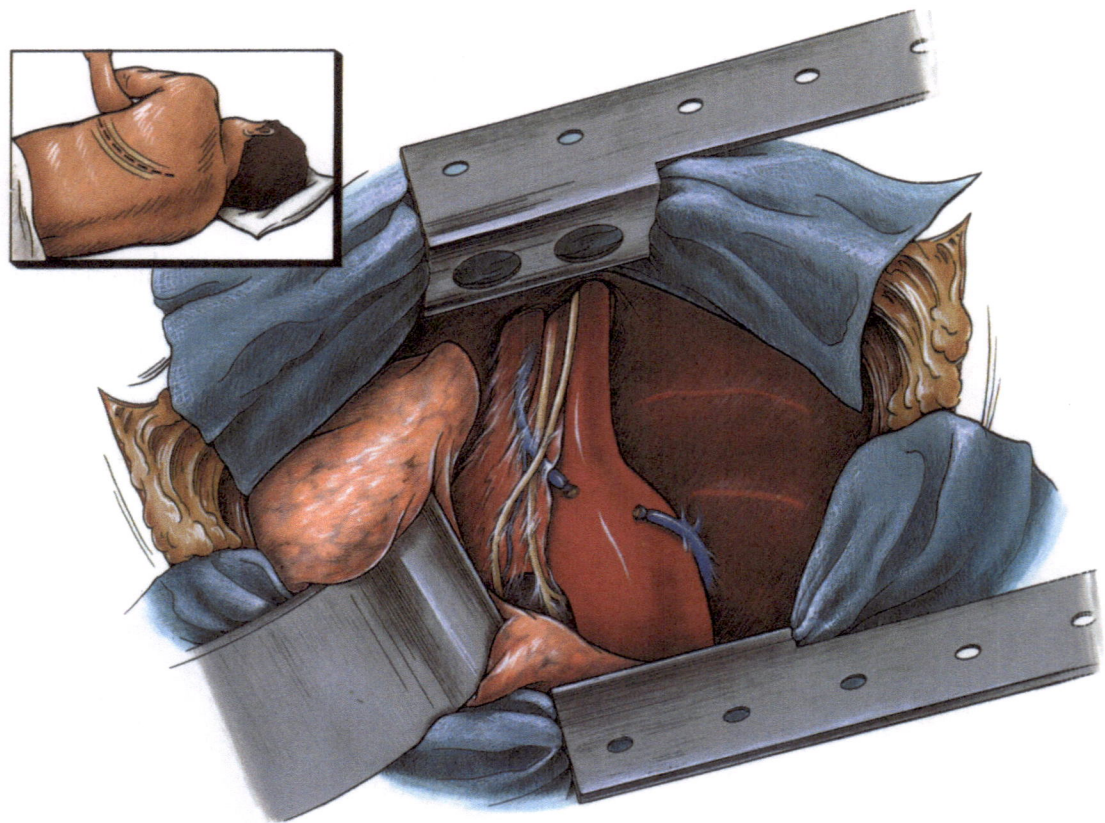

Figure 7.8 Left fourth intercostal approach to the left subclavian artery.

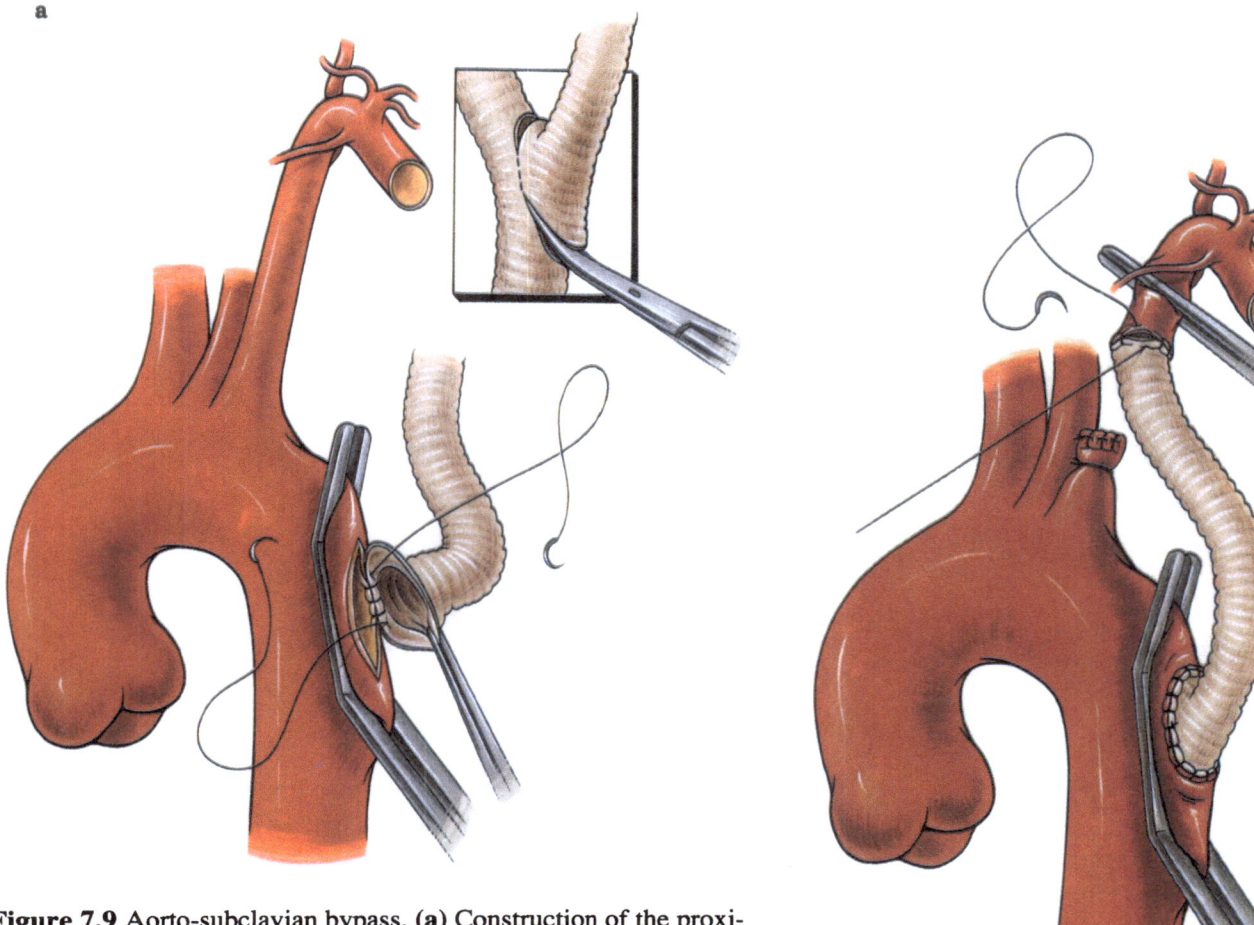

Figure 7.9 Aorto-subclavian bypass. (**a**) Construction of the proximal left anastomosis. (**Inset**) Tailoring the proximal end of a graft from a bifurcated prosthesis to obtain a wider base of implantation into a thick aortic wall. (**b**) Construction of the distal anastomosis.

tation base without compromising the anastomotic lumen. After declamping the aorta, the graft is allowed to distend under pressure so the surgeon can assess the proper length needed to bridge up to the desired level of the SA. The left SA is clamped close to its origin and distal to the VA. The VA itself is separately clamped with a small microsurgical bulldog clamp. The occluded first segment of the SA is cut about 1 cm proximal to the takeoff of the VA. If needed, an endarterectomy of the cut SA may be done with an eversion maneuver to permit clearing the origin of the VA. The graft is anastomosed end-to-end to the distal SA with 5-0 monofilament suture, and flow is reestablished first to the arm and then to the VA. The proximal stump of the SA is handled as described for the IA stump.

Endarterectomy of the left SA is advisable only when the disease does not extend proximally into the aorta. For this procedure a specially designed Wylie clamp permits exclusion clamping of the aorta around the origin of the SA. The SA endarterectomy should not extend into the aortic arch. Tacking sutures may be needed to fix the aortic intima around the origin of the SA. The distal limit of the endarterectomy should be either proximal to or at the level of the VA. The arteriotomy is closed with a continuous 5-0 monofilament suture with or without a synthetic patch angioplasty, depending on the SA size and the quality of the arteriotomy edges. Endarterectomy permits closure of the overlying pleura and avoids direct contact of the lung with the arterial repair, as is the case with an aortosubclavian bypass.

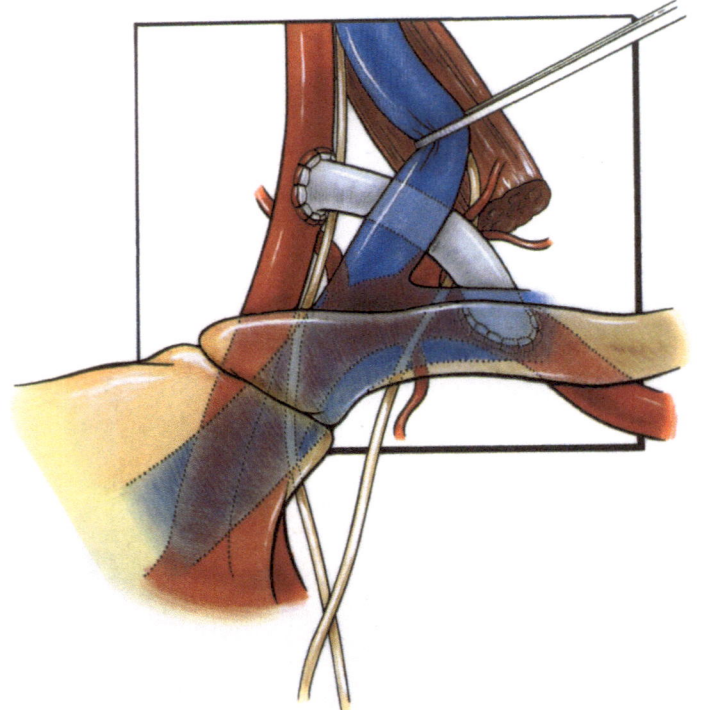

Figure 7.10 Carotid subclavian bypass to the third portion of the latter.

Cervical Bypass

Cervical bypass provides an easy and safe solution for patients with isolated lesions of the CCA or SA, although it is not the best choice for most lesions involving the supraaortic trunks. These bypasses may be classified as ipsilateral and contralateral, or "cross-over."

In earlier years and on general principles, autogenous veins were favored for cervical bypasses. The need for substantial lengths of saphenous vein, which were prone to kinking with neck motion and susceptible to axial rotation, and the gross caliber mismatch between the saphenous vein and the recipient SA discouraged surgeons from its use. As time passed, a favorable experience with the use of synthetic prostheses in these arteries of good caliber and high flow rates gradually established them as the material of choice.

Ipsilateral Bypass

Although it has been mostly superseded by transposition techniques, carotid-subclavian bypass was for years the most common technique for repair of iso-

lated lesions of the proximal SA. There are still circumstances where a bypass is preferable to a transposition, e.g., in individuals with morbid obesity or with a narrow thoracic inlet, where safe exposure of the proximal subclavian artery is difficult. In addition, a bypass is the only acceptable technique to revascularize the SA in patients who have had myocardial revascularization using the left internal mammary artery. In patients with extensive disease of the SA the revascularization of the arm is best handled by a CCA-axillary artery vein bypass.

For a while objections were raised to the technique of carotid-subclavian bypass on the grounds that it might cause a steal from the carotid circulation. These objections can now be discarded on theoretic grounds as well as on the basis of abundant clinical experience. On the other hand, there is no doubt that the use of the CCA for proximal anastomosis of the bypass entails some risk of cerebral ischemia during clamping and, should the bypass occlude later, distal embolization. These risks gave impetus to the development of the cervical "crossover" bypass. We believe crossover bypasses have been overused and offer more inconvenience than advantage; in our experience use of the CCA as a source of inflow for a bypass (or a transposition) has been safe.

The technique of carotid-subclavian bypass is straightforward (Figure 7.10). The operation is done through a supraclavicular incision, and the approach is made by dividing the clavicular head of the sterno-mastoid. The CCA and distal SA are dissected, respectively, on each side of the jugular vein, mobilizing the prescalene fat pad laterally. The division of the scalenus anticus muscle is optional, depending on how much SA is available lateral to it. Traction injury to the vagus and phrenic nerves should be avoided. In this location we use a 7 or 8 mm Dacron or an 8 mm PTFE tube.

After systemic heparinization the distal anastomosis is constructed first. The beveled graft is sewn in end-to-side fashion to the thin wall of the SA using 6-0 monofilament suture. The graft is then tunneled behind the internal jugular vein and in front of the phrenic and vagus nerves, after which it is clamped on the medial side of the jugular vein. The CCA is clamped and an arteriostomy is made in its lateral wall to accommodate the proximal end of the graft. The graft is then cut to the appropriate length and anastomosed to the CCA with continuous 5-0 or 6-0 monofilament suture. With the patient in the head-down position, the distal CCA, proximal CCA, and then the bypass are allowed to back-bleed, with flow being resumed first into the bypass and then into the distal CCA.

The performance of CCA-axillary bypass calls for specific technical steps. The mobility of the shoulder makes a vein graft in this location preferable to a prosthesis. The first step of the operation is to approach the proximal part of the axillary artery in the deltopectoral groove between the clavicle and the pectoralis minor muscle to make sure that it is free of disease. In this part of the artery one can usually find 2-3 cm of length without branches. The segment of saphenous removed from the thigh can be used either in a reversed fashion, or, for optimal caliber matching in a non-reversed manner following valvulotomy. The vein graft is anastomosed to an arteriostomy in the sidewall of the CCA. It is then passed behind the vagus nerve, internal jugular vein and prescalene fat pad, leaving behind it the phrenic nerve and the undisturbed scalenus anticus muscle. The retroclavic-

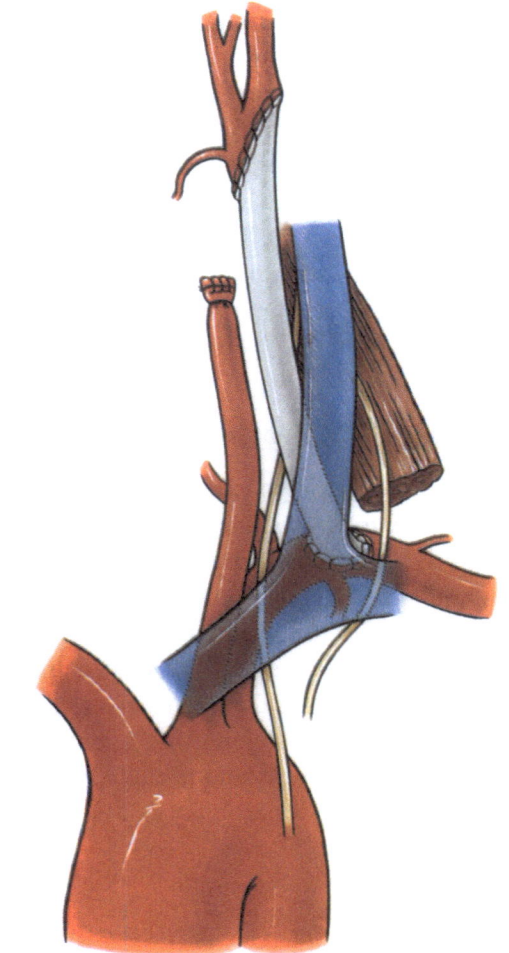

Figure 7.11 Subclavian-carotid bypass for extensive disease of the common carotid artery.

ular tunnel should be large enough to admit two fingerbreadths and should be lateral to the native artery to avoid compression of the graft when the shoulders are extended backwards. The distal anastomosis is done in end-to-side fashion to the axillary artery.

Although we favor transposition techniques to deal with proximal lesions of the CCA, particularly on the left side, a subclavian-carotid bypass permits reconstruction of an extensively diseased CCA (Figure 7.11). The two arteries are approached separately, using the same techniques described for dissecting the distal SA and the carotid bifurcation. After systemic heparinization the proximal end of a 7- to 8-mm prosthetic graft is sewn onto the SA in a manner similar to that described above for the carotid-subclavian bypass. The graft is then tunneled between the two incisions behind the jugular vein and in front of the phrenic and vagus nerves. The distal anastomosis is usually made to the carotid bifurcation as described for aortocarotid bypasses. Concomitant endarterectomy of the carotid artery bifurcation is usually needed (Figure 7.7). In rare cases where the distal CCA and bifurcation are free of disease, the distal anastomosis may be made end-to-end to the CCA.

Contralateral ("Crossover") Bypass

A number of crossover bypasses have been described, including the SA-to-SA, axillary-to-axillary, and CCA-to-CCA, as well as any asymmetric combination of the above. Other than those involving the CCA, these techniques have the theoretic advantage of avoiding clamping of the carotid artery. However, they have long, transverse pathways that result in less than ideal long-term patency rates. Although we do not favor their extensive or primary utilization, each has merit in specific situations, and the techniques of their implantation should be familiar to any surgeon treating cerebrovascular disease.

Crossover bypasses are usually constructed with prosthetic grafts, which in this position fare better than veins. Their typical pathways are either presternal (axillary-axillary) (Figure 7.12) or pretracheal as is used in the SA-SA procedure (Figure 7.13), in some CCA-CCA (Figure 7.14), and in other asymmetric bypasses. We have found that for bypasses involving at least one CCA the retropharyngeal approach (Figures 7.15 and 7.16) allows a shorter route without the risk of compression or erosion of the esophagus. The retroesophageal tunnel is developed by dissecting medially and displacing the carotid and the pharyngoesophageal axis forward until the lamina prevertebralis is identified. The anterior bodies of the cervical vertebrae can be easily palpated. The space between the bodies of the vertebrae and the pharynx easily admits a finger. Dissecting on both sides permits establishment of a tunnel behind the pharynx through which the graft can be run. The distance between the two carotids when using this approach is about 6 cm (Figures 7.16 and 7.17).

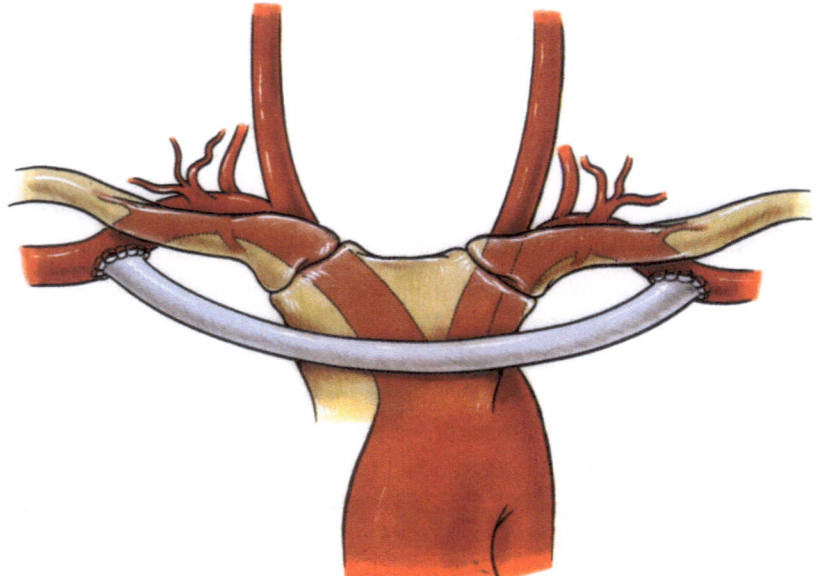

Figure 7.12 Axillary-axillary bypass.

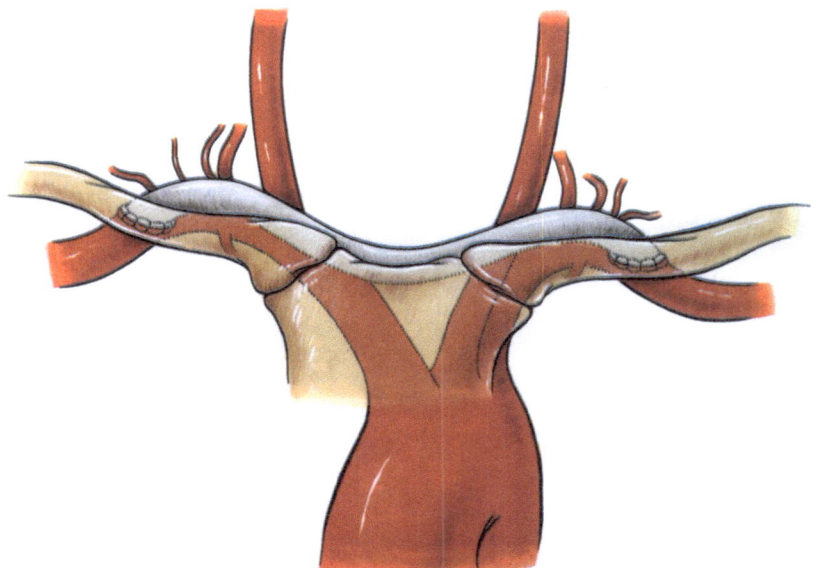

Figure 7.13 Subclavian-subclavian bypass.

Figure 7.14 Three types of intercarotid bypass: high, low, and oblique.

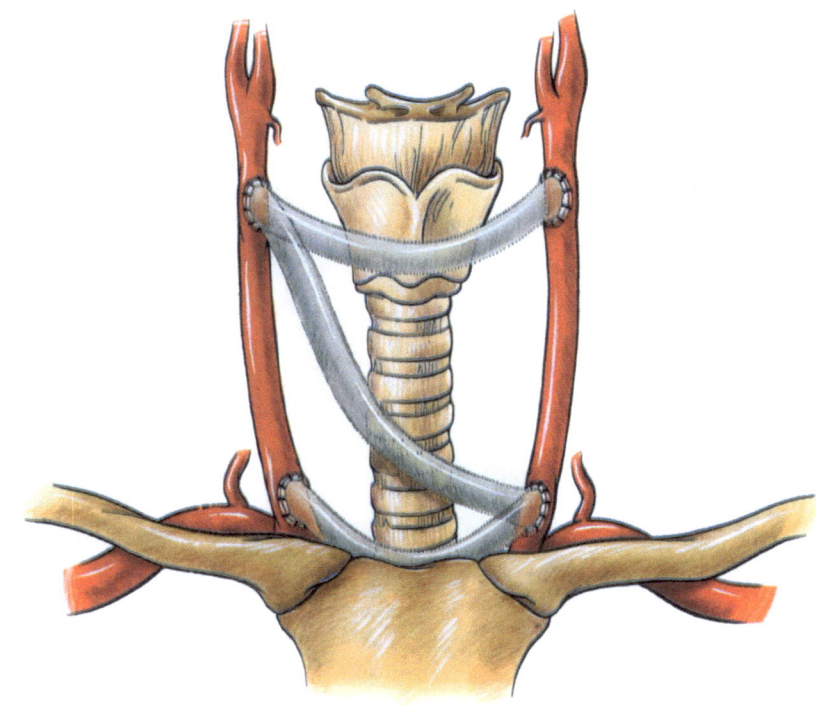

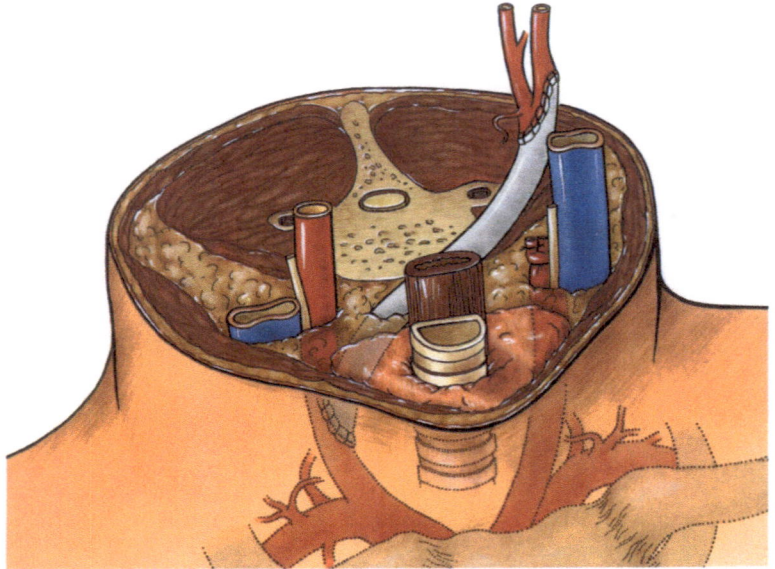

Figure 7.15 Retropharyngeal bypass across the neck.

Figure 7.16 Shorter distance of the retropharyngeal graft when compared with the graft passing in front of the trachea.

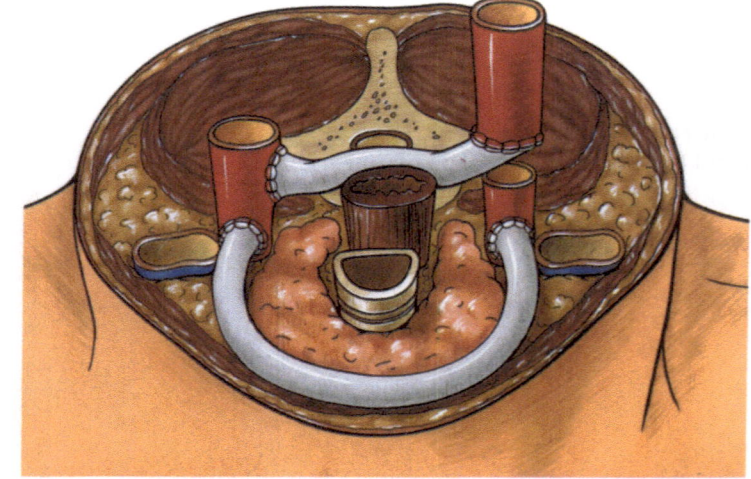

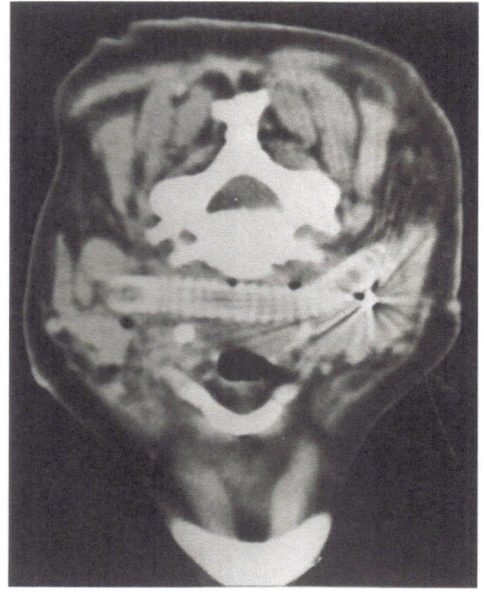

Figure 7.17 Computed tomography scan of a retropharyngeal bypass.

Transpositions

Transposition procedures are particularly well suited to the neck owing to the long, parallel pathways of the neighboring supraaortic trunks, but only recently have these techniques obtained general clinical acceptance. They have gradually replaced cervical bypasses, except in patients with lesions involving the distal portion of the SA or extensive lesions of the CCA where transposition is not a suitable technique. The principle of transposition is to divide an artery distal to the obstructing lesion and anastomose it to a neighboring artery that is free of disease and will act as the new source of blood flow. From a technical point of view, transposition has the appeal of a single artery-to-artery anastomosis at the cost of simultaneous clamping of both donor and recipient arteries.

Transposition of the SA into the CCA is our preferred technique for treating proximal occlusive disease of the SA. This technique is contraindicated in patients who have had myocardial revascularization using the ipsilateral internal mammary artery. The transposition of the SA into the CCA has the drawbacks of any technique that uses the CCA as a source of inflow and, in addition, requires simultaneous clamping of both arteries. Despite these theoretic objections, we have not seen a single ischemic stroke in patients undergoing these procedures whose opposite CCA and ICA were patent. In cases where the opposite ICA is occluded, a crossover bypass may be preferable to avoid clamping the remaining carotid system. If at the time of doing an SA transposition to the CCA there is also a need for a carotid bifurcation endarterectomy on the same side, the transposition may be performed over a shunt inserted through the carotid bifurcation arteriotomy with the proximal end of the shunt low in the CCA (Figure 7.18). After the transposition is done, the shunt can be moved distally to proceed with a standard ICA endarterectomy.

For SA-to-CCA transposition both arteries are approached through a supraclavicular incision between the bellies of the sternomastoid muscle (Figure 7.19). The entire dissection is confined to the space medial to the internal jugular vein, vagus nerve, and prescalene fat pad. The CCA is dissected proximally along its intrathoracic course for as long as is safe. The proximal SA is also dissected toward its origin after the thoracic duct (on the left side) and the vertebral vein are divided. The SA is first looped distally and then proximally to the origin of the VA. The VA is mobilized up to the level where it disappears into the cervical spine. This step may necessitate division of some of its attachments to the sympathetic chain and some of the fibers of the latter that surround the VA. Complete mobilization of the left SA to near the aortic arch is most important. When mobilizing the right SA, the vagus and its recurrent laryngeal branch must be identified and protected.

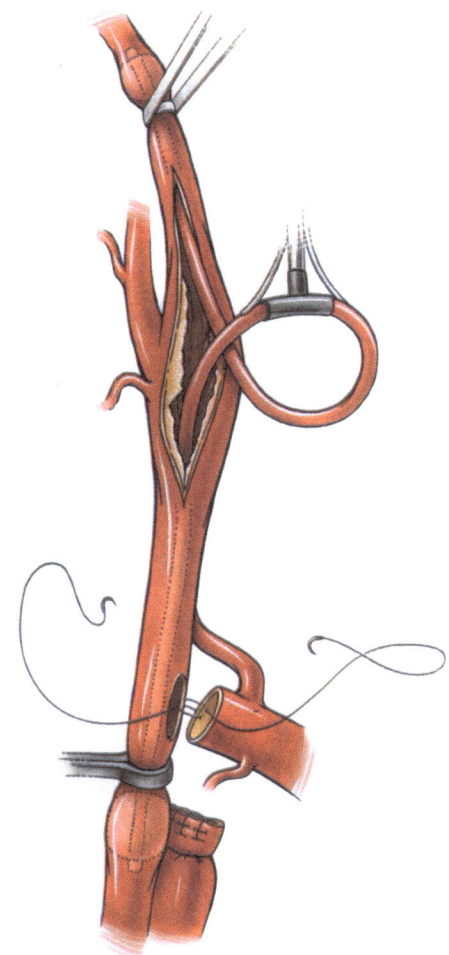

Figure 7.18 Use of a shunt for transposing the subclavian artery to the common carotid artery when the opposite carotid is occluded and there is a need to repair the ipsilateral internal carotid artery.

a

b

c

d

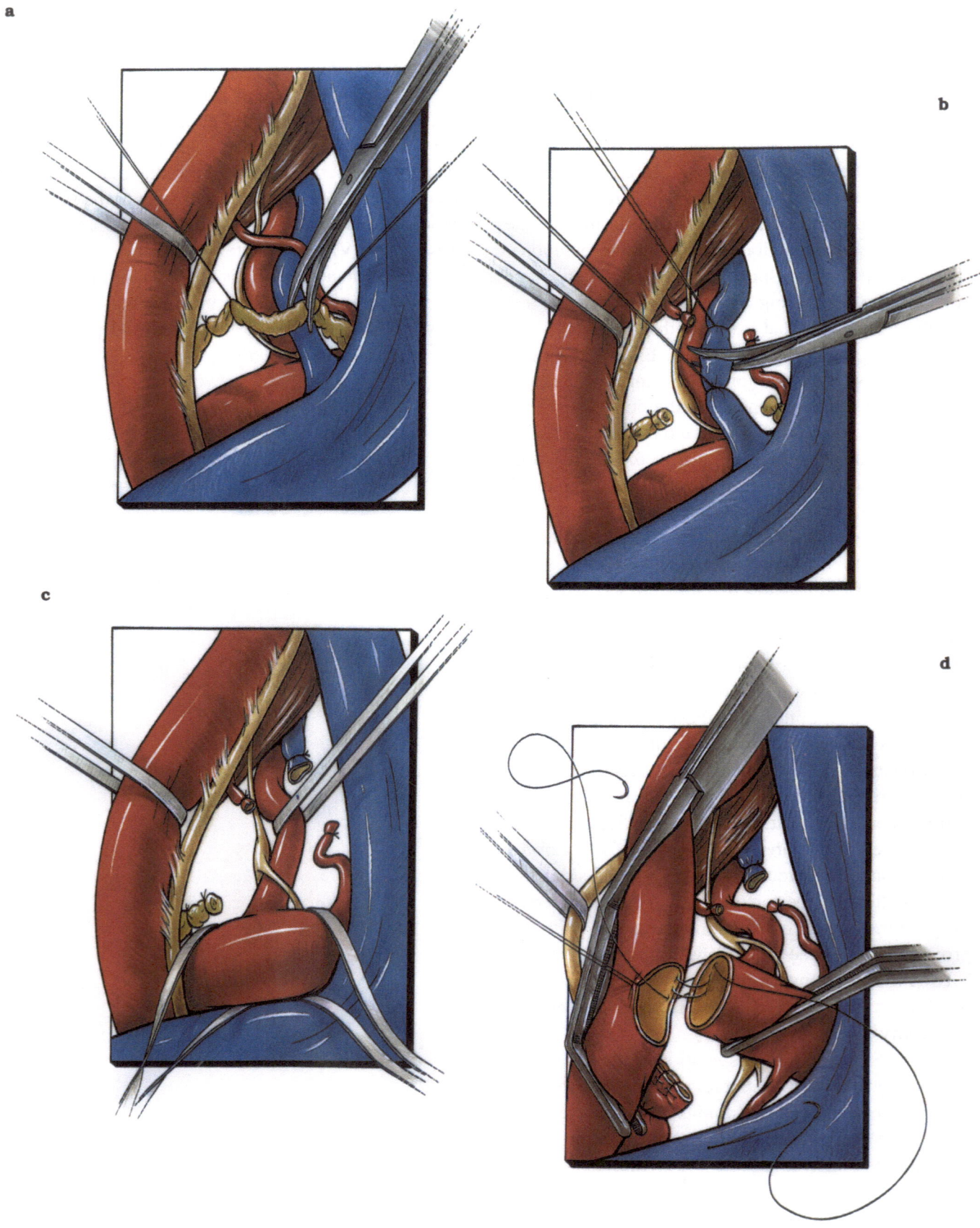

e

Figure 7.19 Left subclavian-to-carotid transposition. (**a**) Approach to both proximal subclavian and common carotid arteries and division of the thoracic duct; (**b**) division of the vertebral vein; (**c**) isolation of the vertebral and common carotid arteries and pre and post vertebral segment of the subclavian artery. (**d**) End-to-side anastomosis of subclavian to common carotid artery. (**e**) Completed operation.

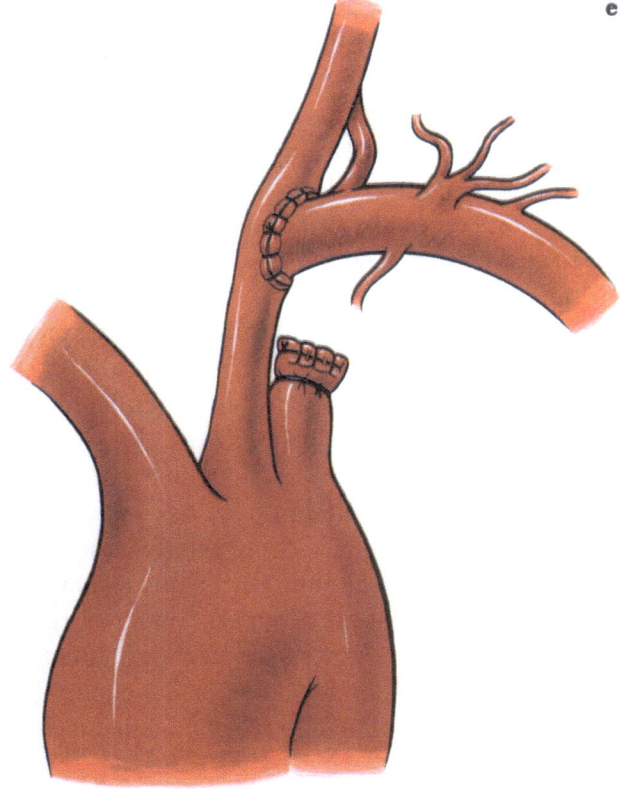

Care is taken not to enter the pleural cavity or stretch the vagus or phrenic nerves.

After systemic heparinization, the proximal SA is clamped using a small Satinsky or similar clamp and ligated with heavy silk suture proximal to the clamp. The VA, distal SA, and occasionally internal mammary artery are clamped, and the proximal SA is divided immediately above the proximal clamp. The proximal stump is carefully oversewn with 4-0 monofilament suture using a small needle to accommodate the limited intrathoracic exposure. The SA is obliquely transected about 1 cm proximal to the origin of the VA. If needed, an eversion endarterectomy of the origin of the VA may be done at this point (Figure 7.20). The anticipated site of anastomosis to the CCA is chosen, bearing in mind that the anastomosis should be low and result in an oblique takeoff of the SA from the CCA without kinking of the proximal VA. Having determined and marked the most appropriate site, the CCA is cross-clamped. An arteriostomy made in its posterolateral wall should accommodate the larger-caliber SA. The anastomosis is done in an open manner with 6-0 monofilament suture. It is important to avoid

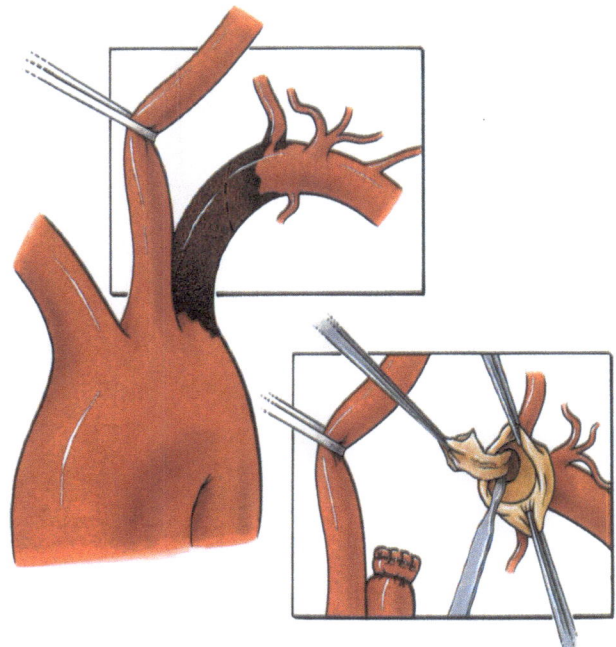

Figure 7.20 Eversion endarterectomy of the ostium of the vertebral artery during a subclavian transposition to the common carotid.

kinking in the VA that may result from doing this anastomosis too high in the CCA, or failing to mobilize the VA adequately before the transposition.

Transposition of the CCA to the SA for treatment of proximal occlusion of the CCA is done less frequently (Figure 7.21). With this technique the CCA is ligated as low as possible and is then transposed and anastomosed end-to-side either to the proximal intrathoracic SA or to the distal retroscalene SA, depending on the local anatomy and personal preference. In the second case, the CCA needs to be mobilized extensively before being tunneled behind the jugular vein to reach the distal SA.

Transposition of a CCA into the opposite CCA (Figure 7.22) is indicated in poor risk patients who have stenosis of the left CCA and extensive disease of the left SA. In these circumstances this technique is preferable to crossover bypass or to a riskier aortocarotid bypass. However it entails simultaneous clamping of both CCAs and can be done only if the right VA has been shown to supply the hemispheres

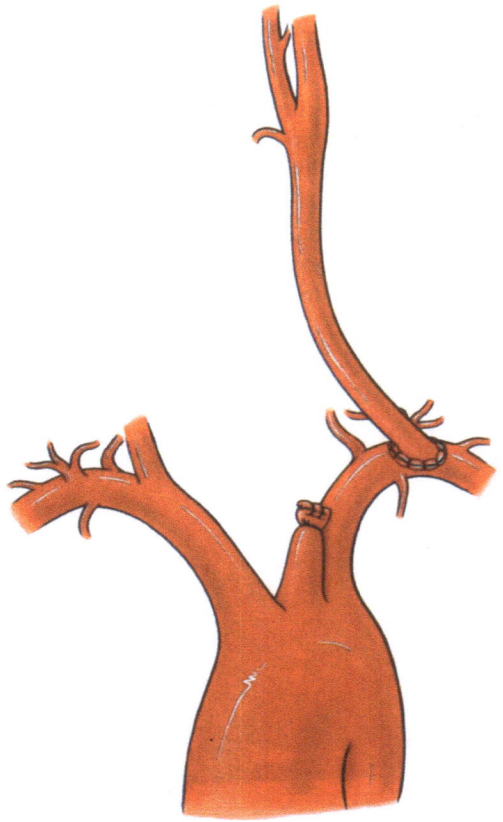

Figure 7.21 Transposition of the common carotid to the subclavian artery.

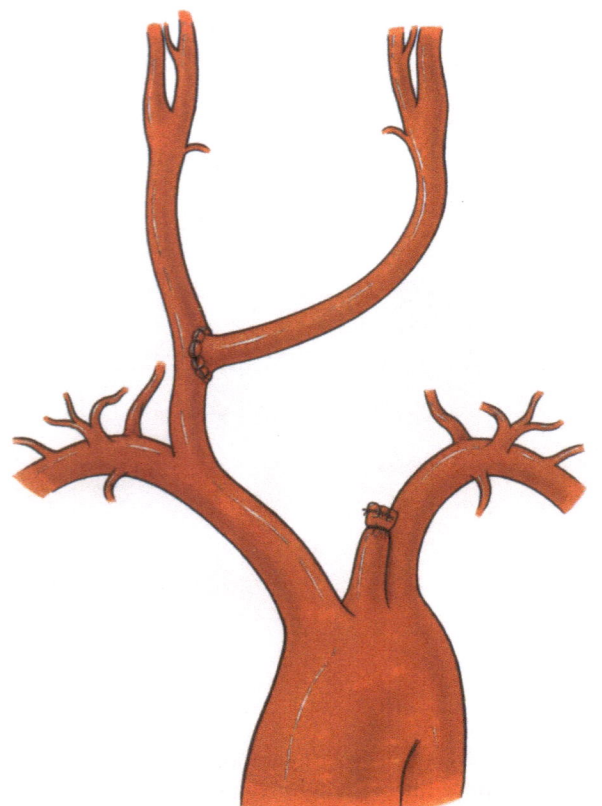

Figure 7.22 Transposition of the left common carotid artery to the right common carotid artery.

Figure 7.23 Transposition of the left common carotid artery to the innominate artery.

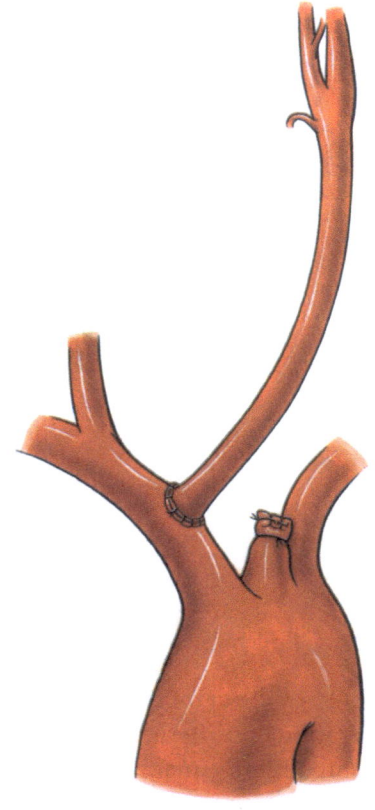

(through posterior communicating arteries) or with the protection of a shunt.

Transposition of the SA into the CCA or vice versa can also be done using an intrathoracic approach. This step is taken during transthoracic reconstruction of multiple lesions of the SAT (see Chapter 10) or if the patient is to undergo a concomitant myocardial revascularization. In the last case, transposing the SA may ensure adequate inflow to the left internal mammary artery. The transsternal route makes this transposition easier. A transthoracic approach is mandatory when the left CCA is being transposed into the IA (Figure 7.23) or if the IA is being transposed into the distal ascending aorta (Figure 6.5). These techniques are seldom used because they are appropriate only under the most unusual anatomic conditions. Furthermore, simultaneous clamping of the IA and left CCA requires ensurance of cerebral protection.

8 Repair of the Internal and External Carotid Arteries

Endarterectomy of the carotid bifurcation is the most common operation done in the arteries supplying the head. Without underestimating the importance of carefully selecting patients, it is likely that differences in surgical technique are an important factor in explaining why some surgical series show mortality and morbidity rates that differ by as much as an order of magnitude.

Methods of Cerebral Protection

Much has been written on the monitoring and protection of the brain during carotid surgery. The longest running argument is, without a doubt, whether to use an intraluminal shunt during carotid cross-clamping. In this controversy surgeons adhere to one of three policies: routine shunting, no shunting at all, and selective shunting. The selective use of the shunt is best done based on preoperative and clinical information such as existence of a previous stroke, knowledge of a contralateral occlusion or intraoperative criteria, e.g., stump pressure, electroencephalographic (EEG) abnormality, behavior of the awake patient, transcranial Doppler findings, or cerebral blood flow data.

It is difficult to assess the worth of any of these methods if we use as final criterion the presence or absence of stroke following the operation. Cerebral ischemia secondary to cross-clamping of the carotid is only one of many causes of operative strokes, and the latter, fortunately, are unusual.

We have been reluctant to endorse a policy of routine shunting for carotid operations because (1) a shunt is obviously unnecessary in most patients; (2) a shunt, once placed, may not function properly, and the only way to determine if it is functioning is to measure blood flow in the brain or through the shunt; (3) the shunt itself may be responsible for dislodgement of debris and embolization, or it may cause intimal injury and eventual thrombosis of the artery; (4) it may be difficult or impossible to place a shunt in certain anatomic circumstances, particularly in high carotid bifurcations or lesions; and (5) the presence of the shunt may increase the difficulty of the operation, particularly in its distal portion.

Selective shunting would be the ideal solution if there was a criterion to determine the need for a shunt that had good specificity and sensitivity in detecting cerebral ischemia and resulting infarction. Such a criterion is not available. In our opinion none of the methods used to determine the need to use a shunt is either safe or practical. The EEG is largely under the influence of the depth of anesthesia and does not monitor the brainstem. The correlation between stump pressures measured in the carotid and cerebral blood flow is poor. Operating on a patient who is awake is a burden to both the surgeon and the patient, and the superiority of regional over general anesthesia has not been demonstrated. Transcranial Doppler is obtrusive at the time of surgery and requires a technician. Additionally, it ignores the brainstem and produces no information on the contralateral hemisphere. Measurement of cerebral blood flow, as propounded by Sundt et al.,[75] is probably the better method of predicting the need for a shunt. It is, however, unavailable in most institutions; more importantly, we do not know the flow threshold level under which shunting is necessary. After all, Sundt et al. shunted roughly 50% of their patients, so the specificity of this method is not good.

One of us (E.K.) has followed a "no shunt" policy in a consecutive series of 2000 patients with results similar to those reported in the best series of the literature by surgeons using different methods of cerebral protection. The only incremental risk factor for intraoperative stroke in this series was the presence of a contralateral ICA occlusion.

Therefore for cerebral protection we rely mainly on the appropriate selection of patients and on meticulous surgical and anesthetic techniques, including precise positioning of the head so as not to interrupt collateral flow, close monitoring and maintenance of blood pressure during the perioperative period, clamping times below 30 minutes, general heparinization, and completion arteriography. Our current indications for shunting are limited to (1) contralateral carotid occlusion and (2) severe stenosis or occlusion of the basilar or vertebral arteries and an incomplete circle of Willis (absence of the anterior communicating artery or the A1 segment).

Exposure of the Carotid Bifurcation

The standard incision to approach the carotid bifurcation runs in front of the sternomastoid muscle, curving posteriorly one fingerbreadth away from the jaw and the tip of the ear lobe to avoid the mandibular branch of the facial nerve and the parotid gland (Figure 8.1). The tip of the parotid is lifted from the surface of the sternomastoid muscle with a hot knife, avoiding the greater occipital nerve. The external jugular vein is divided. The anterior edge of the internal jugular vein is exposed, and the facial vein and any other anterior branch are divided. At the top of the field the internal jugular vein is covered with lymph nodes that obstruct dissection of the anterior edge of the vein. They can be freed first by cutting anterior to them and then following the lower edge of the digastric muscle so as to raise a flap that keeps the lymph nodes reflected posteriorly and held in position by the self-retaining retractor. They can also be cut over a clamp that has been passed over the anterior edge of the vein and up to the lower edge of the digastric muscle. At this level, so long as the surgeon stays on top of the vein and toward its anterior edge, the structures superficial to it can be divided safely.

As the CCA is dissected, the surgeon should separate it from the vagus without handling the nerve itself. If the carotid bifurcation is low, the omohyoid muscle is cut for better exposure of the CCA. A constant arterial loop, a branch of the superior thyroid artery, accompanies the upper edge of the omohyoid and must be divided and ligated with its satellite veins.

The hypoglossal nerve may be covered by the superior branch of the anterior facial vein or by an equally large vein joining independently with the internal jugular vein. The hypoglossal nerve is identified at the top of the field. More often than not the portion of the hypoglossal that overlaps the ICA needs to be mobilized anteriorly. The hypoglossal nerve may occur low and obstruct access to the ICA. If it is unusually low (Figure 8.1), it is probably pulled down by a branch of the ECA (and accompanying veins) that is feeding the sternomastoid muscle or by the occipital artery itself. (An occipital artery seen in the arteriogram to arise from the first centimeter of the ECA anticipates this possibility.) This arterial loop needs to be divided to mobilize the hypoglossal nerve upward and forward. The posterior loop of the ansa hypoglossi, which tethers the hypoglossal nerve, may

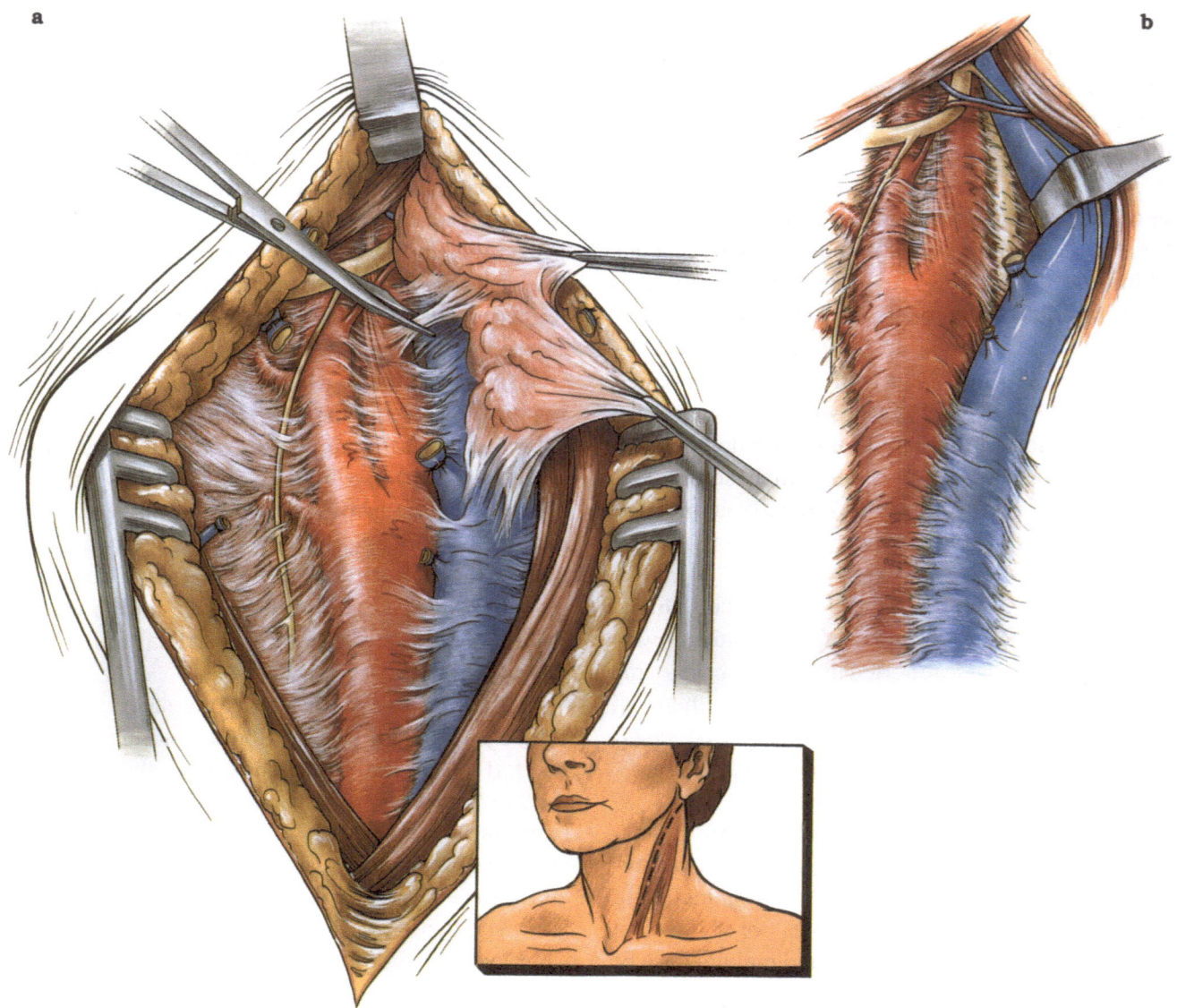

Figure 8.1 Dissection of the carotid bifurcation. **(Inset)** Neck incision. **(a)** Clearing the lymph nodes over the upper portion of the jugular vein. **(b)** Exposure of the internal carotid artery above the bulb. Note the sternomastoid artery and vein tenting down the hypoglossal nerve.

be cut to mobilize the latter anteriorly. The line for dissecting the ICA runs along its posterolateral edge. The dissection of the ICA starts at the upper end of the bulb. The surrounding structures (vagus nerve, internal jugular, hypoglossal nerve) are dissected away from the artery, leaving the carotid bulb undisturbed.

Once cut, the stump of the ansa can be used as a handle on the hypoglossal nerve. Toward the top of the dissection the hypoglossal and vagus nerves meet and share some binding of their sheaths. Using mag-

nification and fine instruments the two trunks can be separated for an additional few millimeters. The nerves should be handled by grasping only the areolar tissue around them.

When dealing with a high bifurcation or a long plaque, the operator may find that these maneuvers have not yet brought into view that bluish-pink arterial wall that is recognized as nondiseased carotid. Additional exposure is obtained by retracting the posterior belly of the digastric muscle. Transection of

(c) Dissection of the internal carotid artery above the bulb and separation of the hypoglossal and vagus nerves to gain additional exposure. The posterior branch of the ansa hypoglossi has been cut and is used to pull the hypoglossal nerve anteriorly, away from the vagus nerve. **(d)** Dissection of the origin of the external carotid artery, close to the wall of the latter.

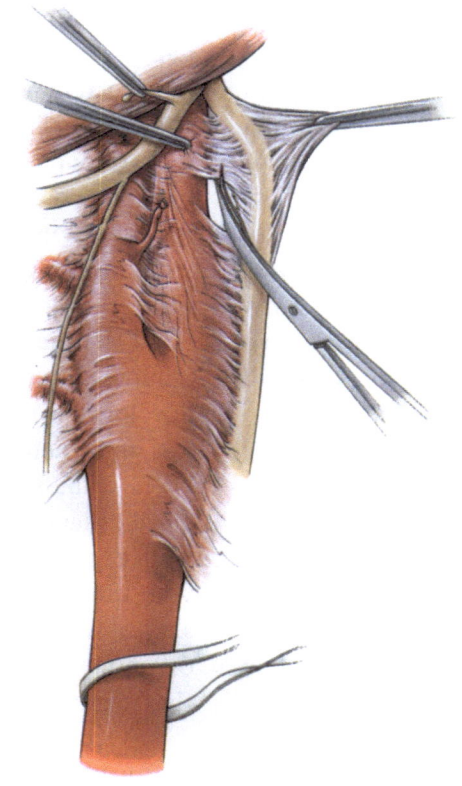
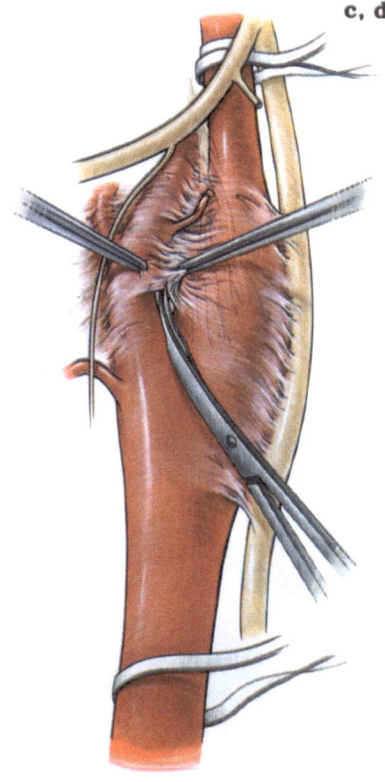

c, d

e, f

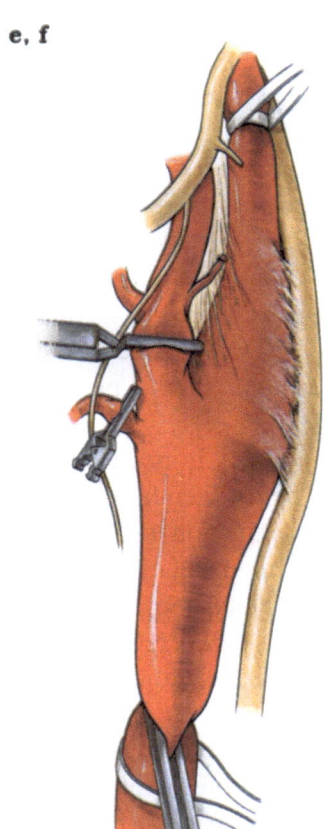
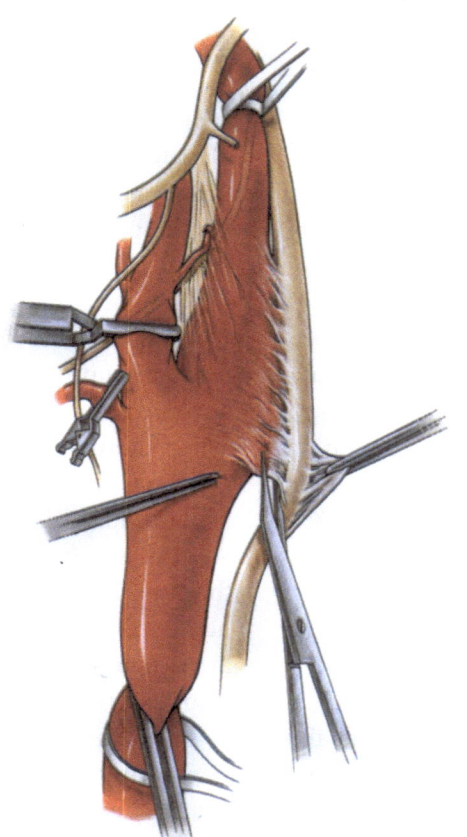

(e) Occlusion of the three components of the bifurcation. Note that the bulb is mostly undissected. **(f)** Dissection of the bulb is completed after cross-clamping. The course of the superior laryngeal nerve below the bulb is outlined.

this muscle is seldom needed provided it is amply mobilized.

As soon as "good" ICA is found, the surgeon dissects it free by holding it in place by its adventitial "hair" while exerting gentle traction on the surrounding tissues away from the ICA in order to dissect them. The ICA is circled with an unweighted Silastic loop. The bulb of the carotid is barely dissected; and the vagus, if it overrides the bulb, is dissected away from it. Without fully mobilizing the bulb, just enough tissue is cleared for the path of the scissors that will open the lumen of the artery.

The origin of the ECA is dissected by staying close to its wall to avoid the external branch of the superior laryngeal nerve anteriorly and the carotid sinus nerve posteriorly (Figure 8.1). The latter is left attached to the wall of the bifurcation and initial portion of the ICA bulb.

Heparin 7000 U is given at this point, and an accelerated coagulation time is obtained 5 minutes later. One of us (R.B.) uses, in addition, 5 mg of dexamethasone and a bolus of dextran (100 ml).

Standard Endarterectomy of the Internal Carotid Artery

Standard endarterectomy of the ICA requires proper magnification. We routinely use 2.5x magnification loops. Once the components of the carotid bifurcation are ·dissected, its two branches are occluded with loops or microsurgical clamps, and the CCA is occluded proximally with a small pediatric vascular clamp (Figure 8.1). Once the ICA is occluded, dissection of the bulb is completed paying attention to the underlying superior laryngeal nerve. This dissection is facilitated by simultaneous traction of the ECA loop anteriorly and the CCA loop (or clamp) downward and posteriorly. The arteriotomy extends over the last 2 cm of CCA, continuing along the posterior wall of the bulb and anteriorly into the ICA to a point beyond the termination of the plaque (Figure 8.2).

If a shunt is to be used, it is inserted at this moment. Balloon shunts with a side venting branch are inserted distally first and then proximally, and then are finally purged. The proximal balloons often do not stay in place, and for safety reasons they require an additional Javid-type clamp or a double loop to retain them in place. Care is taken not to overfill the distal balloon which may injure the distal ICA. A loop under mild tension proximal to the distal balloon avoids retrograde migration of the latter into the arteriotomy. Javid shunts can be inserted in either sequence. The Sundt shunt is inserted proximally first, allowed to bleed, and then inserted distally.

The plane of endarterectomy (external elastic lamina) is sought at the level where the plaque is most developed (Figure 8.2), usually in the proximal bulb, and in the anterior edge of the arteriotomy.

At the proximal end feathering is uncommon, and the plaque is usually cut where it is adherent to the wall (Figure 8.2) leaving a small step that smooths out with time. If the plaque is not adherent, a few U-shaped stitches or, preferably, a running suture with 6-0 monofilament suture will be needed to affix this flap to the artery.

Occasionally a long and eccentric plaque may need to be cut at the termination of the endarterectomy, usually at its proximal end in the CCA. This method leaves a luminal protrusion that exposes the irregular and friable cut section of the plaque (Figure 8.3). In such cases a fine 6-0 or 7-0 suture can be used to elevate the endarterectomized surface so it is continuous with the intima. The suture can be interrupted or continuous; the latter eliminates the gap between stitches. The bite on the endarterectomized layer needs to be as deep as the height of the cut section of the plaque, so the resulting flow surface does not step down abruptly, and the cut end of the plaque is covered.

Alternatively, when a shunt is not used, the proximal clamp is placed where the endarterectomy should end (as determined by palpation) (Figure 8.4). After dissecting the plaque to the level of the clamp, the artery is crushed immediately above it with a hemostat and the specimen delivered into the arteriotomy by squeezing the plaque within the artery using the fingers.

To ensure that there is no problem (usually a flap) with the termination of the proximal end: (1) one can inspect the termination from inside by pulling the proximal clamp upward and everting the endar-

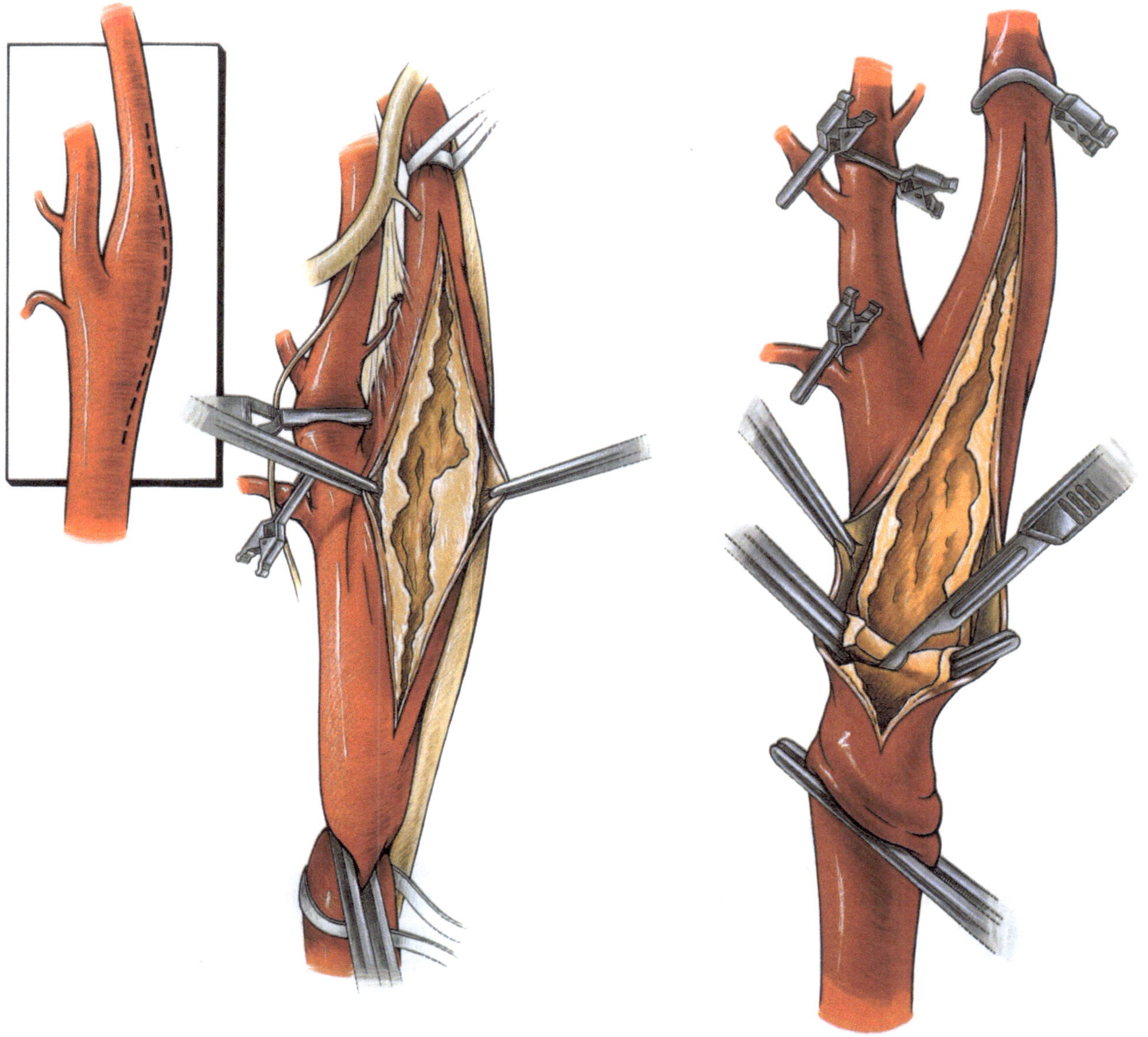

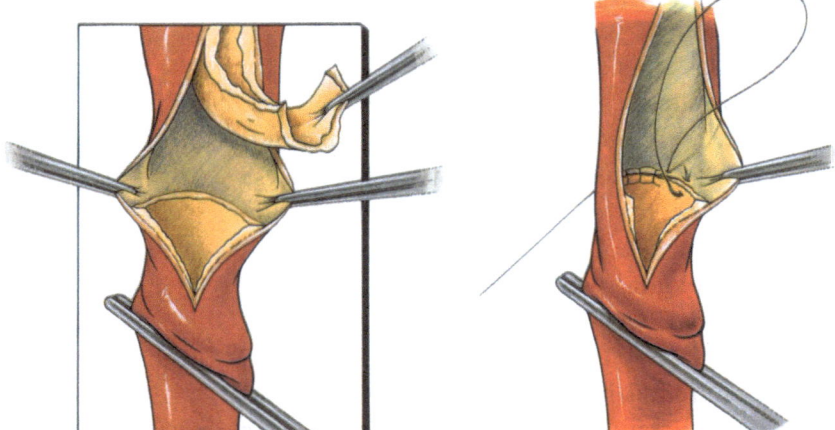

Figure 8.2 Steps for endarterectomy of the proximal portion of the carotid bifurcation. (**a**) Arteriotomy on the common and internal carotid arteries. (**b**) Cutting the proximal end of the plaque over a right-angle clamp. (**c**) Proximal end of the plaque may be well fixed to the artery, or (**d**) it may require some tacking sutures.

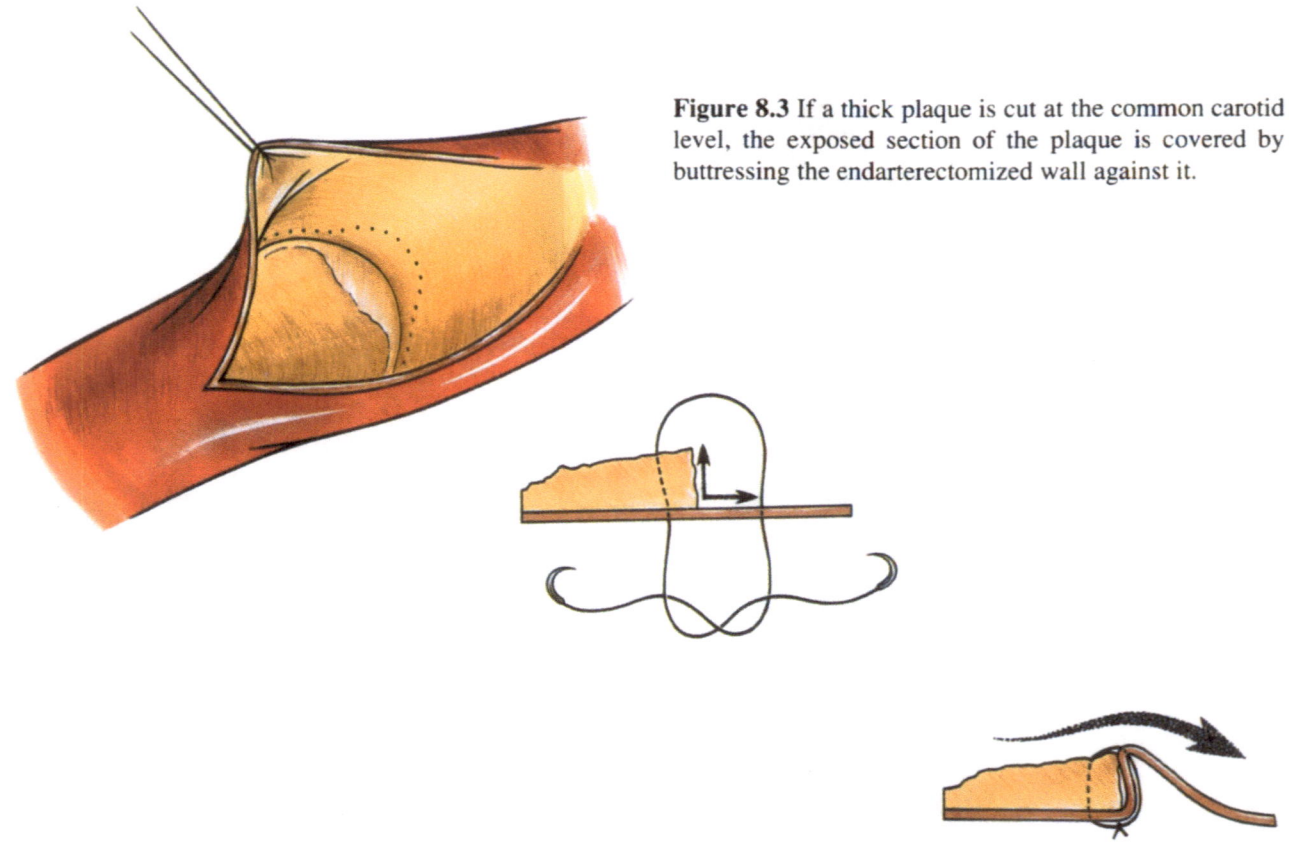

Figure 8.3 If a thick plaque is cut at the common carotid level, the exposed section of the plaque is covered by buttressing the endarterectomized wall against it.

terectomized segment; (2) after moving the proximal clamp farther down and prolonging the arteriotomy proximally, the flap can be repaired from inside by recutting it or affixing it with sutures; (3) without prolonging the arteriotomy and after moving the proximal clamp farther below, one can also cut the CCA transversely, free the plaque circumferentially in the distal CCA, or perform an eversion endarterectomy and follow with an end-to-end anastomosis after tacking the intima (Figure 8.5). This maneuver is seldom needed.

Once its proximal end is freed, the rest of the plaque can be handled in a number of ways. The plaque may be circled above the level of the ECA takeoff and cut about 1 cm from its distal end in the ICA. The proximal two-thirds of the plaque is now attached to the ECA. The endarterectomy of the ECA component of the bifurcation lesion requires freeing the plaque around its orifice in a more superficial plane (immediately below the plaque) than is fol-

lowed for the rest of the endarterectomy. The plaque is gently pulled while the spatula dissects the wall away. Previous inspection of the ECA would have suggested whether to expect a "feathering" termination: An eccentric plaque limited to the orifice of an otherwise supple ECA trunk would feather off with gentle traction and axial rotation. A concentrically indurated wall throughout the trunk of the ECA requires cutting the plaque off slightly above the orifice of entrance of the ECA under direct vision. This maneuver is helped by pulling on the ECA trunk toward the arteriotomy and everting its wall away from it. If the quality of the endarterectomy of the ECA is in question, usually because of a flap (seen either as a subadventitial hematoma after reestablishing flow or on the intraoperative arteriogram), it is better to do a separate arteriotomy in the ECA to affix the distal intima or to obliterate the opening of the ECA with an occluding clip affixed with a suture. Thrombus forming in a flap at the ostium of the ECA

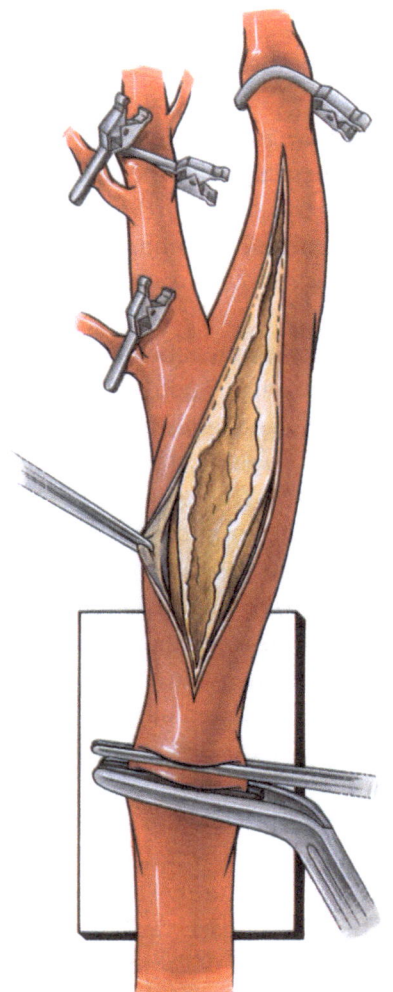

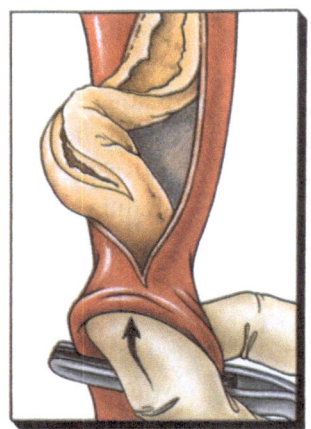

Figure 8.4 Termination of the proximal endarterectomy by "crushing" the plaque and (**inset**) squeezing it distally.

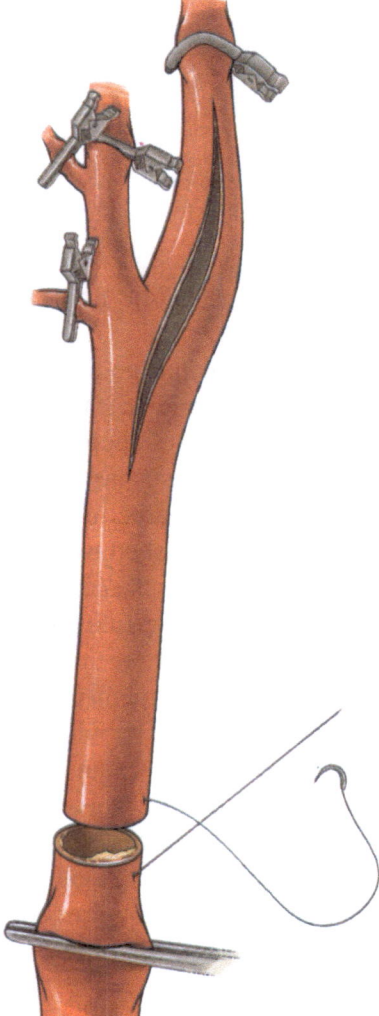

Figure 8.5 Rarely, transection and reanastomosis of the common carotid artery is necessary to obtain a good proximal termination to the endarterectomy. The long component of the distal common carotid plaque can be cleared by eversion. Any remaining plaque in the proximal common carotid artery is attached to the wall by the anastomosing suture.

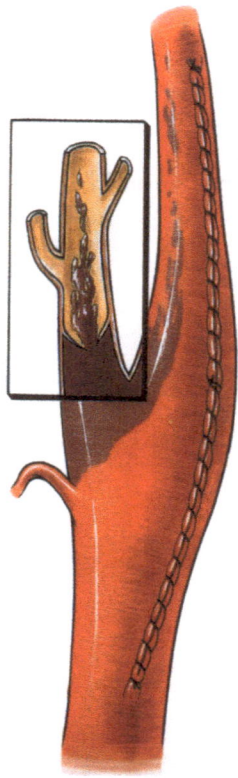

Figure 8.6 Thrombus in the external carotid artery secondary to a flap may embolize the internal carotid artery.

may project into the lumen of the bifurcation and embolize the ICA (Figure 8.6).

The distal third of the plaque going into the ICA is the most critical. It is best handled if the plaque has been freed of all other attachment points and pivots around its ICA end. The ideal distal termination of an endarterectomy is done by feathering the plaque (Figure 8.7), which is accomplished by abandoning the deep (external elastic) plane near the end of the plaque and entering the more superficial layer immediately below the plaque. To make the transition into this superficial plane the plaque is gently pulled along the axis of the artery (not lifting it) with mild axial rotation while the surgeon's other hand pushes the ICA wall posteriorly (Figure 8.8). This maneuver is done on both edges, and the distal end of the plaque is removed. It is also possible to cause a clean pressure fracture of the end of the plaque by pressing with a spatula on the distal end while pulling the plaque

axially. The technique of eversion endarterectomy may also be used to free the distal attachment of the plaque.

The remaining surface is debrided of smooth muscle fibers by lifting them up with the dissecting spatula and pulling them transversely (Figure 8.9). Smaller debris can be identified by rubbing the surface with fine gauze or with a Q-tip wetted in heparinized saline.

Prior to closure a decision must be made about whether to patch the arteriotomy. Patch material can be autogenous vein, usually saphenous but less commonly internal or external jugular (Figure 6.4) or synthetic (Figure 8.10): polytetrafluorethylene (PTFE) or Dacron. Currently our indications for patching are the presence of: (1) a small carotid bulb; (2) an arteriotomy that goes beyond the bulb in patients with a small ICA; (3) transverse tears along the arteriotomy edges or at its end, (4) mild angulation caused by elongation of the artery after endarterectomy; and (5) a fibrotic restenosis, limited to the origin of the bulb, from a previous endarterectomy.

Whether a patch or simple closure is used, we start at both ends and continue toward the middle using 7-0 or 6-0 monofilament sutures. The closure is facilitated by pulling the CCA downward to correct excess length in the posterior wall of the arteriotomy. We do not tie the suture at its completion but, rather, remove the needles from the suture and, after irrigation with heparinized saline (Figure 8.11), hold the two ends untied during back-bleeding until flow has been reestablished. This step is done with the patient in slight head-down position to avoid air bubbles that may be trapped below the ICA occlusion point. Delaying the tying of the suture until flow is reestablished and the carotid is expanded by pressure results in more harmonious coaptation of the arterial wall. Flow is resumed first to the ECA (Figure 8.11); the ICA bulb is then milked toward the origin of the ECA and finally opened to flow.

Because most complications from endarterectomy are of a technical nature, it makes sense to ensure the correctness of the procedure after its completion. We have no experience with ultrasonography

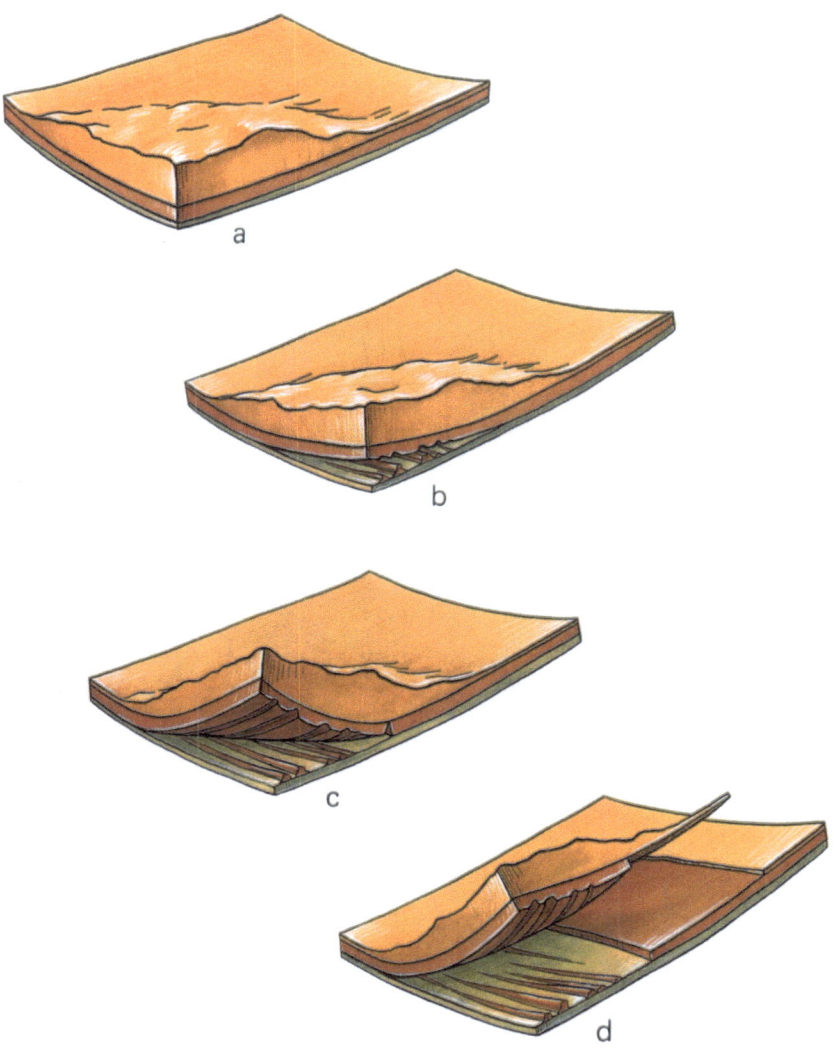

Figure 8.7 Feathering of a plaque (**a**) requires transitioning from the outer lamina plane (**b**) to the internal lamina. This maneuver requires fracturing the media (**c**). The overlying thin intima feathers off (**d**). The underlying media is generally bound to the wall and requires no fixation sutures.

and little with angioscopy, but we have found that an intraoperative arteriogram gives reliable information about the completeness of the reconstruction. It is not an encumbering step when using a C-arm with digital equipment, which produces good pictures with a few milliliters of dye. The injection is done retrogradely in the CCA with all the clamps open. The problems most commonly found are (1) intimal flaps in the ECA; (2) mild stenosis at the upper end of the arteriotomy; (3) a proximal intimal flap, usually at the site of clamping or looping or at the site of lodgement of the proximal balloon of an intraluminal shunt; and (4) spasm of the ICA. The spasm is relieved by intraadventitial and topical papaverine infiltration. Reexploration after noting any of these findings is a matter of personal judgment.

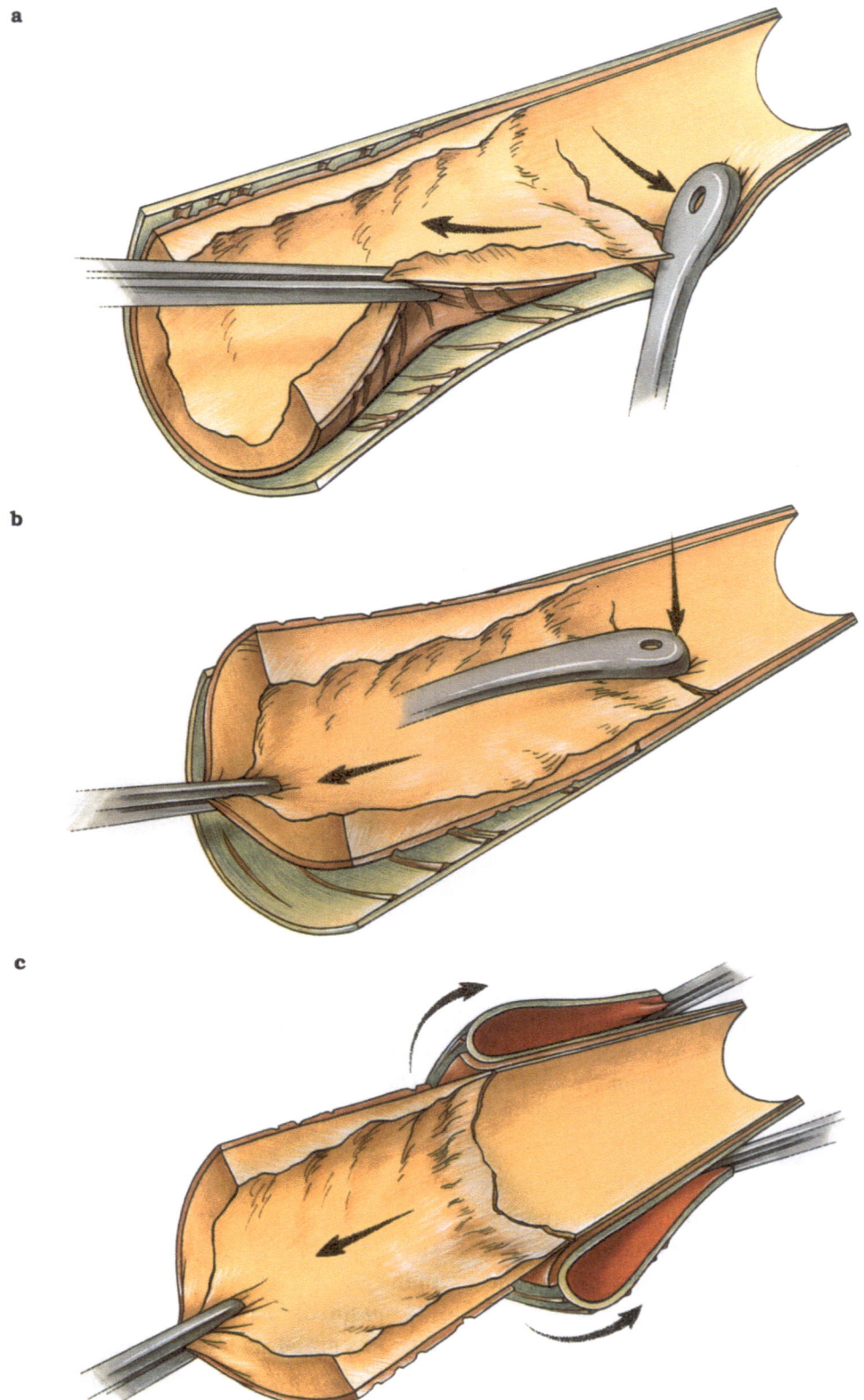

Figure 8.8 Three techniques to clear the distal end of the plaque. (**a**) Traction and counterpressure with axial rotation. (**b**) Pressure fracture combined with gentle traction. (**c**) Eversion: this eversion technique is standard when the bulb has been transected.

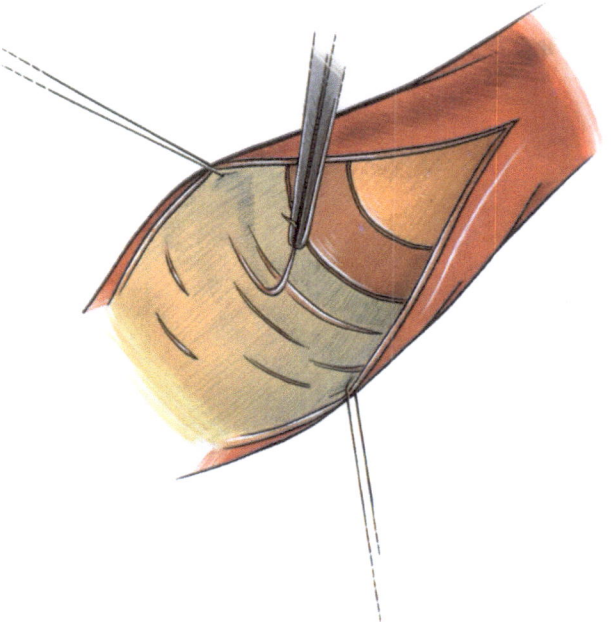

Figure 8.9 Remaining bits of media are removed by pulling them transversely.

Figure 8.10 Closure of the arteriotomy with a prosthetic patch.

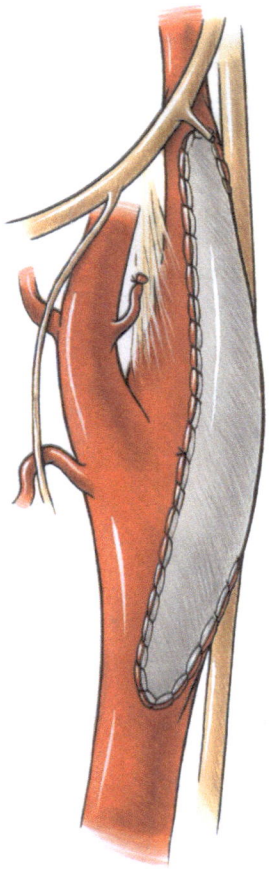

a, b

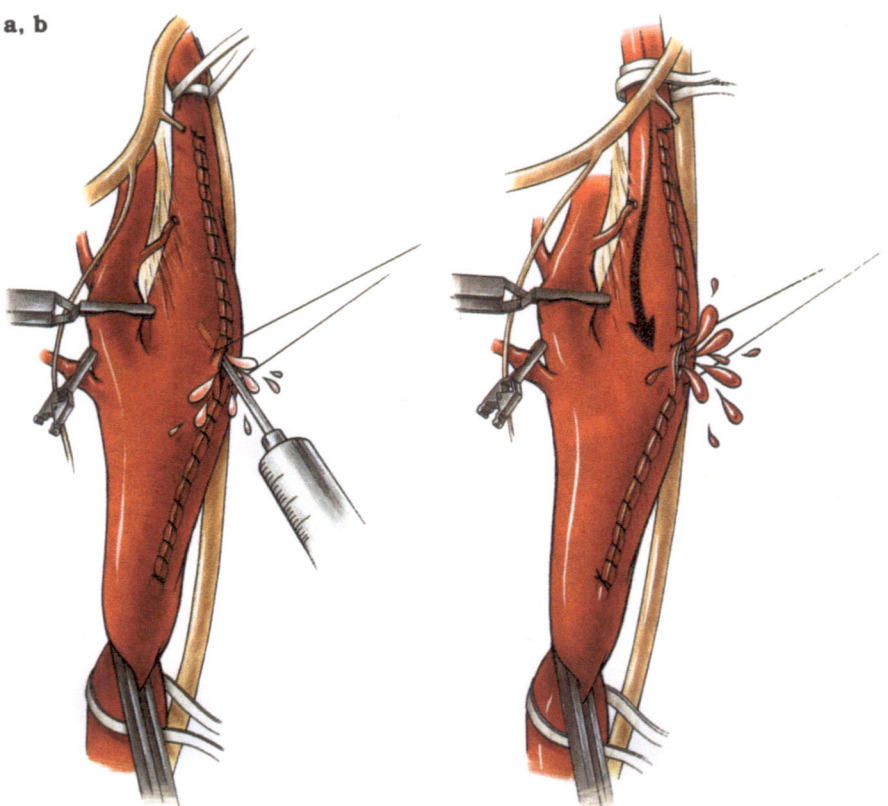

Figure 8.11 (**a**) Irrigation of the endarterectomy surface with heparinized saline and dextran. Backbleeding of the (**b**) internal,

(**c**) external and (**d**) common carotid arteries.

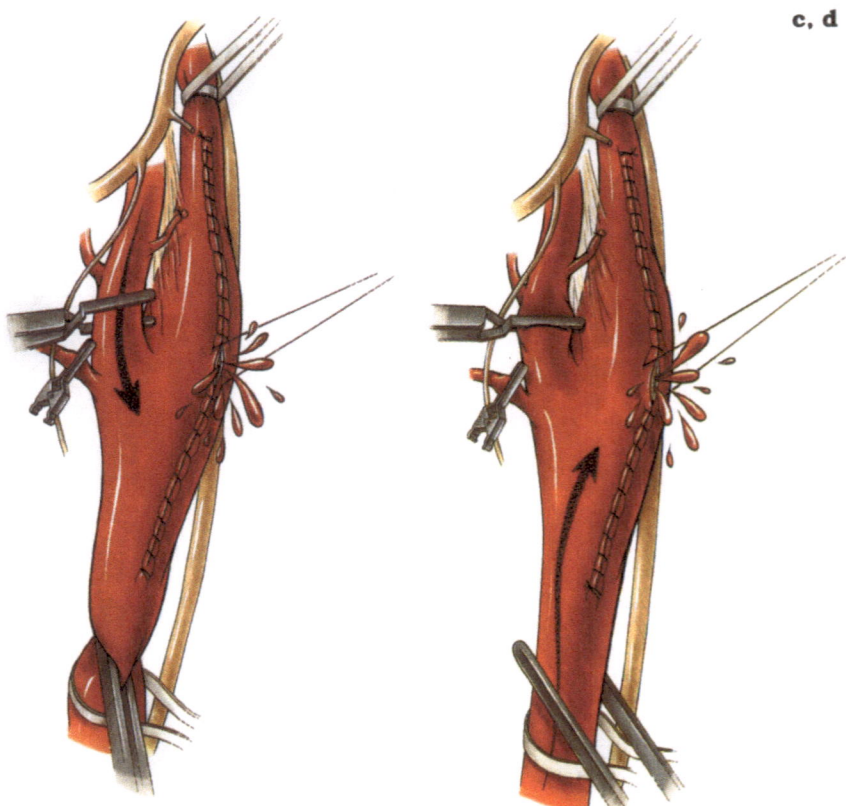

c, d

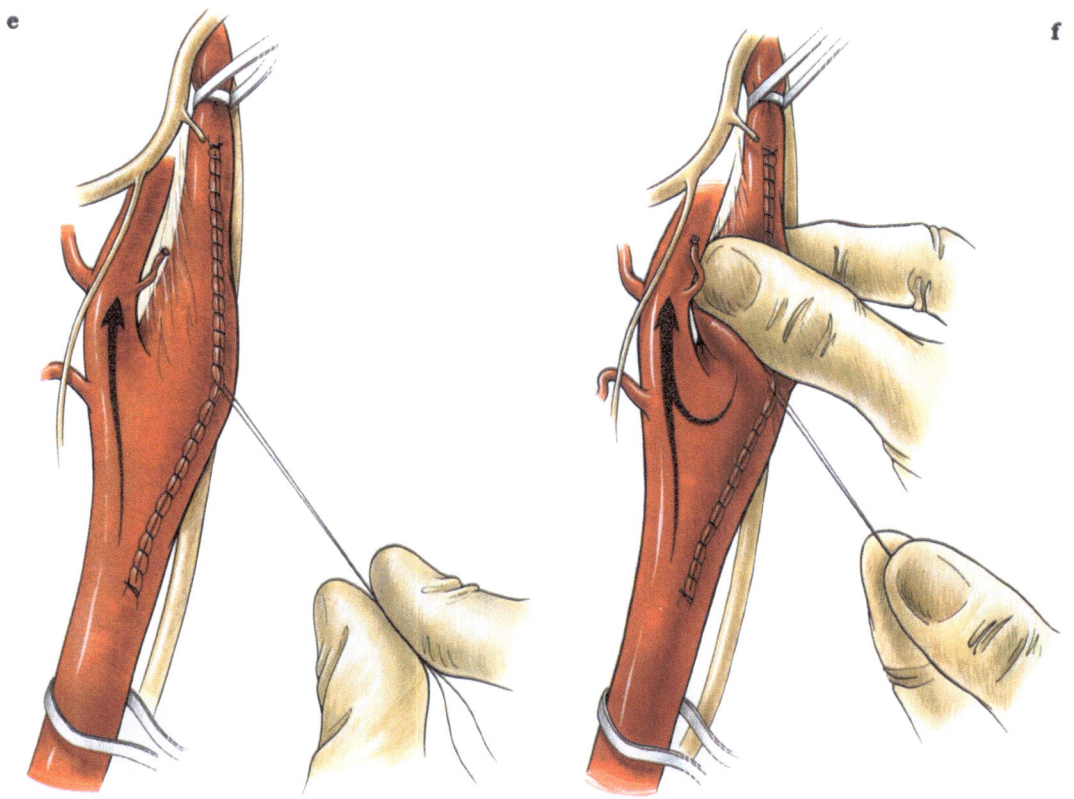

(e) Resumption of flow into the external carotid (f) Retrograde milking of the bulb into the external carotid. (g) Release of the internal carotid and tying of the suture.

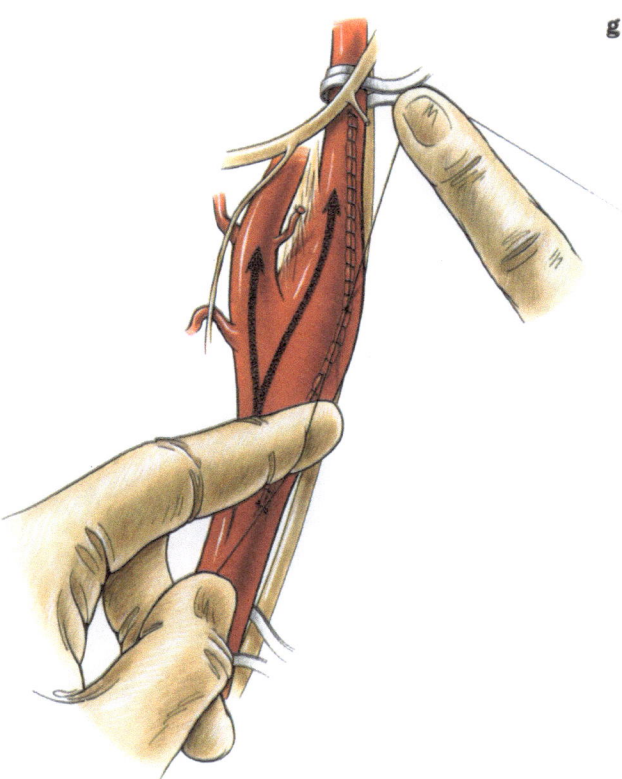

a

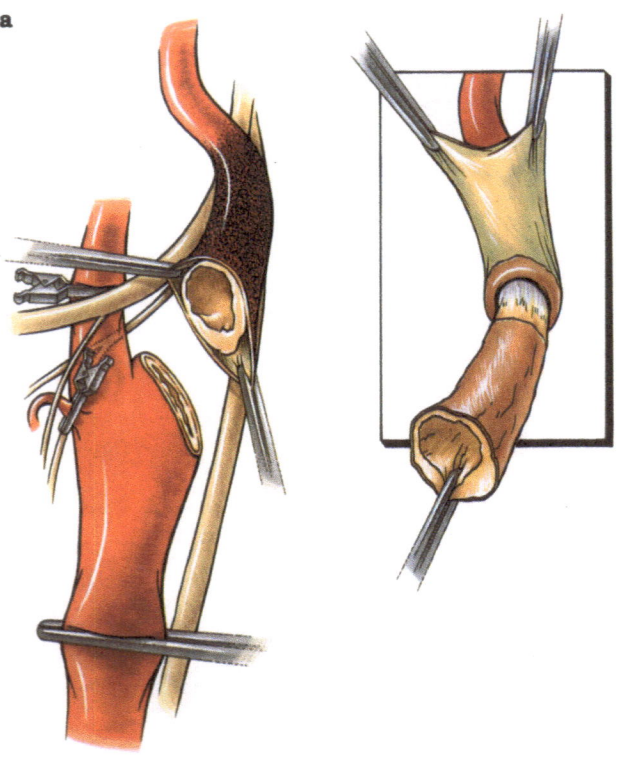

b, c

d

Figure 8.12 Eversion endarterectomy of the internal carotid artery. (**a**) Initiation of the eversion of the plaque in the bulb. (**Inset:** Feathering of the plaque.) (**b**) Prolongation of the arteriotomies. (**c**) Endarterectomy of the common and external carotid components of the plaque. (**d**) Any excess length is trimmed, and the bulb is reanastomosed to the enlarged common carotid opening. In this case, the hypoglossal nerve has been transposed behind the internal carotid.

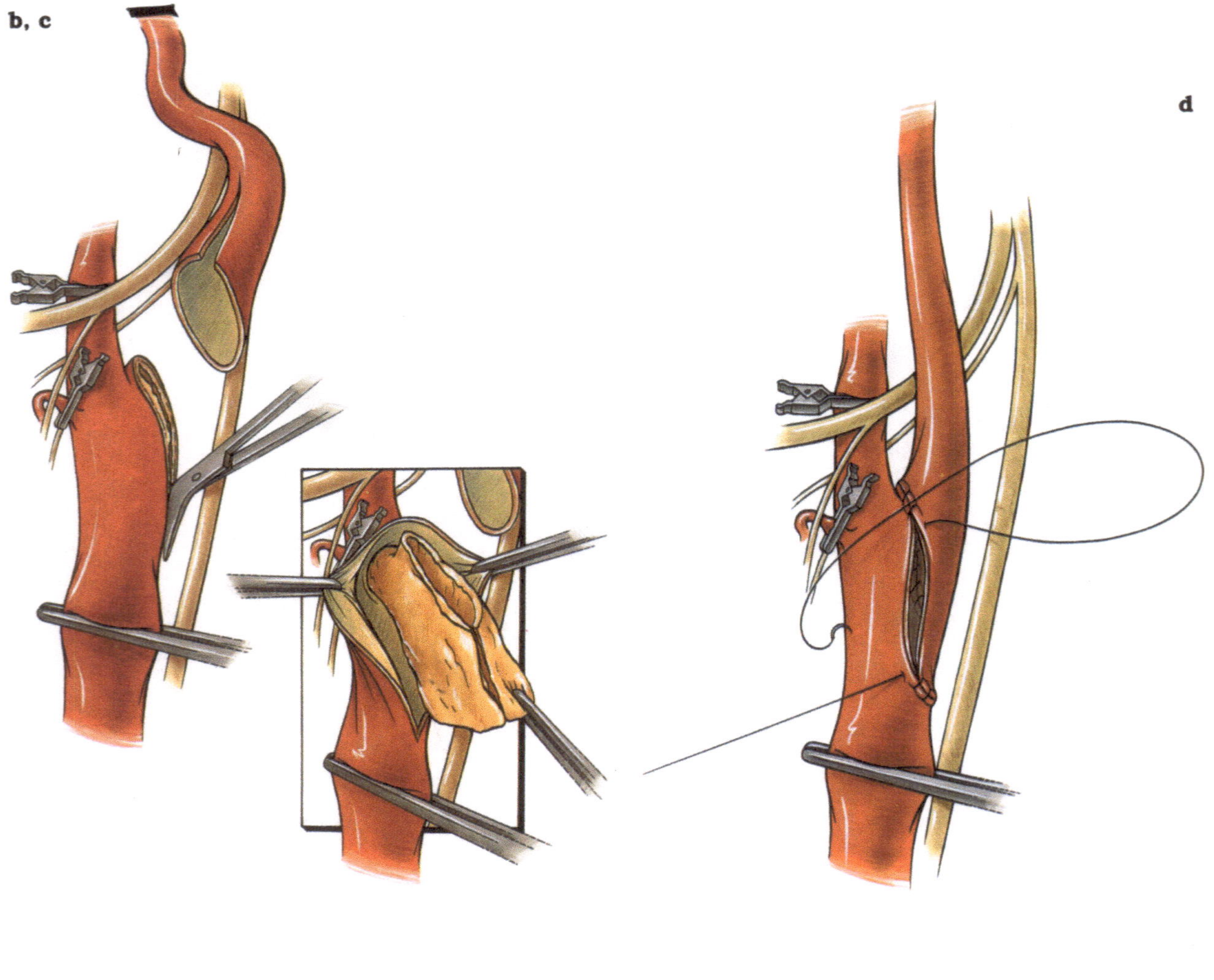

Eversion Endarterectomy of the Carotid Bifurcation

Eversion endarterectomy is a particularly suitable technique in patients with redundancy of the cervical ICA. It is the standard technique for one of us (RB).

After clamping the three components of the carotid bifurcation the intercarotid nerve is infiltrated with bupivacaine (Marcaine) and severed at the crutch of the bifurcation, which is cleared by dissection. The origin of the carotid bulb is cut at an oblique angle (Figure 8.12), taking care not to injure the superior laryngeal nerve, which runs behind the carotid bulb. After dissecting the plaque around the cut edge at the deep endarterectomy plane, the edges are everted while gentle axial traction is exerted on the plaque. The transition zone develops as feathering of the intima occurs. The artery is kept everted until all the circular bits of media are removed and a good distal end to the endarterectomy is ensured; then the eversion is reduced.

Because this technique is preferably used in patients with some elongation of the cervical ICA, the cut origin of the bulb in the CCA is prolonged with a posterior arteriotomy. This method facilitates endarterectomy of the common and external carotid arteries and provides a lower takeoff to the ICA to correct its redundancy. Endarterectomy of the CCA and ECA is done in the same manner as described for the standard endarterectomy technique. The anterior wall of the ICA is slit to match the length of the arteriotomy of the CCA. The resulting junction amounts to an angioplasty of the carotid bulb. If the hypoglossal nerve is low or if it is anatomically convenient, it is transposed behind the ICA.

If the technique of eversion endarterectomy is used in a patient with little redundancy of the ICA, the reanastomosis and angioplasty of the bulb are done by what is known as "advancement" of the bifurcation. For this technique the extra length created by slitting the anterior wall of the bulb is matched by extending the arteriotomy of the CCA into the ECA (Figure 8.13).

In patients with a plaque that does not extend high in the carotid bulb but with substantial disease of the distal CCA, eversion endarterectomy is done through the CCA to allow better clearing of the disease in this vessel (Figure 8.14). In this case once the components of the bifurcation are clamped, the crutch of the latter is dissected clean and any extra adventitial tissue is excised. The CCA is transected below the bifurcation. The plaque in the proximal 2 to 3 cm of the CCA is cleared by eversion. Distally eversion of the bifurcation is facilitated by having dissected the periadvential tissue from it and severed the intercarotid nerve and the superior thyroid artery.

Figure 8.13 If eversion endarterectomy is done in a patient without redundancy of the internal carotid, the angioplasty of the bulb is achieved by opening the posterior wall of the external carotid artery ("advancement" of the bifurcation).

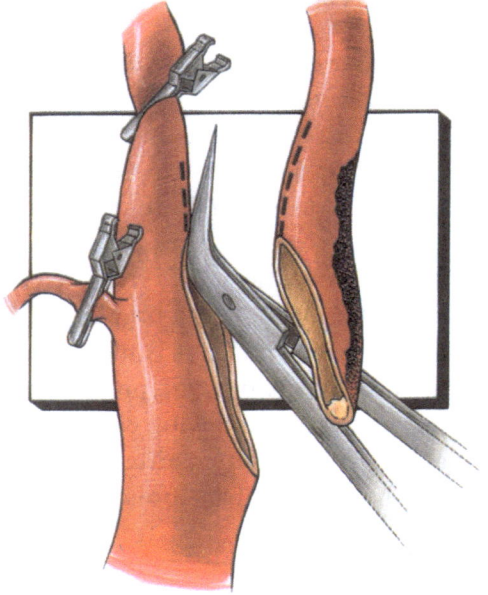

a   b

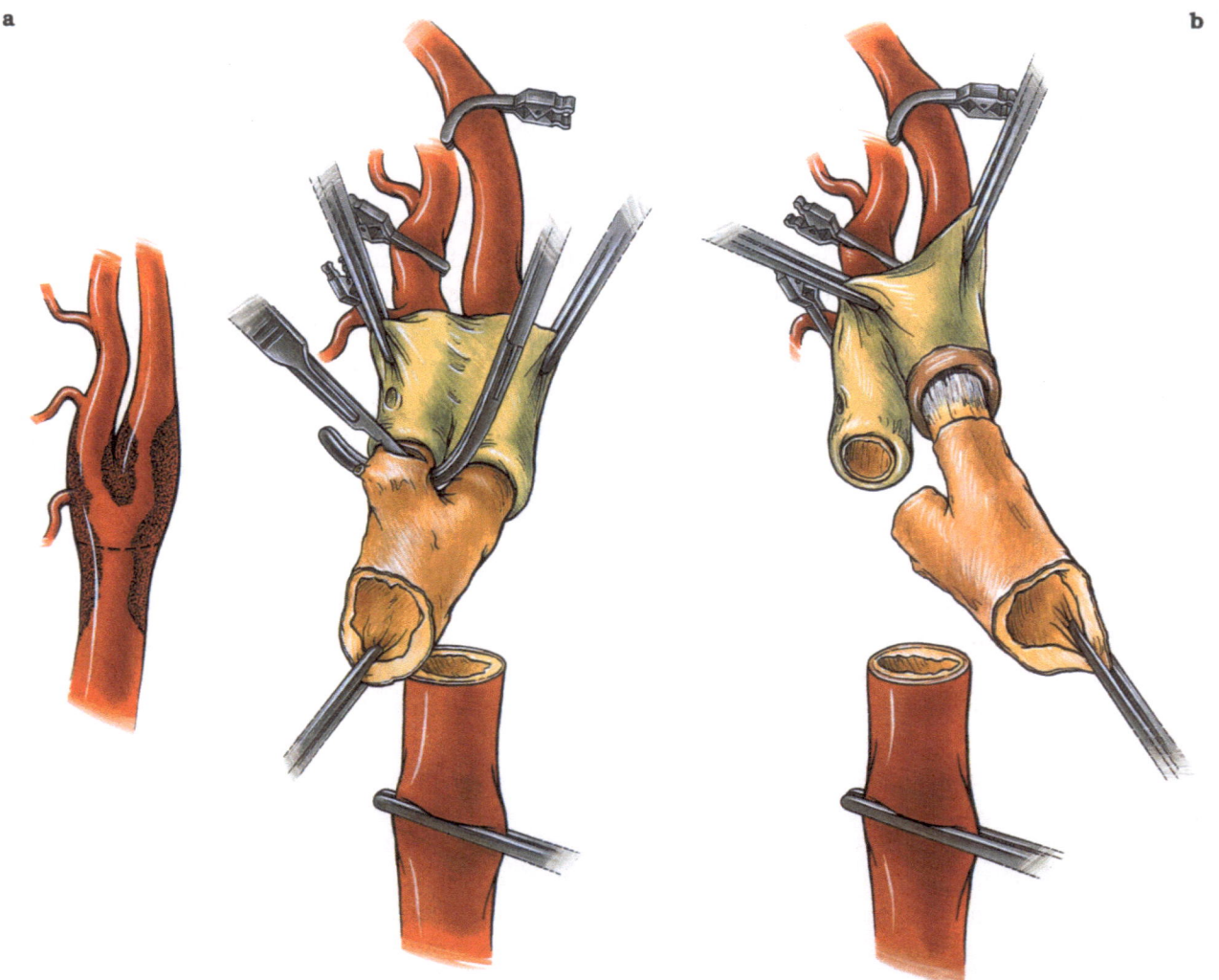

The ECA is everted first, amputating the intima around the superior thyroid artery ostium and everting the main ECA if it should taper, or dividing a circumferential plaque close to the wall of the ECA. The final maneuver is eversion endarterectomy of the ICA.

The eversion is not allowed to reduce until good feathering of the plaque and debridement of the media fibers are ensured. The CCA is then sutured end-to-end with continuous 6-0 polypropylene. An intraoperative angiogram following eversion endarterectomy of the carotid bifurcation usually shows an artery that has a normal anatomic appearance.

Correction of Redundancy

The shapes generated by redundancy of the ICA are conventionally classified as coils, kinks, and loops (Figure 8.15). Most redundant carotid arteries do not cause problems. Symptoms, however, may arise from (1) concomitant atheroma; (2) a critical, usually intermittent obstruction caused by a kink; and (3) an intimal lesion that has developed at the site of the kink.

Correction of a redundant ICA can be achieved by a number of methods (Figure 8.16). Shortening of the CCA is used on rare occasions when there is

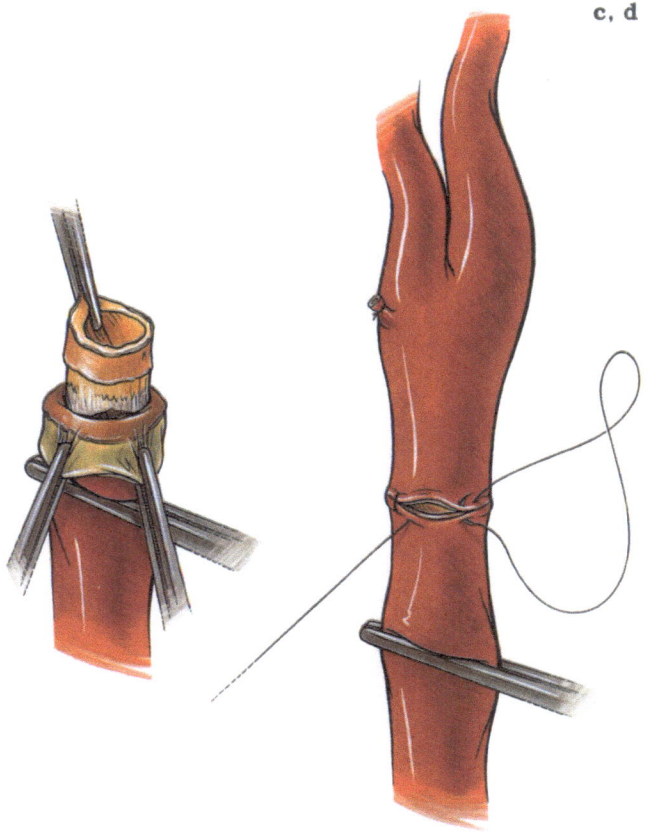

Figure 8.14 Eversion endarterectomy of the carotid bifurcation through the common carotid artery. (**a**) External carotid artery is cleared. (**b**) Eversion of the internal carotid artery. (**c**) Common carotid artery is everted to clear 2 to 3 cm. (**d**) Common carotid is reanastomosed.

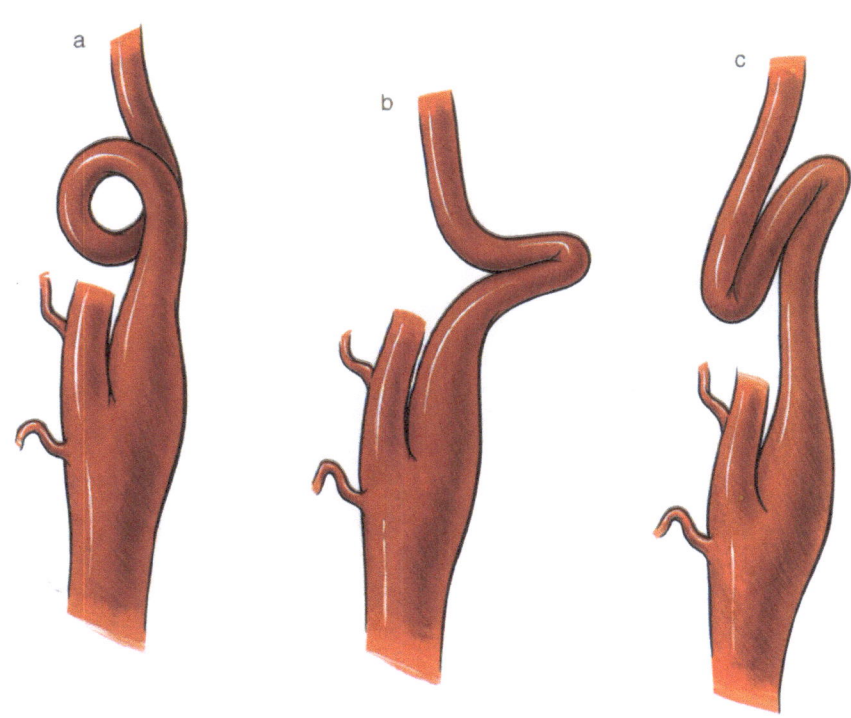

Figure 8.15 Three types of redundancy of the internal carotid artery. (**a**) Coil. (**b**) Kink. (**c**) Loop.

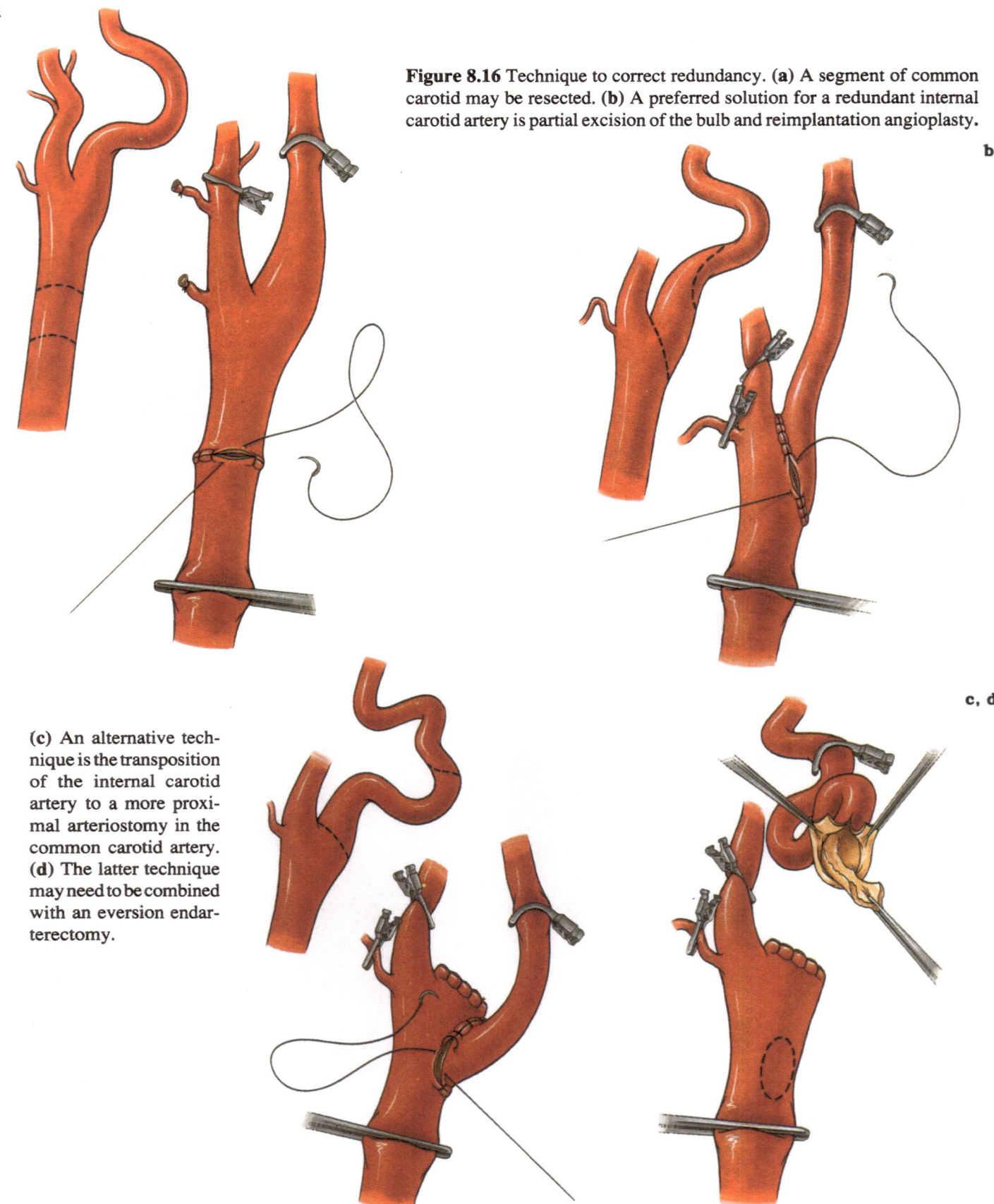

a

Figure 8.16 Technique to correct redundancy. (**a**) A segment of common carotid may be resected. (**b**) A preferred solution for a redundant internal carotid artery is partial excision of the bulb and reimplantation angioplasty.

b

c, d

(**c**) An alternative technique is the transposition of the internal carotid artery to a more proximal arteriostomy in the common carotid artery. (**d**) The latter technique may need to be combined with an eversion endarterectomy.

unwanted elongation after an ICA endarterectomy. To lower the bifurcation, the superior thyroid and often the facial artery must be divided. Segmental resection of the ICA restores anatomic normalcy and is the technique of choice when there is a localized aneurysm of the ICA. When dealing with a redundant carotid, we prefer oblique transection of the ICA origin, with open or eversion endarterectomy if indicated, and, depending on available length, reattachment of the shortened ICA to the distal CCA or transposition of the bulb to the more proximal CCA. If there is severe intrinsic disease of the ICA above the bulb, which is unusual, our preference is an exclusion vein graft bypass (see below).

Elongation occurs naturally in the carotid artery, but it is also a consequence of the mobilization of the bifurcation and the thinning of the arterial wall that follows endarterectomy. It is uncommon for a spontaneously elongated artery to be the source of symptoms, although occasionally a kink in a carotid artery may be aggravated by rotation of the neck to the point where blood flow is critically diminished, symptoms develop, and a repair is indicated. The indications for operating on an elongated ICA are (1) associated severe or symptomatic plaque of the carotid bifurcation; (2) a critical stenosis caused by a kink, (often bilateral and in conjunction with VA occlusive disease); (3) TIA symptoms without evidence of intracranial carotid or cardiac disease; and (4) a severe kink in the territory of a grossly elongated carotid. In these patients there may be small intimal lesions in the redundant ICA, too distal to be seen on ultrasound scans and difficult to resolve visually on the arteriogram.

Bypass of the Internal Carotid Artery

Some surgeons, notably Cormier,[76] have proposed the bypass technique as the primary operation for most carotid artery disease. For us the indications for ICA bypass are as follows: (1) some reoperations; (2) high-lying lesions; (3) nonatherosclerotic disease such as radiation arteritis, advanced forms of fibromuscular dysplasia, or aneurysms when simpler opera-

tions are not feasible; and (4) perioperative complications such as tears during endarterectomy or severe buckling after reestablishing flow in an already elongated carotid.

The best material for ICA bypass is saphenous vein of normal appearance with a diameter of 4 mm or more. If the vein is fibrosed or smaller, or there is neck fibrosis (due to multiple operations or radiotherapy), we use 6 mm thin-walled PTFE, provided the repair goes no higher than the lower edge of the digastric muscle. If the repair must be done above this level, where the wall of the carotid becomes even thinner, we prefer to use a segment of superficial femoral artery, which is in turn replaced with PTFE. Preoperatively, it is necessary to assess the superficial femoral artery with either ultrasonography or arteriography before choosing it as an autograft. A note of caution is made regarding the use of autogenous material in necks with extensive fibrosis following radiotherapy. Synthetic material appears to withstand external compression better and to be less susceptible to encroachment by scarring.

The technique of ICA bypass is straightforward. The distal anastomosis is end-to-side to the ICA, although eventually a proximal clip will make it function as an end-to-end junction (Figure 8.17). The end-to-side anastomosis is easier to construct and avoids the problem of axial rotation, angulation, or partial intussusceptions of the smaller recipient artery into a large vein graft occasionally seen in end-to-end anastomoses. The proximal anastomosis is done posterolaterally and low in the CCA where the artery tends to be of better quality. One needs to cut the omohyoid muscle and sometimes the sternothyroid muscle to expose the low CCA. Care should be taken not to injure the vagus, which occasionally rides on the anterior wall of the CCA at this low level. If the bulb of the ICA is intact, as happens in the case of some distal cervical ICA aneurysms, the proximal anastomosis can be made end-to-end to a transected carotid bulb.

When using a vein, one should be certain it contains no valves in order to avoid problems with retrograde purging or late stenoses at valve sites. If valves present problems with the venting of the bypass before reestablishing flow, we place the proxi-

a, b   **c**

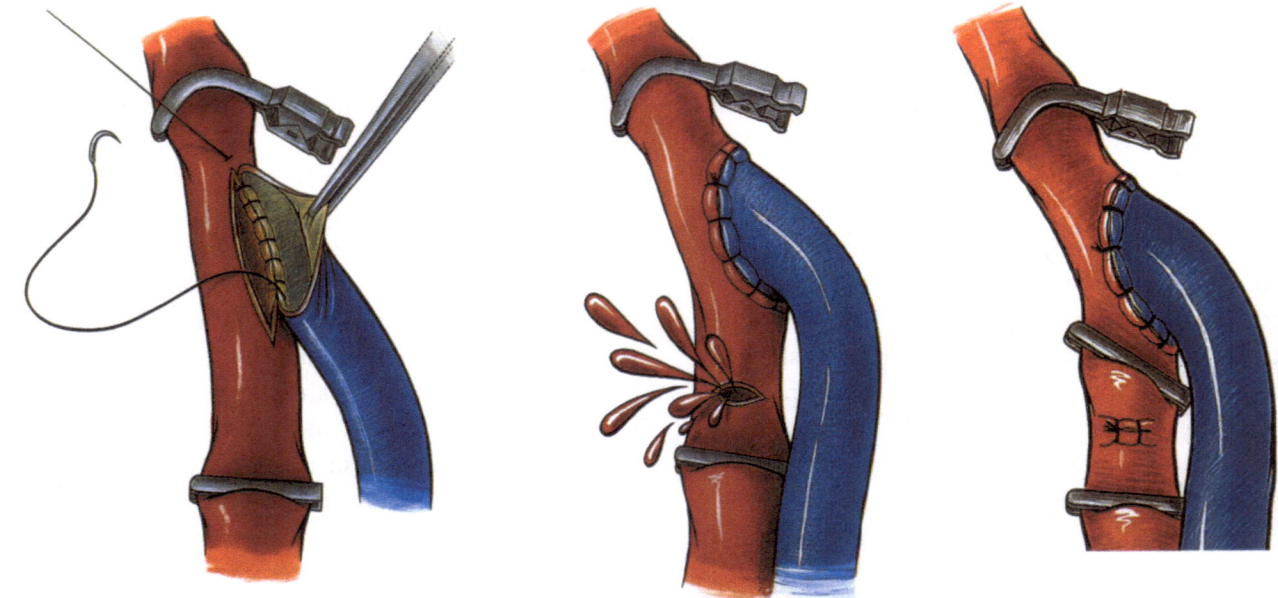

Figure 8.17 Bypass to the internal carotid artery. (**a**) The distal anastomosis is constructed as end-to-side. (**b**) Anterograde bleeding of the vein graft and retrograde bleeding from the internal carotid is accomplished through a small arteriotomy below the anastomosis. (**c**) Anastomosis becomes functionally an end-to-end one by precise application of a second clip below the heel of the anastomosis.

mal ICA clip 1 cm below the distal anastomosis. A small incision in the ICA immediately above this clip permits anterograde purging of the vein graft and retrograde purging of the distal ICA. A second hemoclip closer to the anastomosis excludes the arteriotomy used for venting. Purging of a valved vein graft can also be done by passing a catheter from below before completing the proximal anastomosis.

Steps to Enlarge Distal Exposure

During the course of a carotid operation, the surgeon may need to extend the exposure distally because of a high bifurcation or a plaque that extends beyond the usual limits. This need to expose the ICA high in the neck may be anticipated before the operation through arteriographic information, or it may arise unexpectedly during a carotid reconstruction.

The main obstacle to approaching the high cervical ICA is the ramus of the mandible. This anatomic structure can have differing configurations: Those that are long and posterior cause difficulties even with the exposure of a carotid that bifurcates at

the usual level. Other mandibular rami have a gentle curvature forward and permit access to the ICA high in the neck.

If the need for a high carotid access is anticipated, the operation should be done with nasotracheal intubation, which permits full teeth occlusion and therefore forward displacement of the angle of the jaw (Figure 8.18). Nasotracheal intubation also facilitates preoperative anterior subluxation of the condyle, a maneuver that may be needed in particularly unfavorable configurations. Subluxation should be coupled with wiring of the teeth to prevent its spontaneous reduction during the operation and subsequent deterioration of the exposure.

In cases where the need for a high approach is anticipated, the ICA is approached from behind the internal jugular vein (Figure 8.19). We routinely use this approach for distal VA reconstructions: It gives good, comfortable exposure of the deep spaces of the neck up to the level of C1. The steps are as follows. The incision is made anterior to the sternomastoid muscle. The external jugular vein is divided, and the posterior aspect of the parotid gland is lifted from the sternomastoid muscle. The anterior edge of the stern-

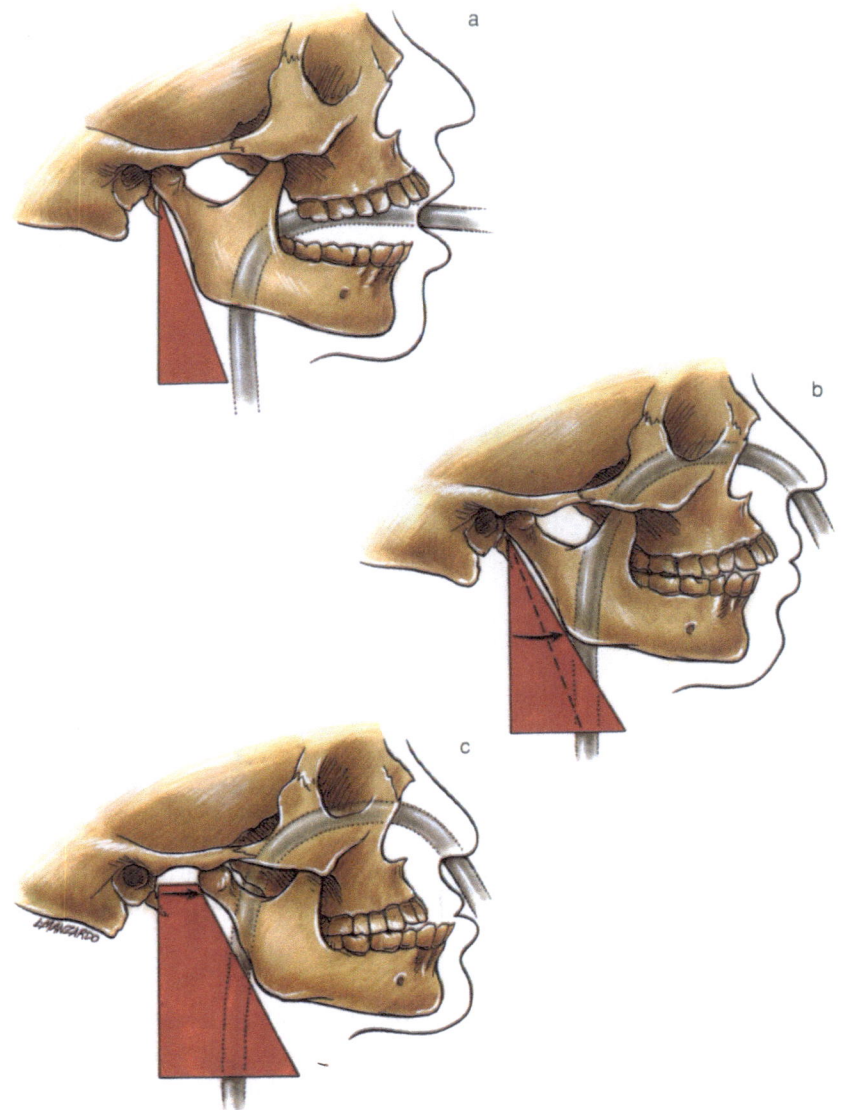

Figure 8.18 Nasotracheal intubation and anterior subluxation increase distal exposure of the cervical internal carotid artery.

omastoid muscle is dissected, and its tendinous edge is followed to its insertion on the mastoid process. Often the posterior auricular nerve must be cut. The spinal accessory nerve is located between the jugular vein and the sternomastoid muscle and is dissected upward. The jugular vein is displaced anteriorly, ligating a rare, small branch that may arise from its posterior edge. The sympathetic chain is left undisturbed, and the vagus and hypoglossal nerves are lifted up and moved medially with the jugular vein. After cutting the posterior belly of the digastric muscle, the occipital artery, which lies behind the muscle, is exposed and cut close to the mastoid process. The

superior laryngeal nerve is identified. It anchors the vagus toward the midline and sometimes must be dissected gently for 1 to 2 cm in order to flip the vagus anteriorly and over the ICA. The transverse process of C1 can be easily palpated, and from this level down to the carotid bifurcation continuous exposure of the ICA is available without the encumbrance of any other structure. If the styloid process causes any difficulty with exposure of the distal ICA, it can be excised with a fine rongeur.

If the ICA needs to be exposed at the base of the skull, between C1 and the temporal bone, the approach to it should be anterior to the jugular vein and

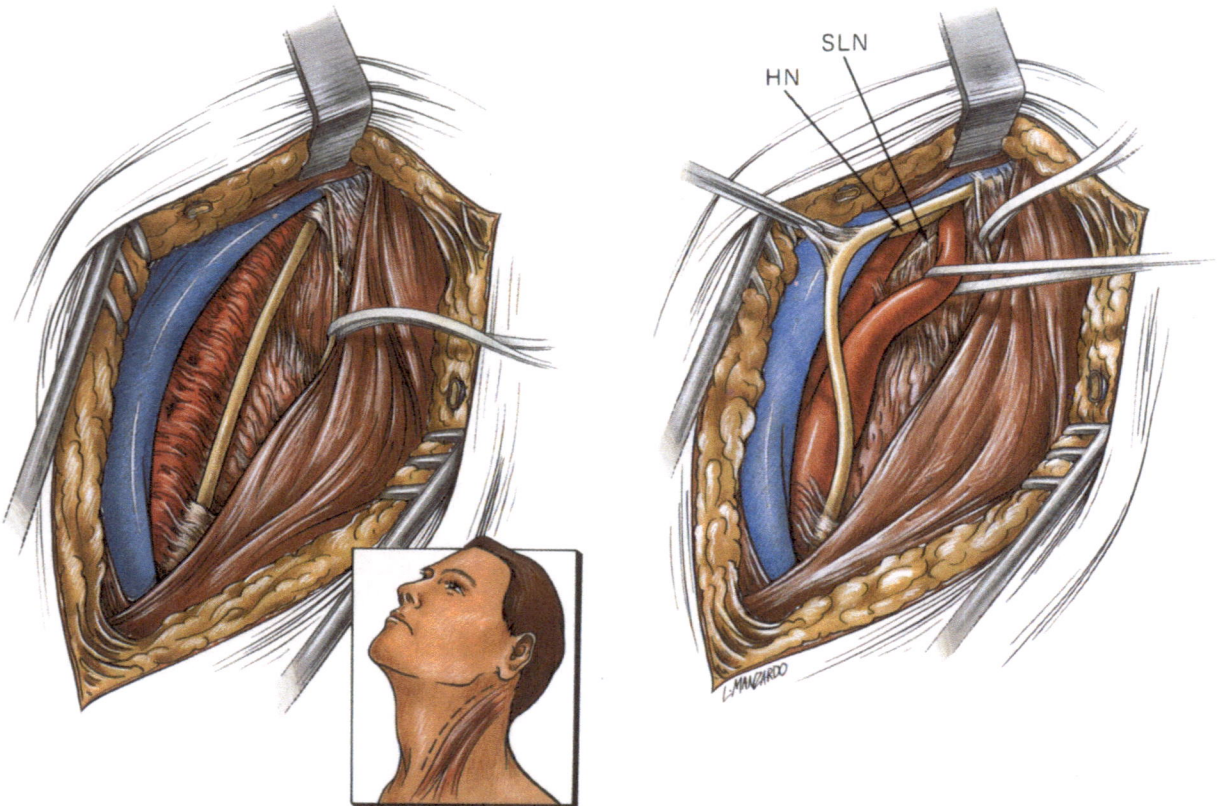

Figure 8.19 Exposure of the cervical internal carotid artery by the retrojugular approach. (**a**) Accessory spinal nerve is slung by a loop. (**b**) Vagus is flipped with the internal jugular vein over the internal carotid artery. HN = hypoglossal nerve; SLN = superior laryngeal nerve.

above the hypoglossal nerve. This step can be done as a continuation of the retrojugular approach.

The digastric muscle is freed and retracted upward. The hypoglossal nerve is freed and displaced anteriorly. The occipital artery is divided near the point where it runs over the hypoglossal nerve if the origin of the former is low in the ECA. All anterior branches of the anterior jugular vein are divided. We occasionally find it expedient to divide the internal jugular vein closing its stump with running 6-0 polypropylene suture plus a tie. This technique improves exposure at the top of the dissection.

As the ICA is followed, at this point posterior to the ECA, the bony ridge of the styloid process is found anterior to the mastoid (Figure 8.20) and the styloid-based muscles and ligaments are seen. The glossopharyngeal nerve is identified. It may be splayed into two trunks as it crosses over the ICA. With the glossophar-

yngeal nerve isolated, the styloid process is exposed with a 0.25 inch periosteal elevator as it generally obstructs the path to the ICA. The styloid process is removed with precise bites of a rongeur under direct vision to avoid damaging the facial nerve behind the styloid, and the styloid muscles are divided. With a malleable retractor pushing the internal jugular vein (or its stump) posteriorly, the ICA can then be exposed up to the vertical portion where it enters the temporal bone.

Should an unanticipated need for extended distal ICA exposure arise during the course of a carotid operation, the standard exposure anterior to the jugular vein, as described for the carotid bifurcation (p. 109) can be extended as follows. (1) The lymph nodes lying on top of the jugular vein and below the digastric muscle can either be cut or reflected as a posterior flap, as was described for the exposure of the carotid bifurcation. The already identified hypoglossal nerve can now be displaced anteriorly by cutting the posterior loop of the ansa, which tethers it posteriorly. (2) The sternomastoid (and occasionally the occipital) artery that may hold the hypoglossal nerve down is divided. (3) The hypoglossal and vagus sheaths share some connections, so these two nerves are carefully separated under loop magnification. This step allows a few additional millimeters of mobilization of the hypoglossal nerve forward and upward. (4) The digastric muscle is cut or partially resected, with care being taken not to injure the glossopharyngeal nerve, which crosses over the ICA deep, and cephalad, to the muscle. (5) The occipital artery below the lower edge of the digastric muscle is also cut. The vagus at this point may lie anterior to the carotid. (6) Dissection of the cervical portion of the ICA may be carried out, displacing the vagus forward and dissecting behind it. This technique requires freeing it from the carotid

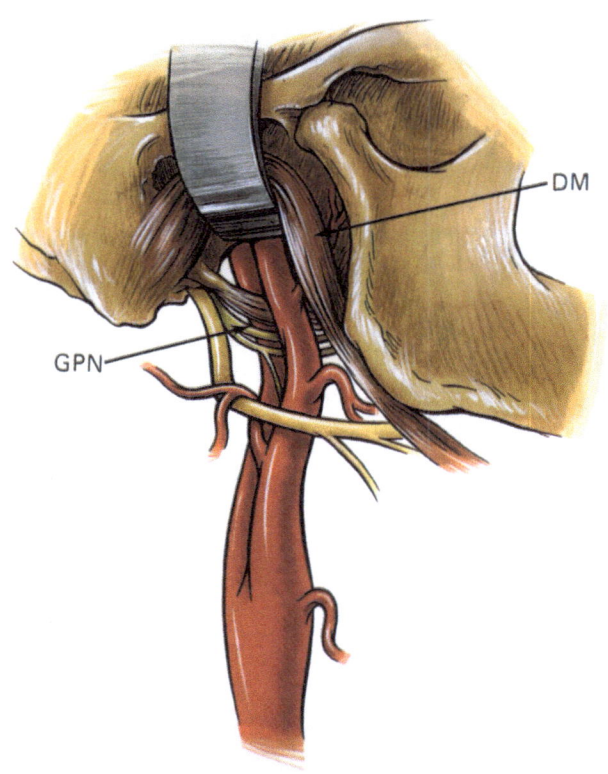

Figure 8.20 Anterior cervical approach to the distal cervical internal carotid artery above the level of C1. GPN = glossopharyngeal nerve; DM = digastric muscle.

bulb, where it lies posterior to the artery, and transposing it on top of the ICA, avoiding injury to the superior laryngeal nerve. (7) The ICA may also be dissected above the hypoglossal and vagus confluent. (8) Additional exposure may be obtained by identifying the styloid process, exposing it with a Key elevator, and removing it with a rongeur. The exposed cervical ICA may be further dissected by gentle traction on its adventitial coat. This maneuver straightens out any existing tortuosity and provides additional length. The jugular vein and the vagus nerve are retracted away and posteriorly from the carotid, using narrow, malleable neurosurgical retractors.

If it is difficult to separate the hypoglossal-vagal confluent or to mobilize the hypoglossal nerve anteriorly, the carotid bulb can be cut below the hypoglossal nerve and the free ICA is transposed anterior to it. With the ICA freed and anterior to the hypoglossal nerve, some additional distal dissection is possible.

Control of the distal cervical ICA with a clamp as one approaches the temporal bone may be difficult; the use of an occluding catheter is a better solution. The occluding catheter is introduced in the ICA at the carotid bulb or above it. This segment of ICA is isolated between a double loop distally and a cross-clamp proximally at the carotid bulb. The balloon catheter is introduced through an arteriotomy at this lower ICA level where handling is safer. The proximal ICA remains clamped at all times to avoid distal embolization as the distal balloon is advanced to the petrous ICA. Some back-bleeding is allowed while testing the intracranial occluding balloon to clear any debris that might have been carried upward by the latter. If the cervical ICA is tortuous, placement of the occluding balloon catheter may be facilitated by dividing the ICA through the bulb and transposing it anterior to the glossopharyngeal and hypoglossal nerves. This step allows one to straighten the extracranial ICA.

The arteriotomy of the ICA will be longitudinal if one does not plan to transect it but, rather, chooses to do an end-to-side anastomosis (to be converted later into a functional end-to-end by ligating the ICA proximal to the distal anastomosis). In the case of a need for an end-to-end distal anastomosis, the ICA is divided by cutting first the wall anterior to the occlud-

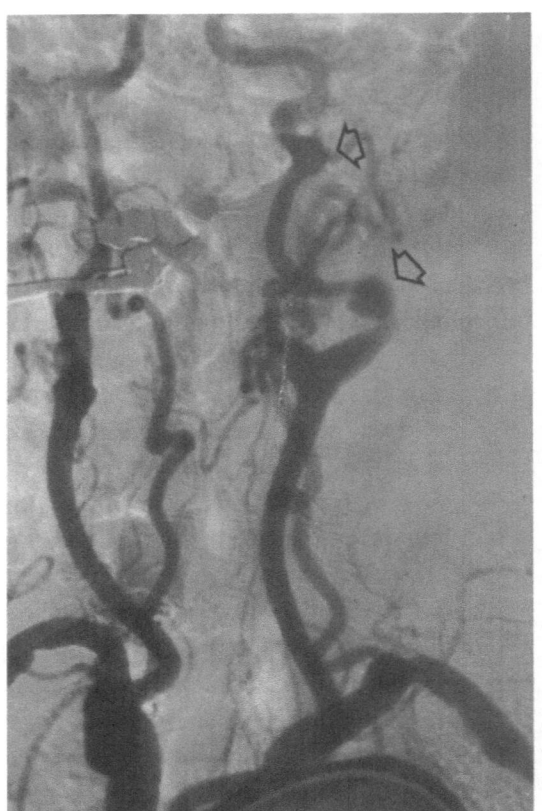

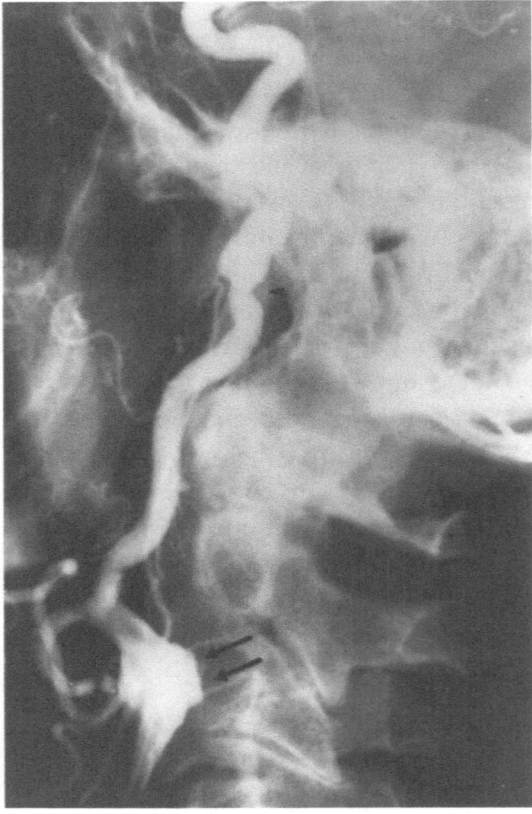

Figure 8.21 Two dysplastic aneurysms of the internal carotid artery (open arrows) **(a)** were repaired by a transpetrosal transposition of the external to internal carotid arteries **(b)**. Closed arrows point to the stump of the internal carotid bulb.

ing catheter and inserting two stay sutures of 7-0 monofilament suture to gain control of the stump, then dividing the posterior half of the artery. Loss of control of the artery or balloon at this point may have grave consequences. A short occluding catheter is better than a standard embolectomy catheter because the latter may become tangled in the instruments and inadvertently pulled out. Under these circumstances, catheter reinsertion for control of back-bleeding may be risky or impossible.

Neither of these approaches allows exposure of the last centimeter of cervical ICA. To do a repair at the level of the temporal bone ridge involves a petrosectomy and transposition of the facial nerve, and requires a combined approach with a neurootologist (Figures 8.21 and 8.22) (see Chapter 11).

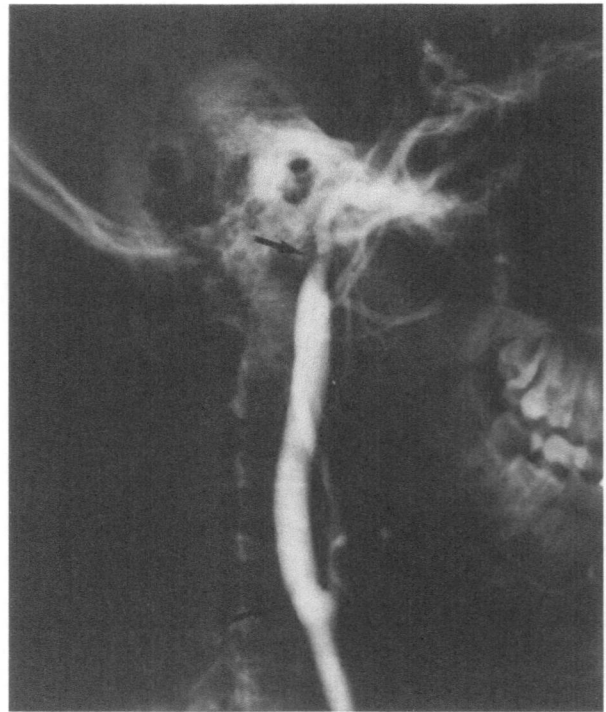

Figure 8.22 Transpetrosal internal carotid reconstruction using a saphenous vein graft.

Reconstruction of the External Carotid Artery

Most operations on the ECA are done on carotid bifurcations where the ICA has occluded and the compensatory collateral circuit of the ECA is being hampered by a severe stenosis at its origin. A less frequent indication is when the stump of the occluded ICA is presumed to be the source of embolization to the eye or brain through the ECA pathway. Exceptionally, in patients with bilateral occlusion of both VAs, the ECA supplies blood to the posterior circulation by means of anastomoses between the occipital and distal VA. In these patients, if the ECA is stenosed or occluded, reconstructing it improves flow to the posterior circulation.

The approach to the ECA varies, depending on whether the ICA is occluded, diseased, or normal. With an occluded ICA, which is by far the more common situation, access to the bifurcation is the same as that used for a standard endarterectomy. The simplest technique (Figure 8.23) is to dissect the bifurcation in the standard manner except that the dissection goes further distally on the ECA and is restricted to the bulb of the ICA. The ECA is dissected up to its bi- or trifurcation, usually at the level of the facial or lingual artery takeoff. The hypoglossal nerve is displaced superiorly. After heparin is administered, the arteries are clamped using small occluders for each of the three branches of the ECA trunk. The ascending pharyngeal artery, whose origin in the posterior wall of the ECA is not always obvious, may back-bleed and require separate control. An arteriotomy from the distal CCA to the ECA gives access to the plaque. The endarterectomy includes the distal CCA, the proximal bulb of the occluded ICA, and the ECA. The ECA plaque seldom feathers distally (as in the ICA) and usually requires a sharp cut at the level where the ECA branches out. The origin of the previously occluded carotid bulb, now soft after its proximal endarterectomy, is obliterated with one or two large hemoclips, obliquely placed from the outside, that obliterate the cul-de-sac at the origin of the thrombosed ICA. The clips are anchored to the ICA by a couple of 5-0 sutures.

An alternative method of repairing the ECA involves excising the ICA bulb and using it as an autogenous patch (Figure 8.23). For this technique the bifurcation is approached in the same manner. The thrombosed ICA is severed above the bulb. After heparin administration and clamping, the ICA bulb is cut flush with its origin. The CCA and ECA are opened from the orifice of the ICA along their posterior walls. If an endarterectomy of the bifurcation is needed, it is continued with the ECA endarterectomy up to the trifurcation of the latter. There is usually some excess wall that needs to be excised around the cut origin of the ICA. The arteriotomy is closed with a patch made from the occluded ICA, which has been opened lengthwise and endarterectomized. The resulting shape is that of a tapered tube.

The wall of the occluded ICA can also be cut to result in a flap with which one can patch the ECA (Figure 8.23). It requires excising a substantial amount of wall from both the flap and the bifurcation to avoid an excessively wide angioplasty. We have used all three methods and see no advantage of one over the others.

Endarterectomy of the orifice of the ECA is, of course, part of the standard technique of carotid endarterectomy. In some cases the lesion extends far enough in the ECA that it cannot be cleared satisfactorily from within the bifurcation, and a separate arteriotomy of the ECA is needed (Figure 8.24). The latter is usually not made contiguous with the CCA-ICA arteriotomy in order to avoid a three-corner closure if a patch is not used in the longer arteriotomy. Closure of the separate ECA incision usually requires a patch.

If the surgeon anticipates the need for patching the main arteriotomy into the ICA, the secondary opening on the ECA can be made as a side cut from the previous one, and the closure may be done with a Y-shaped patch (Figure 8.24). Suturing of this patch must start at the crotch of the Y with the length of its three branches trimmed as the apices are reached.

In some cases an open endarterectomy of the external carotid artery is required during the course of an internal carotid endarterectomy. This situation occurs when the external carotid is seen to be the main supply to the vertebrobasilar system via occipital collaterals. When it is not possible to ensure proper

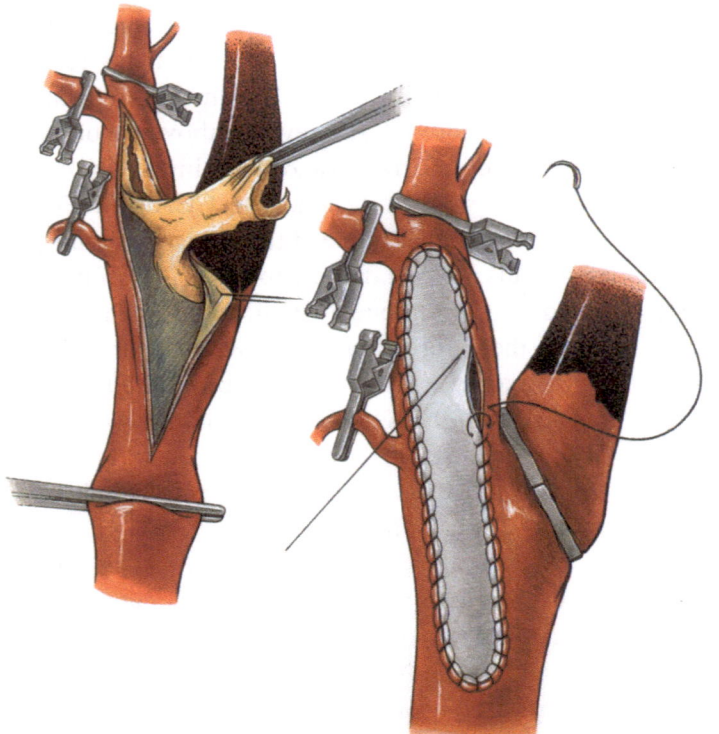

Figure 8.23 Isolated patching of the external carotid artery origin. (**a**) As part of an endarterectomy of the distal common and external carotid arteries, excluding the internal carotid artery cul-de-sac.

(c) Fashioning the closure with a flap tailored from the wall of the internal carotid bulb after amputation of the chronically occluded internal carotid artery.

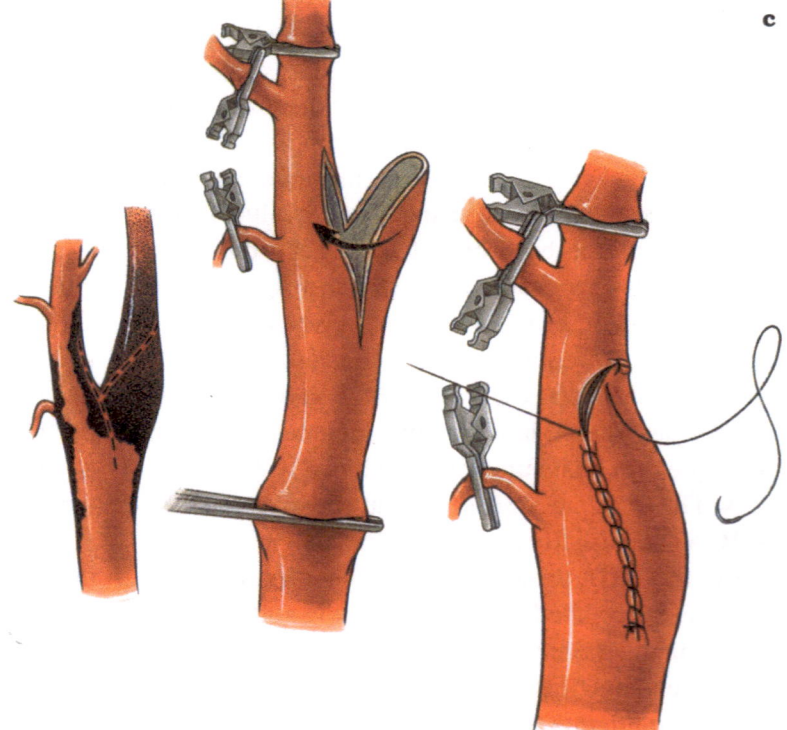

c

b

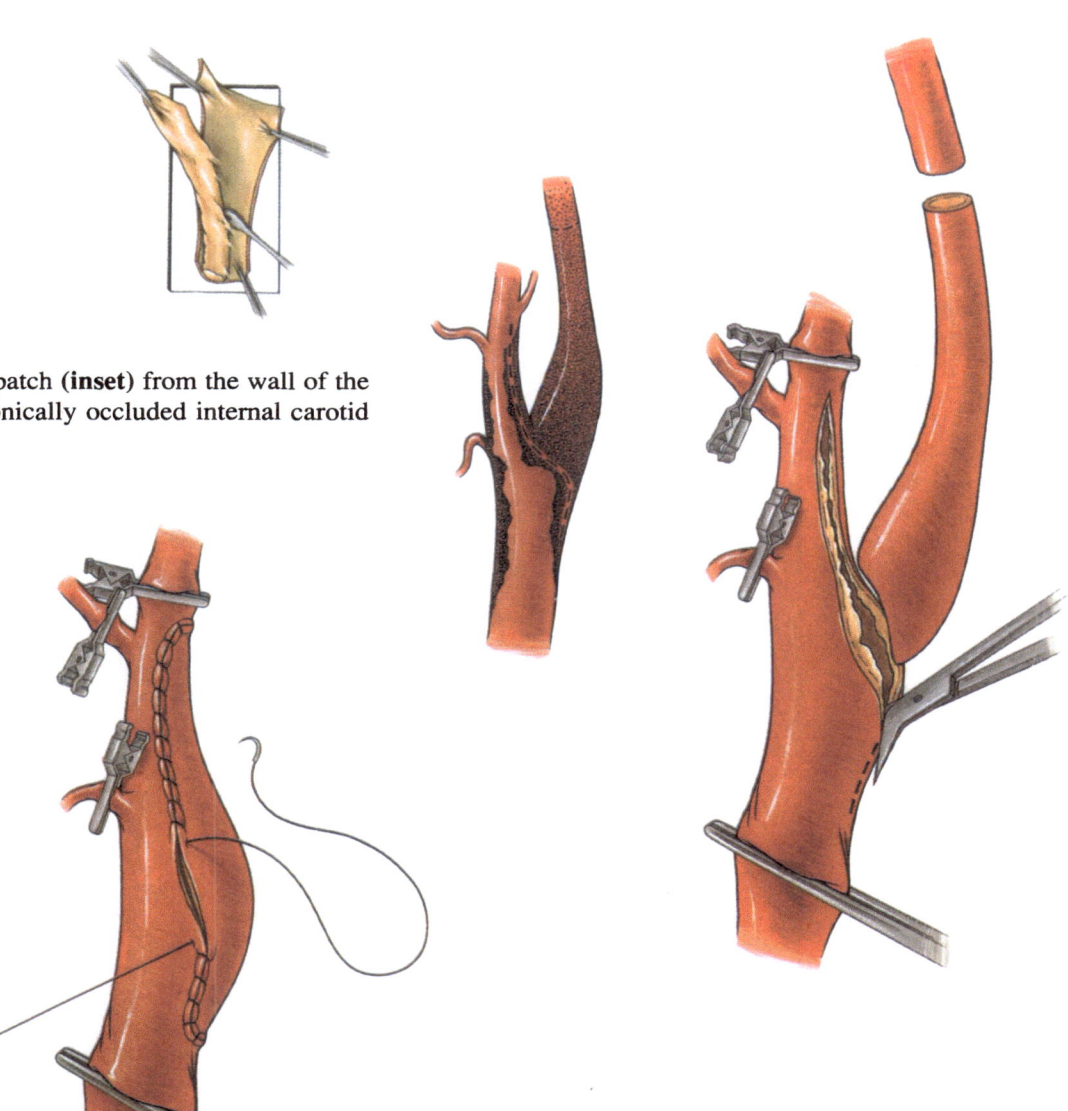

(**b**) Fashioning the patch (**inset**) from the wall of the amputated and chronically occluded internal carotid artery.

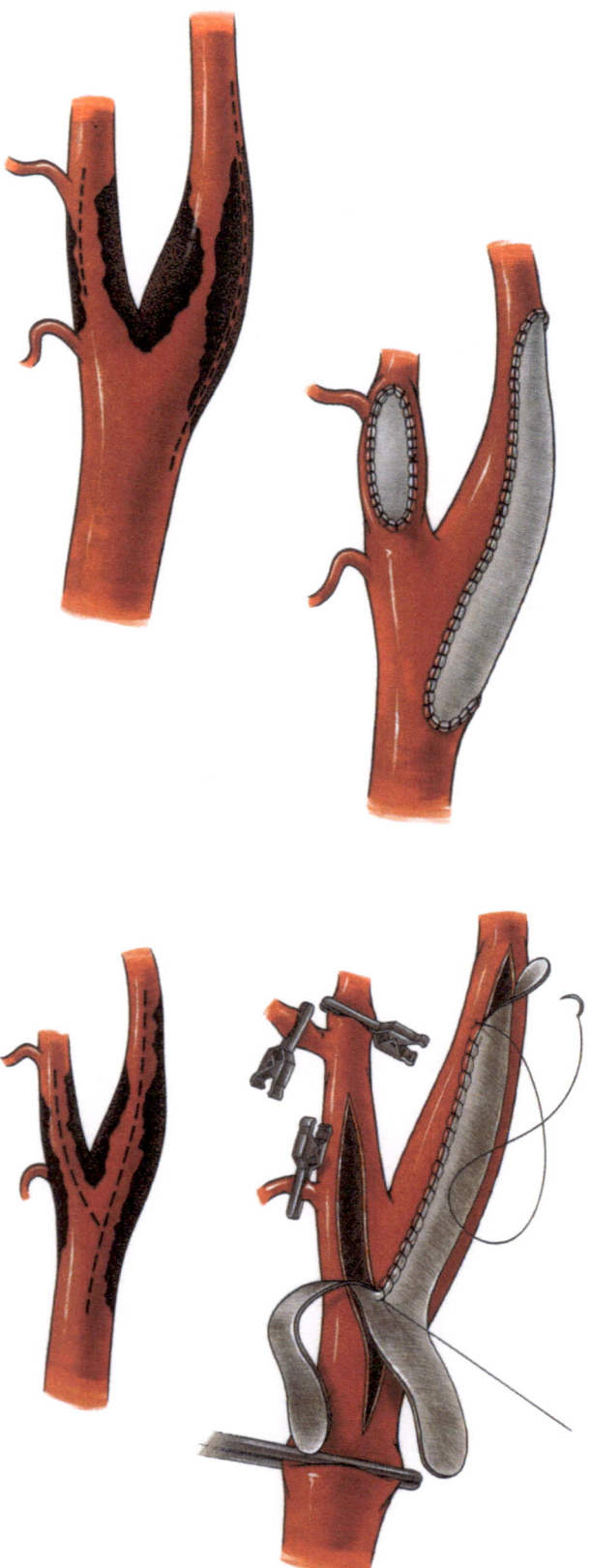

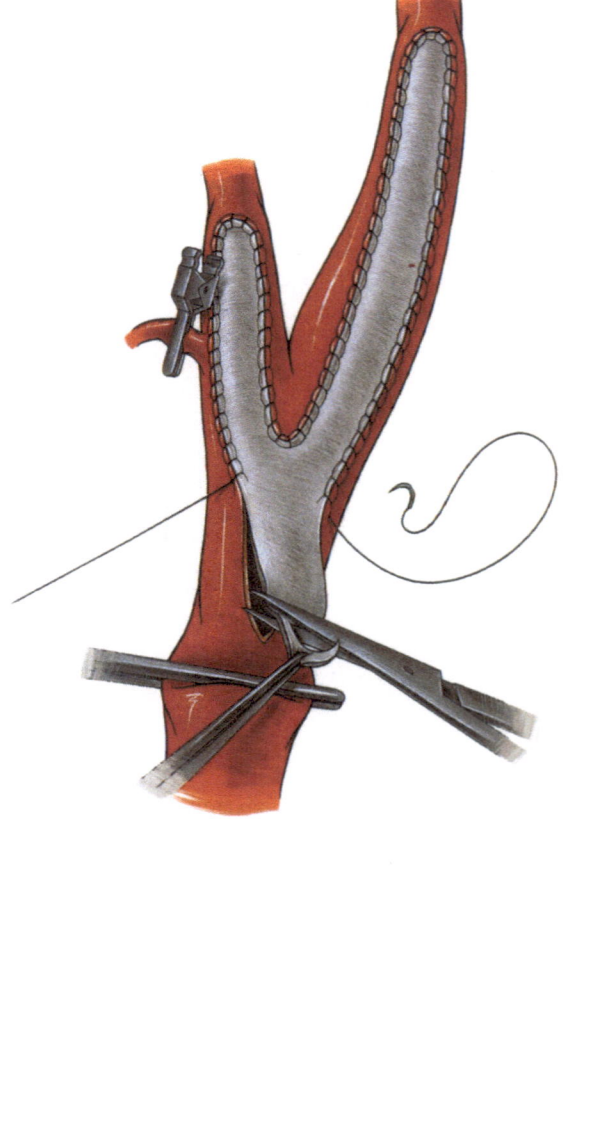

Figure 8.24 (a) Separate endarterectomy of the external carotid artery requires a separate patch. **(b)** Alternatively, if the secondary arteriotomy of the external carotid has been made from the primary arteriotomy, a Y patch is inserted.

Figure 8.25 Mutual patching of the external and internal carotid artery origins after open endarterectomy of each vessel. This technique is usually referred to as "advancement" of the bifurcation. **(a)** The posterior wall of the external carotid and the anterior wall of the endarterectomized carotid bulb are opened for the same length. **(b)** Closure starts in the lowest point of the posterior arteriotomy and **(c)** is completed on the anterior wall.

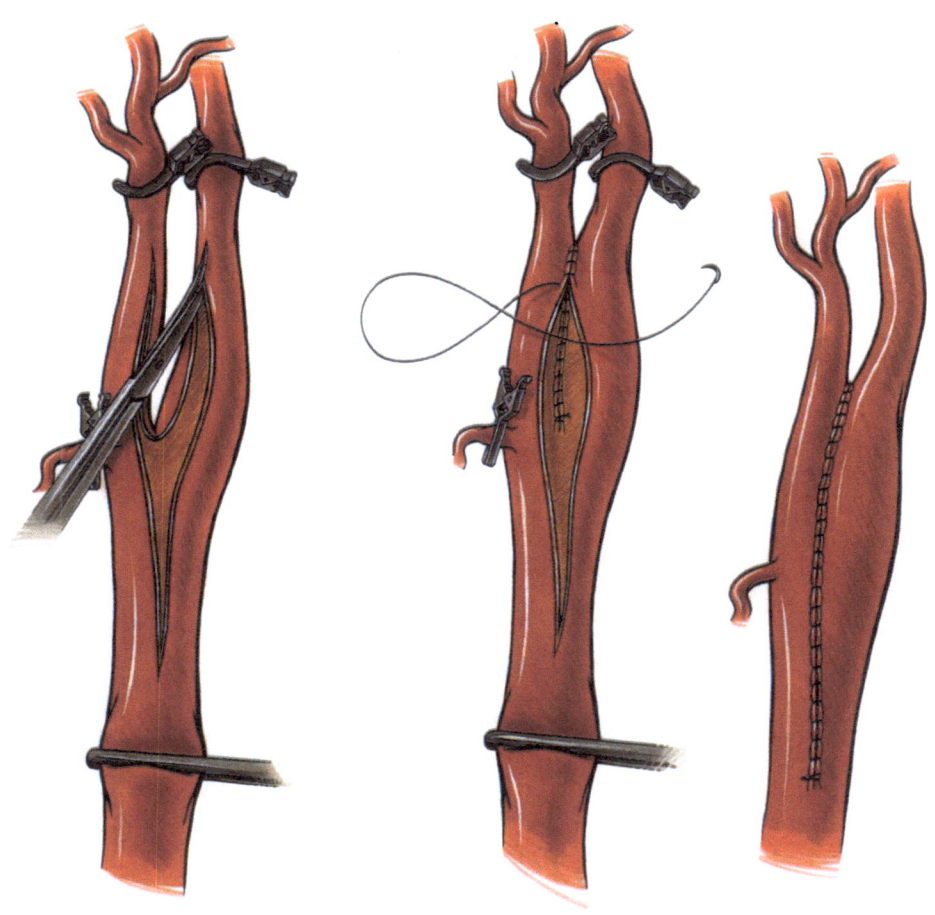

clearing of the external carotid using the standard technique for endarterectomy of the bifurcation, we favor the use of the technique known as "advancement" of the bifurcation. It permits an open endarterectomy of both external and internal carotid arteries and autogenous patching of each arterial origin with the opposite artery (Figure 8.25). In this technique the carotid baroceptor nerves are cut, and the crotch of the bifurcation is cleared. The arteriotomy in the common carotid wall leads straight into the crotch of the bifurcation, where it splits into a T as it follows first the posterior wall of the ECA and then the anterior wall of the carotid bulb. The arteriotomies into the ECA and ICA have the same length.

Closure starts in the posterior wall at the lowest point. The continuous 7-0 monofilament suture is run upward from inside the artery, and once the apex of the angioplasty is approximated, it is continued downward, closing the wall that faces the surgeon. A second suture line is started at the lower point of the incision to finish the closure somewhere in the middle third of the arteriotomy.

This technique of mutual arterioplasty of the origins of the external and internal carotid arteries can be used to provide autogenous patching of a small bulb when a synthetic patch is not desirable. Prerequisites for this technique are the presence of an external carotid trunk of sufficient length to match the opening in the bulb and a close bifurcation angle. This technique cannot be used when the bifurcation angle is wide and the bulb exits the bifurcation in a posterior oblique direction or if the ECA divides early

In the exceptional circumstance where an ECA supplying the vertebrobasilar system (through occipital to vertebral artery anastomoses) becomes stenotic and thus the source of symptoms, isolated endarterectomy of the ECA involves the orifice of the artery and requires clamping of the bifurcation (with or without an ICA shunt) and patch closure of the ECA.

9 Repair of the Vertebral Artery

Even though access to the vertebral artery (VA) is feasible at any level, only two sites are generally used for its reconstruction (Figure 9.1). Proximal reconstructions of the VA are done in its first segment, which extends from its takeoff to the transverse process of C6. Distal reconstructions are done in the third segment, which extends from the top of C2 to the atlantooccipital membrane. Within this segment, the VA is specifically isolated between the transverse processes of C1 and C2. It is better to reconstruct the artery in this third segment when treating occlusive disease involving the second segment of the VA. The approach to the second segment is fraught with difficulties caused by venous bleeding, narrow spaces between the transverse processes, and the danger of traumatic and ischemic injury to the nerve roots of the brachial plexus. (Access to the second segment of the VA for traumatic injuries is discussed in Chapter 11) On rare occasions the artery must be exposed in the upper half of its third segment, between the transverse process of C1 and the occipital bone.

For reconstruction of the VA we use autogenous bypasses or transposition techniques. Prosthetic replacements should be avoided.

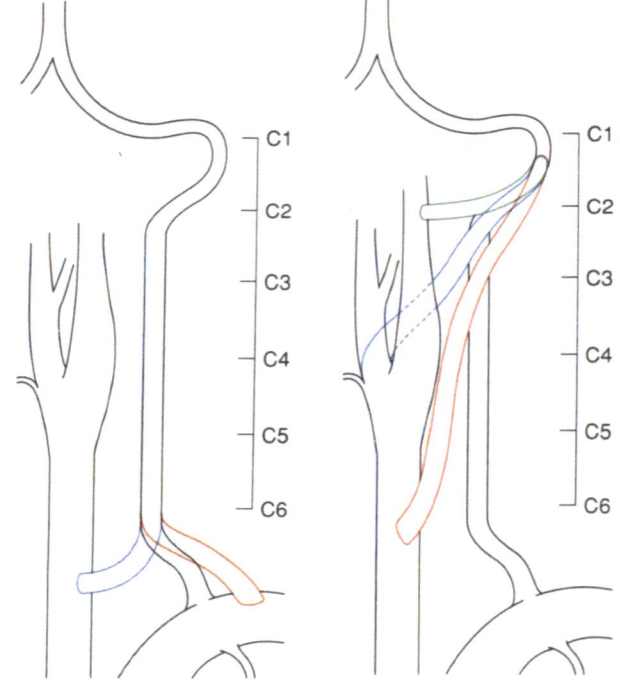

Figure 9.1 Most common techniques for proximal (**a**) and distal (**b**) vertebral artery reconstruction.

Reconstruction of the Proximal Vertebral Artery

The approach to the proximal VA depends on the technique chosen for repair (Figure 9.2). The most frequent procedure is transposition of the VA to the CCA, for which the supraclavicular intersternocleidomastoid approach is best. Rarely, a proximal VA reconstruction is done by transposition to another subclavian site or a subclavian-vertebral bypass. The latter techniques require exposure of the second portion of the SA after dividing the scalenus anticus muscle.

Transposition of the Vertebral Artery to the Common Carotid Artery

Transposition of the VA to the CCA (Figure 9.3) is our technique of choice, and we use it in more than 90% of proximal reconstructions of the VA. It is a simple technique, requiring only one anastomosis and minimal dissection, and it has excellent patency rates. Reservations we had years ago about simultaneously clamping the common carotid and VA are no longer justified with few exceptions discussed below.

A roll is placed under the patient's shoulder. The head is slightly hyperextended and turned to the opposite side with its weight supported by padding. The incision starts at the head of the clavicle and runs obliquely up for 6 to 8 cm. The two bellies of the sternocleidomastoid are separated and the small vessels that run between them cauterized. The jugular vein is identified between the two muscle bellies and retracted laterally, together with the vagus nerve. The vagus is left attached to the adventitia of the vein, and the retractor is placed on the vein without touching the vagus. The CCA is dissected and its adequacy as a donor source is assessed by palpation.

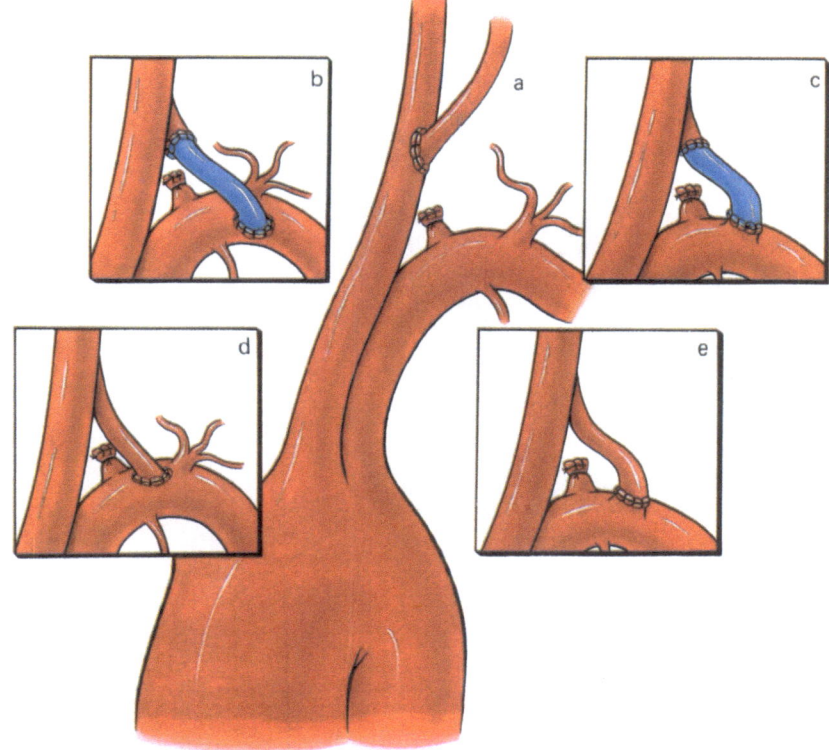

Figure 9.2 Modalities for reconstructing the proximal vertebral artery. (**a**) Transposition to the common carotid artery is the usual technique. A subclavian vertebral bypass may take origin in the subclavian artery (**b**) or in the divided thyrocervical trunk (**c**). A redundant vertebral artery may be transposed to a new subclavian site (**d**) or to the divided thyrocervical trunk (**e**).

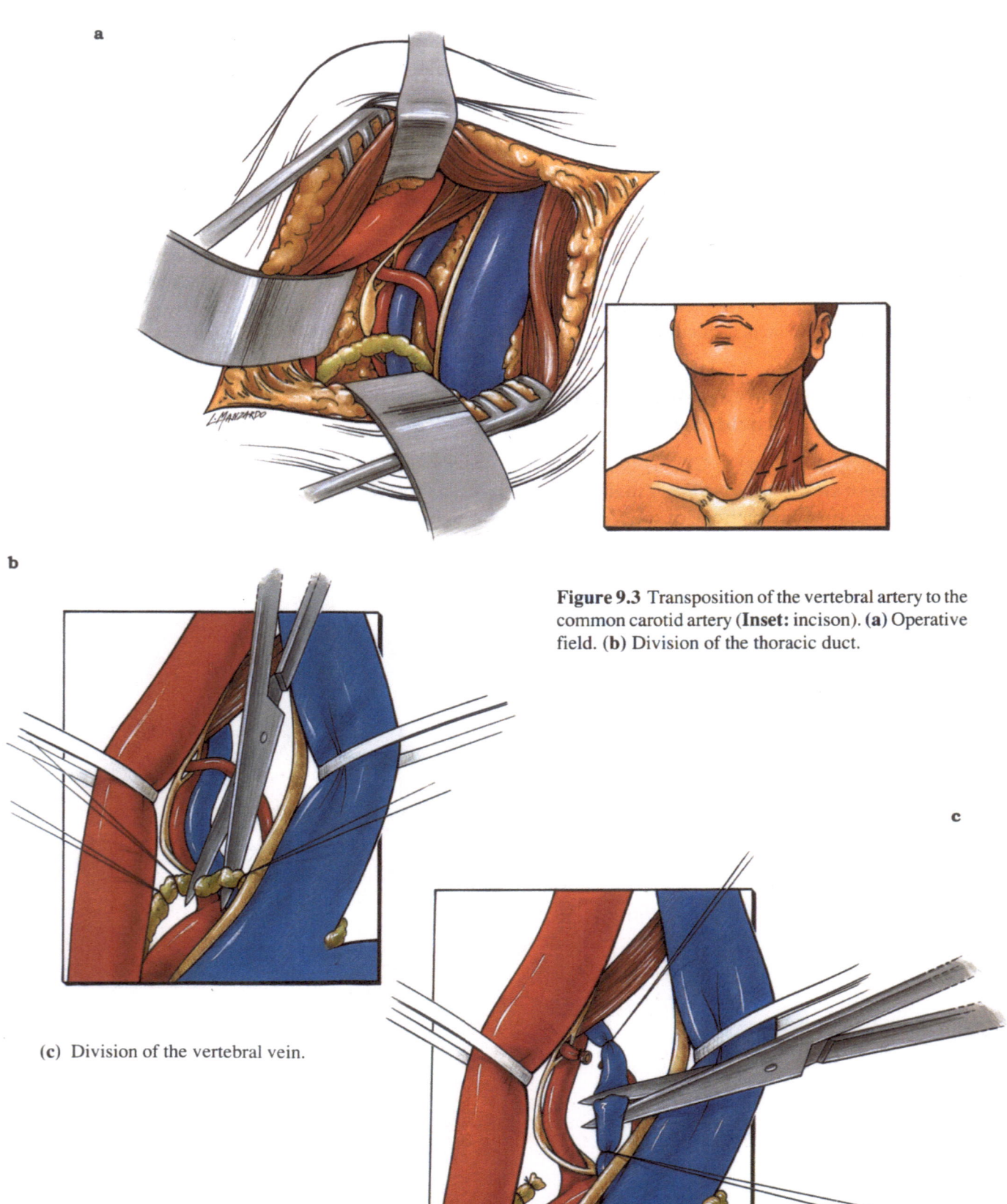

a

b

Figure 9.3 Transposition of the vertebral artery to the common carotid artery (**Inset:** incison). (**a**) Operative field. (**b**) Division of the thoracic duct.

c

(**c**) Division of the vertebral vein.

d

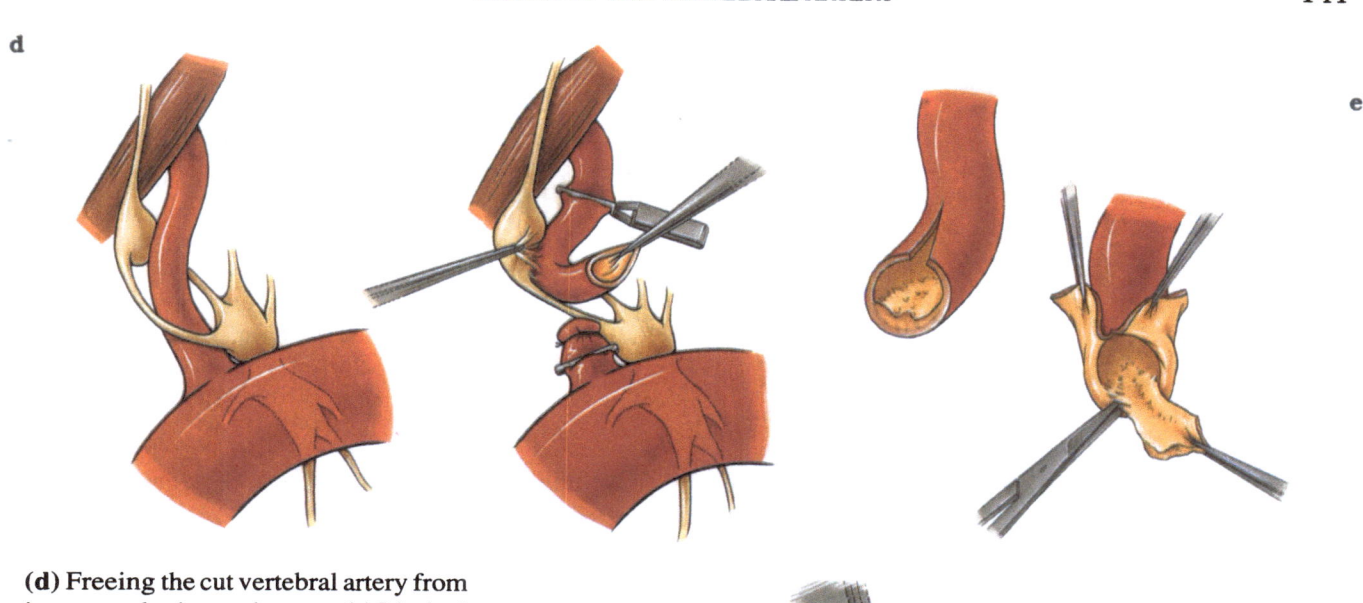

e

(**d**) Freeing the cut vertebral artery from its sympathetic attachments. (**e**) Limited eversion endarterectomy of the plaque remaining in the VA may be necessary. (**f**) Transposition of the proximal vertebral artery to the common carotid artery. The anastomosis is done with open technique.

f

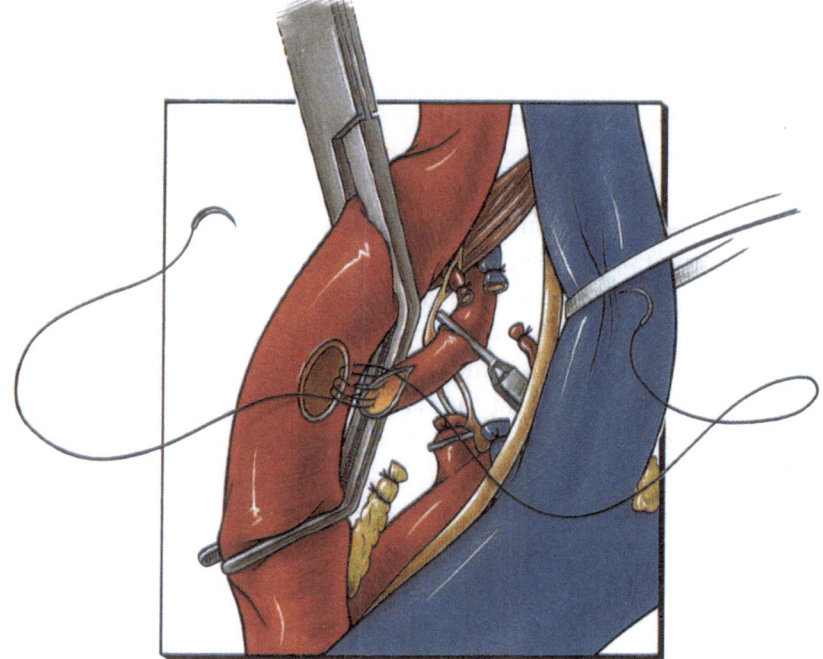

The surgeon moves temporarily to the patient's head and begins to dissect into the mediastinum, clearing the moximal CCA as far as possible. Soft, malleable, neurosurgical retractors are used to gently retract the CCA and internal jugular vein.

On the left side the thoracic duct must be identified; on the right there are two or three small accessory ducts. The thoracic duct emerges from behind the left CCA and runs transversely into the confluent of the jugular and subclavian veins. It is first ligated and then cut. Occasionally two or three trunks enter the jugulosubclavian confluent separately.

The vertebral vein is deep to the thoracic duct. Generally the inferior thyroid artery crosses the field transversely over the vertebral vein. If so, it is divided. The vertebral vein is also divided at the point where it is seen as a single trunk. By now the surgeon will have already noted the sympathetic chain running behind the CCA. The chain can be used as a reference point to identify the VA, as the stellate ganglion at the bottom of the chain is in close relation

Top view

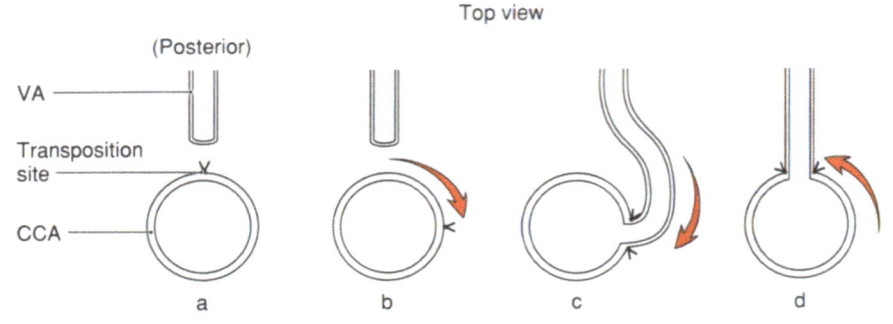

(Posterior)

VA

Transposition
site

CCA

a   b   c   d

(Anterior)

Figure 9.4 (a-d) Transposition of the vertebral artery to the common carotid artery. Rotation of the common carotid artery to construct the anastomosis with the VA in a lateral plane. After release of the clamps the anastomosis resumes a location posterior to the common carotid artery (CCA).

to the origin of the artery. The intermediate or middle ganglion, seen higher up, often rests on the VA itself.

The VA lies behind the vertebral vein and may be tortuous, in contrast to the vein, which is straight. The artery is identified and encircled with a loop above the point where the sympathetic fibers cross it. Frequently the intermediate (or less frequently the stellate) ganglion is attached to the anterior surface of the VA, and its rami impede lateral access to the artery. It is best to loop the VA again near its origin below the point where it is crossed by the sympathetic fibers. During this dissection, it is important to avoid damage to the sympathetics to prevent a Horner's syndrome. The portion of the VA adherent to the intermediate ganglion is left undissected until later, after the origin of the artery has been divided. The artery is dissected proximally down to its origin from the SA and distally up to the point where the tendon of the longus colli crosses over it, just before it disappears into the transverse process of C6. At times the tendon of the longus colli is located more laterally in the transverse process of C6, covering the VA for a centimeter or two before the artery enters the foramen in the bone. Dividing this tendon permits freeing the artery further. Care should be taken to secure or cauterize a small vein draining into the vertebral vein, which runs under the edge of the tendon of the longus colli muscle.

In a few patients it is difficult to find the upper third of the VA's first segment if the artery enters the spine at the transverse process of C7 and, in order to do so, runs a transverse, shorter course in the neck. This variation may be anticipated from preoperative arteriographic evidence, but other times it comes as a surprise to the surgeon. When confronted with an abnormal entry at C7, the VA is dissected, and an assessment is made to see if it will easily reach the CCA without kinking. If it appears that it will not reach, there are two alternatives for reconstruction: One solution is to resect the anterior portion of the transverse process of C7 using a rongeur (with bone wax on hand to control bleeding) to free additional length of VA. The other is to perform a bypass from the SA to the VA before it penetrates at C7.

With the VA dissected, the neighboring CCA is cleared of adventitia at the site elected for transposition. The patient is given systemic heparin. The VA is clamped as high as possible with a microsurgical clip. Proximally, a large hemoclip occludes its takeoff from the SA. The VA is divided above the hemoclip and its stump is suture-ligated with 6-0 monofilament suture. The artery is then pulled from under the sympathetic chain, and the adhesions that remain between it and the VA are divided. The distal free end of the VA is brought into apposition to the site chosen for anastomosis in the CCA, and, if needed, excess length is trimmed. A small cut in the anterior wall of the VA provides a beveled end for anastomosis.

It may be that after division of the VA from its origin some of the stenosing plaque remains in its posterior wall. This situation can be easily dealt with by an eversion endarterectomy so long as one stays in the superficial plane that leads to a good feathering off of the distal end of the plaque.

Next the CCA is axially rotated (Figures 9.3 and 9.4), bringing its posterior wall into the lateral position. A baby Satinsky clamp works well to cross-clamp and hold the CCA down next to the VA. An ellipse of CCA wall is removed with an aortic punch, and the VA is anastomosed to this arteriostomy with a continuous open 7-0 monofilament suture. When the suture is two-thirds completed, it is pulled to bring the vessels together. The distal and proximal carotid and the distal VA are back-bled into the wound. Flow is resumed first into the VA and then into the distal carotid.

Reconstruction of the Proximal Vertebral Artery from the Subclavian Artery

The second portion of the SA must be exposed if a transposition to the CCA is not possible because the latter is severely diseased or cannot be clamped safely or, occasionally, because of a short first VA segment. The incision required to expose the second portion of the SA (Figure 9.5) is similar to the one previously described, except that the clavicular head of the sternocleidomastoid is cut and the omohyoid and prescalene fat pad are retracted upward and laterally. The phrenic nerve is dissected from the surface of the scalenus anticus as it curves from an anterior to a medial location on the muscle. The scalenus anticus is divided low, and the second portion of the SA is exposed. Arteriograms may provide some guidance as to the best site for reimplantation, but examination

and palpation are also necessary to find the best spot in the SA. Occasionally, the thyrocervical trunk may serve as implantation site after division of its branches (Figure 9.2).

When a vein graft is used for bypass, the distal anastomosis is done first (Figure 9.6). This anastomosis may be constructed end-to-end. The VA is cut 1.5 cm proximal to its point of disappearance under the longus colli. The proximal end of the artery is ligated, and its distal end is spatulated to allow construction of the distal anastomosis to the saphenous vein graft. Alternatively, it may be made end-to-side and converted later to a functional end-to-end construction by occluding the VA with a clip proximal to the anastomosis. Once the distal anastomosis is completed, the graft is trimmed to an appropriate length, with the surgeon bearing in mind that redundancy will result in a kink. At the site elected for implantation, an aortic punch should be used to make an opening to anastomose either the VA or the proximal end of a saphenous vein graft. Prior to completing the proximal anastomosis, which is done with 7-0 monofilament suture, the distal and proximal SA, as well as the VA, are back-bled before the sutures are tied and flow is reestablished first into the distal SA then into the VA.

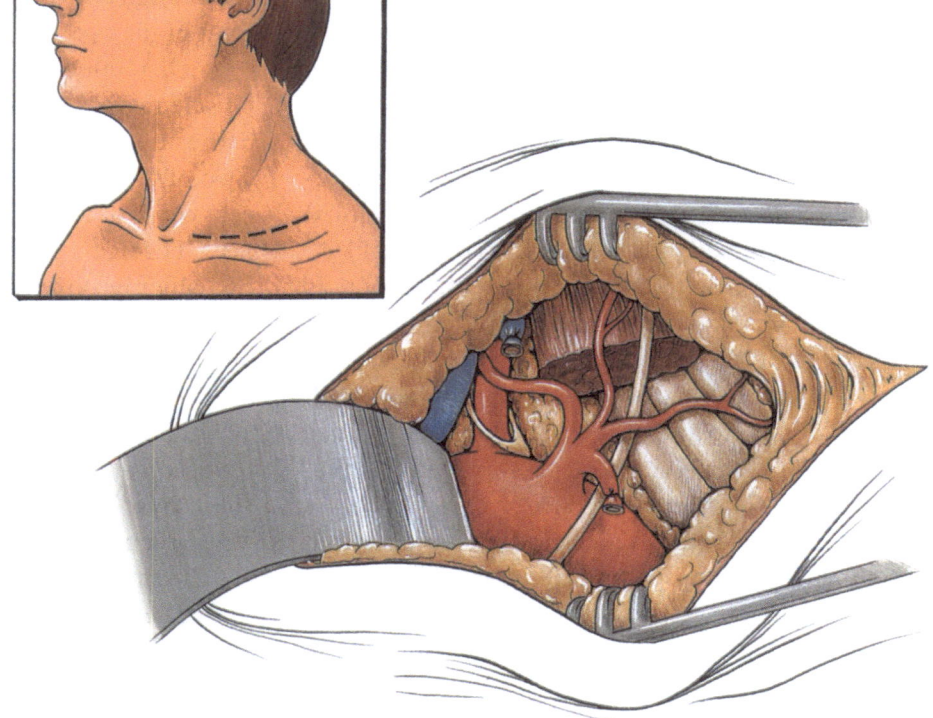

Figure 9.5 Exposure of the retroscalene segment of the subclavian artery.

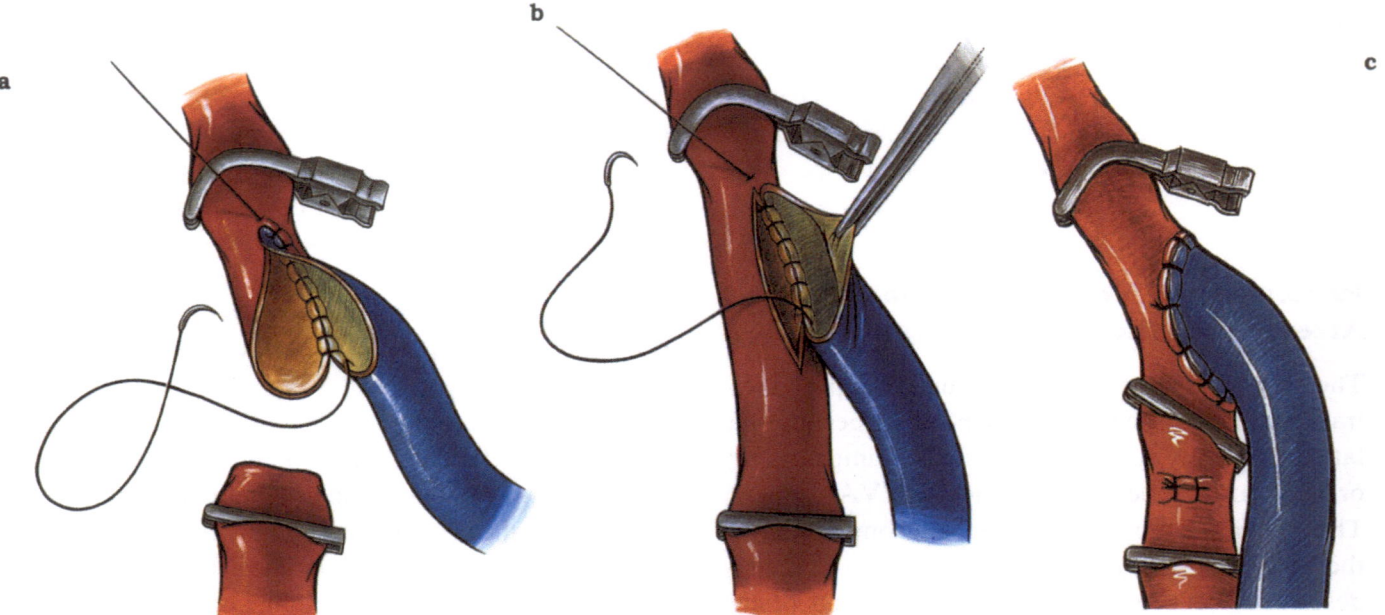

Figure 9.6 Distal anastomosis of a subclavian-vertebral bypass may be end-to-end (**a**) or end-to-side (**b**). The latter is later converted to end-to-end (**c**) by applying a hemoclip in the proximal vertebral artery.

Reconstruction of the Distal Vertebral Artery

For reconstruction of the distal VA, the artery is approached between the transverse processes of C1 and C2. The common techniques of reconstruction (Figure 9.1) include bypass from the CCA to the distal VA, transposition of the ECA to the distal VA, and transposition of the distal VA to the ICA by end-to-side anastomosis. Rarely, a hypertrophic occipital artery may be directly anastomosed to the distal VA.

The approach to this segment of the VA is through an incision anterior to the sternomastoid muscle (Figure 9.7). The tip of the parotid gland is elevated after the external jugular vein is transected. Division of the greater auricular nerve is sometimes necessary for exposure. The accessory spinal nerve, which may be found about two fingerbreadths below the mastoid tip, is isolated between the sternomastoid muscle and the posterior wall of the internal jugular vein. This nerve usually carries a small complement of vessels around it. The nerve is exposed distally by

lifting or cutting the digastric muscle. As the nerve crosses over the jugular vein, a finger can palpate the sharp, bony prominence of the transverse process of C1 through the vein wall. This point marks the upper limit of the operative field.

Dissection of the anterior edge of the levator muscle reveals the anterior ramus of C2 exiting underneath and dividing usually into three branches. Two of them form loops that anastomose with adjacent cervical nerves.

The distal VA can be approached from here in two slightly different ways. When the approach is over its lateral wall, the levator scapula is cut. The other technique approaches the artery anteriorly with resection of the anterior intertransversarium muscle and retraction of the anterior edge of the levator posteriorly. The anterior ramus of C2 can be seen to curve over the anterolateral wall of the underlying VA, which runs perpendicular to it. The nerve is then cut and the VA exposed.

There are several vena comitantes that share adventitial connections with the VA and become larger over the anterior and posterior walls of the artery. These veins are gently dissected away from the artery. Small veins crossing in front are handled by unipolar coagulation or by elevating and tying them with 7-0 ligatures before cutting them. As the veins are separated from the artery, the latter can be inspected searching for collaterals entering it from behind. If a collateral is seen, it is occluded with a microclip as far away from the artery as possible. There is considerable variation in the length of the artery between the transverse process of C1 and C2 and in the degree to which the adventitia of the artery may be attached to the periosteum of the uncinate joints under it. The segment of artery between C1 and C2 is mobilized, and held with a fine Silastic loop.

If the choice is to do a *CCA-to-distal VA bypass* (Figure 9.8), the vein should be obtained from the thigh. Preoperative ultrasound mapping helps to select a segment of saphenous with a diameter greater than 3.5 mm and preferably without valves. The distal anastomosis is constructed first and can be made end-to-end or end-to-side (Figure 9.9). If there is enough length of artery for an end-to-side anastomosis, as is usually the case, the latter is easier to perform. It also avoids the problems of axial rotation of the artery, which may occur with an end-to-end anastomosis. The end-to-side anastomosis is done in an open manner, using continuous 7-0 monofilament suture or 8-0 monofilament suture. Once the anastomosis is completed the end-to-side anastomosis is made into a functional end-to-end junction by ligating or clipping the VA below the anastomosis. This method is our preference because it is technically easier and safer.

In some cases, however, the space between C1 and C2 is short, or the artery may have been damaged during dissection. In these cases an end-to-end anastomosis below the point of entrance into C1 may be necessary. If so, the distal end of the artery is occluded with a microsurgical clip. If the VA is to be cut across for the end-to-end anastomosis, its proximal end is first looped with a 5-0 monofilament suture with a small bite taken from the wall of the artery and the periosteum and muscle surrounding it. The artery is then occluded with a hemoclip and the 5-0 monofilament suture tied after dividing the artery. The loss

of the proximal end of the artery can be a source of severe hemorrhage, which may be difficult to control, as the divided VA may retract and disappear into the transverse process of C2. The free distal end of the artery may be anastomosed end-to-end to a saphenous vein graft with 3.5× loop magnification using continuous 7-0 or 8-0 monofilament suture.

The vein graft is then passed under the jugular vein into the proximity of the previously dissected distal CCA. The CCA is cross-clamped away from the bifurcation where atheroma is often present that could be crushed by the occluding clamp. The graft is anastomosed to an arteriostomy that can be made with an aortic punch in the posterior wall of the CCA or by excising a triangle from the wall of the CCA. Prior to completing the suture, the vessels are back-bled and flow is resumed, first into the distal VA and then into the CCA. If there are any valves in the vein graft preventing adequate black-bleeding before resumption of flow, the graft may be bled forward and the distal VA backward through a small VA arteriotomy proximal to the distal end-to-side anastomosis. After bleeding the two vessels, the clip distal to the arteriotomy converts the anastomosis into an end-to-end one and isolates the arteriotomy between the two occluding hemoclips. An additional suture is placed to close the arteriotomy for additional safety.

When there is no adequate saphenous vein a *transposition of the ECA to the distal VA* at the C1–C2 level may be used (Figure 9.9). For this technique the distal VA is exposed as described above, and the ECA is dissected from its origin to the point where it gives off the internal maxillary artery. The branches of the ECA are divided, skeletonizing the artery above and below the hypoglossal nerve and underneath the digastric muscle, which is, in turn, divided. Once an adequate length of ECA is obtained (and rechecked with a measuring suture that follows the anticipated path), the ECA is clamped at its origin and its distal end divided. The end of the ECA is pulled from under the hypoglossal nerve and then tunneled under the jugular vein into proximity with the VA. The distal ECA is prepared for the anastomosis using the standard principles of microsurgical technique: using fine instruments and removing the artery's adventitial coat. The

a

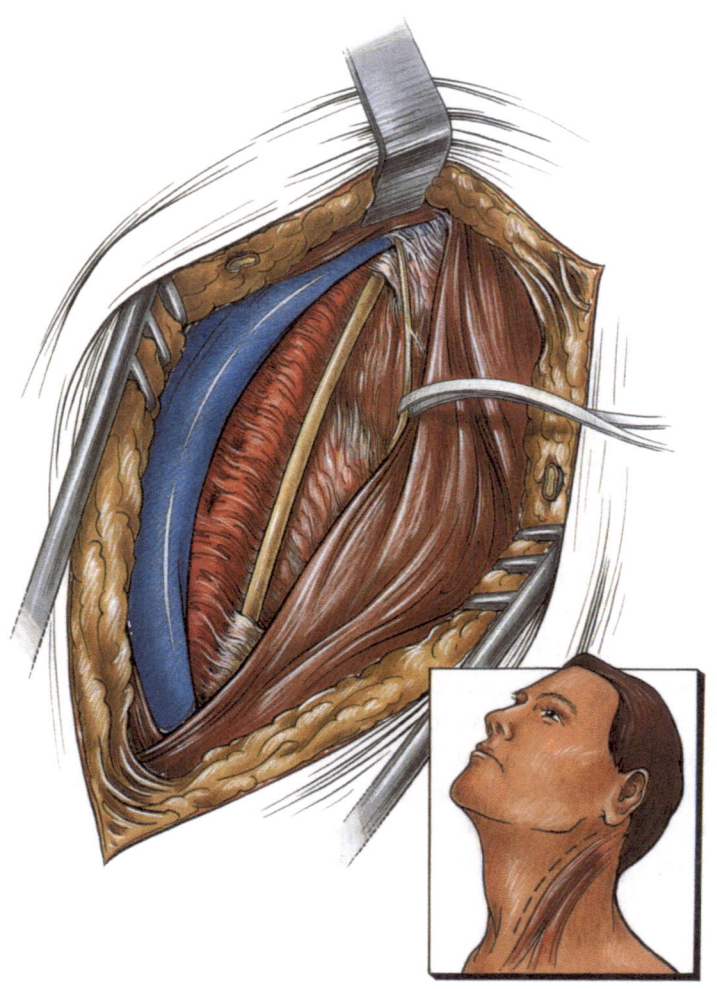

b

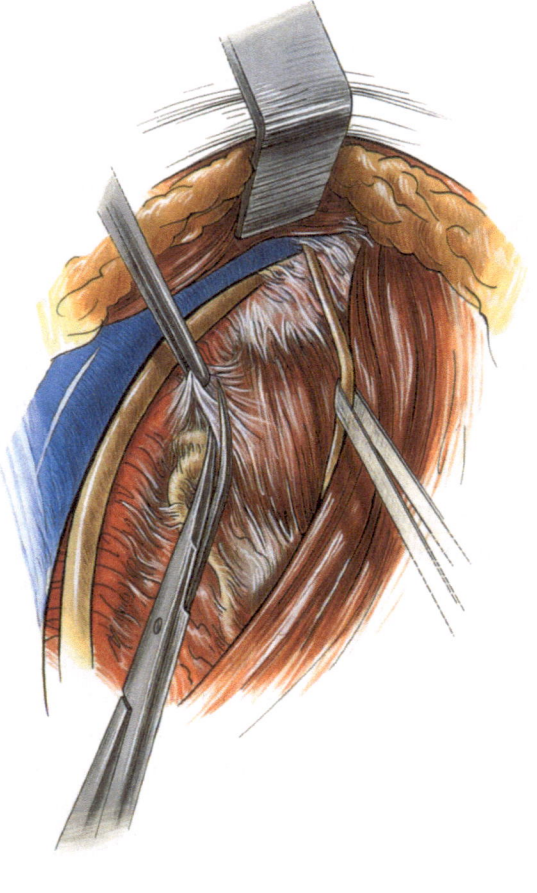

c

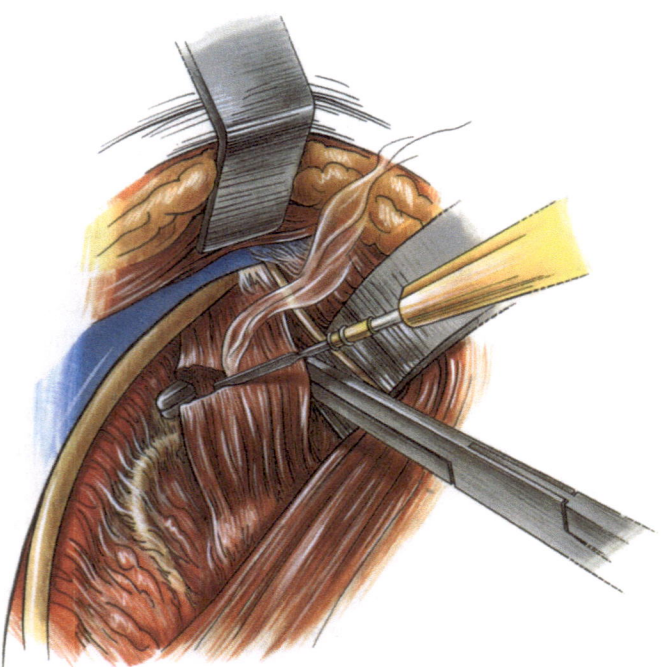

Figure 9.7 Approach to the distal vertebral artery. (**Inset**) Incision. (**a**) Dissection of the spinal accessory nerve and fibrofatty tissue covering the levator scapula. (**b**) Dissection of the anterior edge of the levator scapula showing the anterior ramus of C2. (**c**) Division of the levator scapula.

d

e

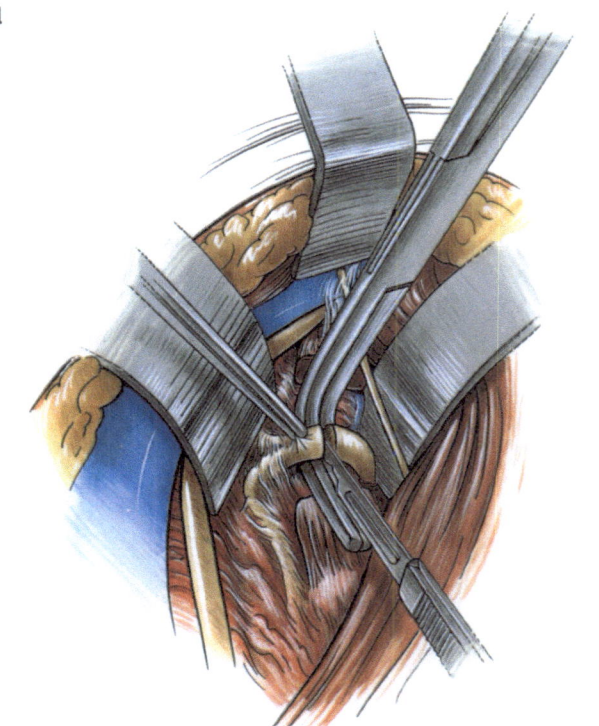

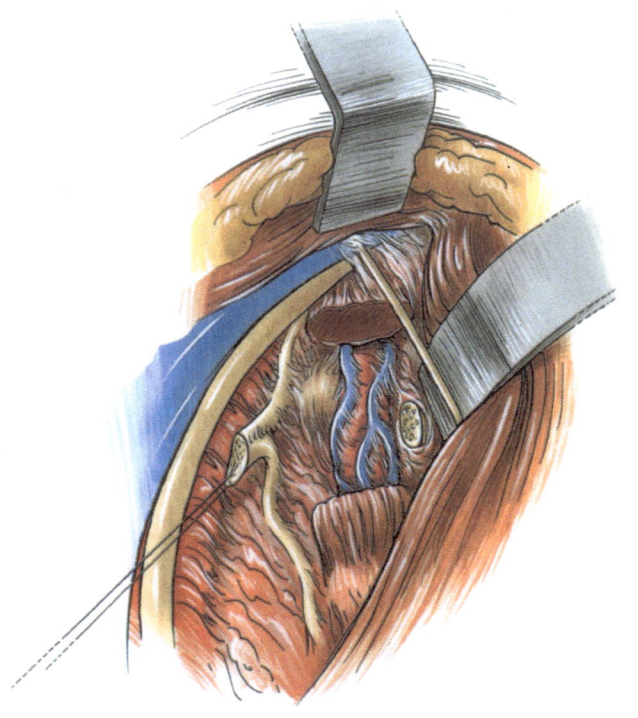

f

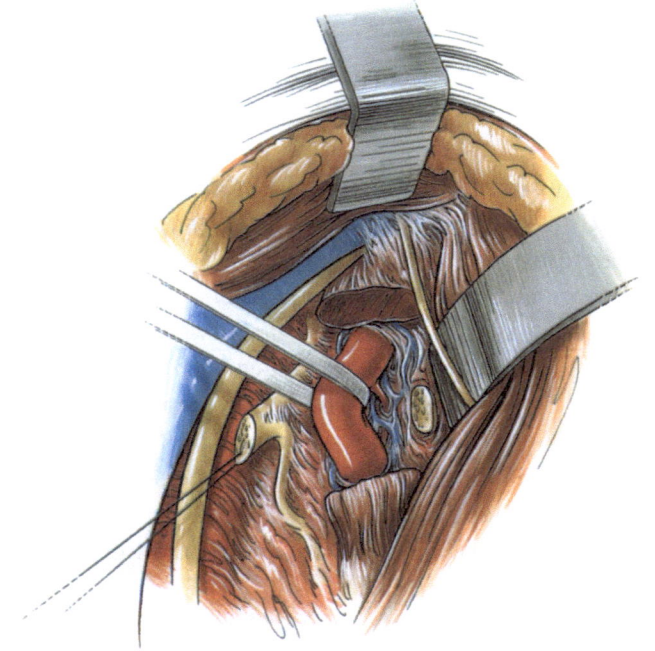

(d) Division of the anterior ramus of C2. (e) Exposure of the vertebral artery and overlying vertebral venous plexus at the C1–C2 space. (f) Distal vertebral artery slung after dissecting away the vertebral veins.

a   b

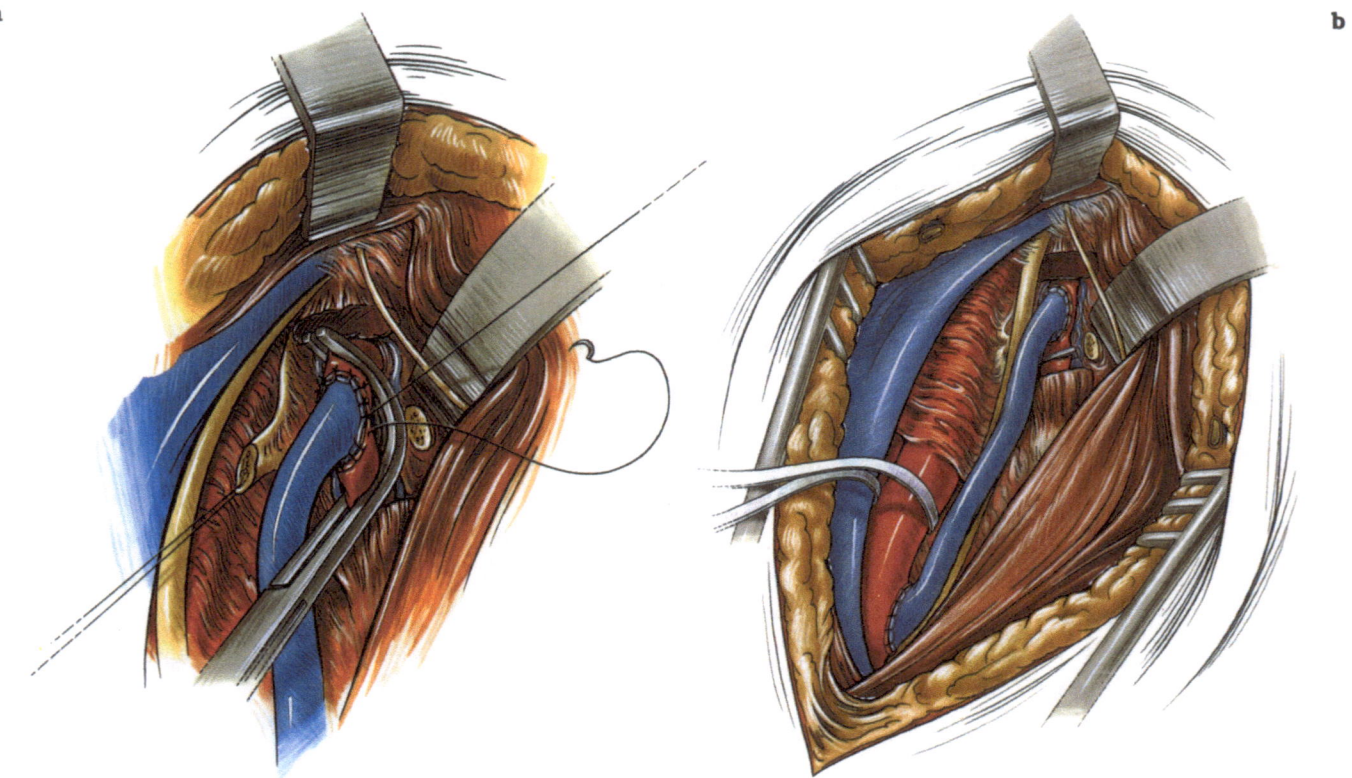

Figure 9.8 Common carotid to distal vertebral artery vein bypass. (**a**) Distal end-to-side anastomosis is performed first. (**b**) Completed procedure.

anastomosis can be either end-to-side and later converted into a functional end-to-end by a proximal clip or, if the exposed vertebral or the dissected external carotid are short, an end-to-end anastomosis.

For *transposition of the occipital artery to the distal VA* (Figure 9.10), the latter is exposed in the manner described above. The large occipital artery is found underneath the digastric muscle. The artery is freed, and its small branches are ligated and divided. Its end is prepared using the same technique described for the ECA, and the distal anastomosis is done in the same manner.

Transposition of the distal VA into the ICA is a technique that simplifies the operation and does not require use of a saphenous vein graft (Figure 9.11). This technique, however, should not be used in patients with contralateral CCA/ICA occlusion. We dissect the VA within the C1–C2 interval, trying to take advantage of any tortuosity and to gain as much length as possible by mobilizing the artery from its periosteal attachments. The ICA should be mobilized

from the bulb up to the C1 level, using the same approach as is described Chapter 8. Spasm of the distal cervical ICA during dissection is frequent and should be treated by topical application of papaverine. The VA is clipped and transected at the exit of the C2 transverse process to avoid the loss of any arterial length. The proximal stump is secured to the C2 process and adjacent muscles with a 5-0 transfixion suture. The natural curve of the VA within the C1–C2 interval provides an easy reach to the posterolateral aspect of the ICA, to which it is anastomosed with a continuous 7-0 monofilament running suture. In the rare case where the VA is not long enough in the C1–C2 interspace to allow from anastomosis to the ICA, the lateral wall of the transverse process of C2 can be resected to gain extra length from the proximal VA.

Occasionally the anatomic circumstances require *unusual techniques*. There may not be enough redundancy in the VA at C1–C2 to easily reach the ICA. In this case if there is redundancy of the ICA it is better to use this extra length of the ICA to reach the

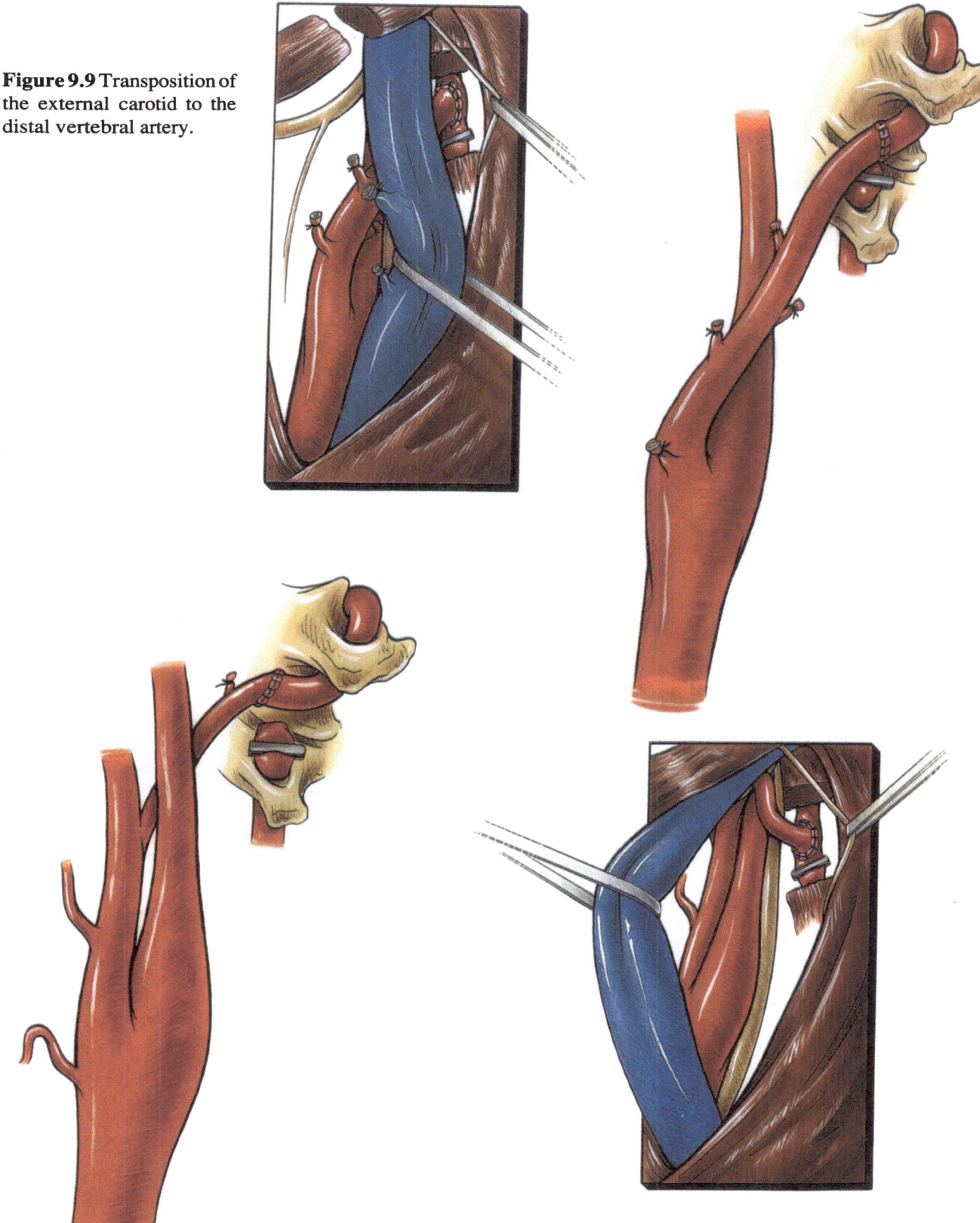

Figure 9.9 Transposition of the external carotid to the distal vertebral artery.

Figure 9.10 Transposition of the occipital to the distal vertebral artery. Anastomosis may be end-to-end or end-to-side.

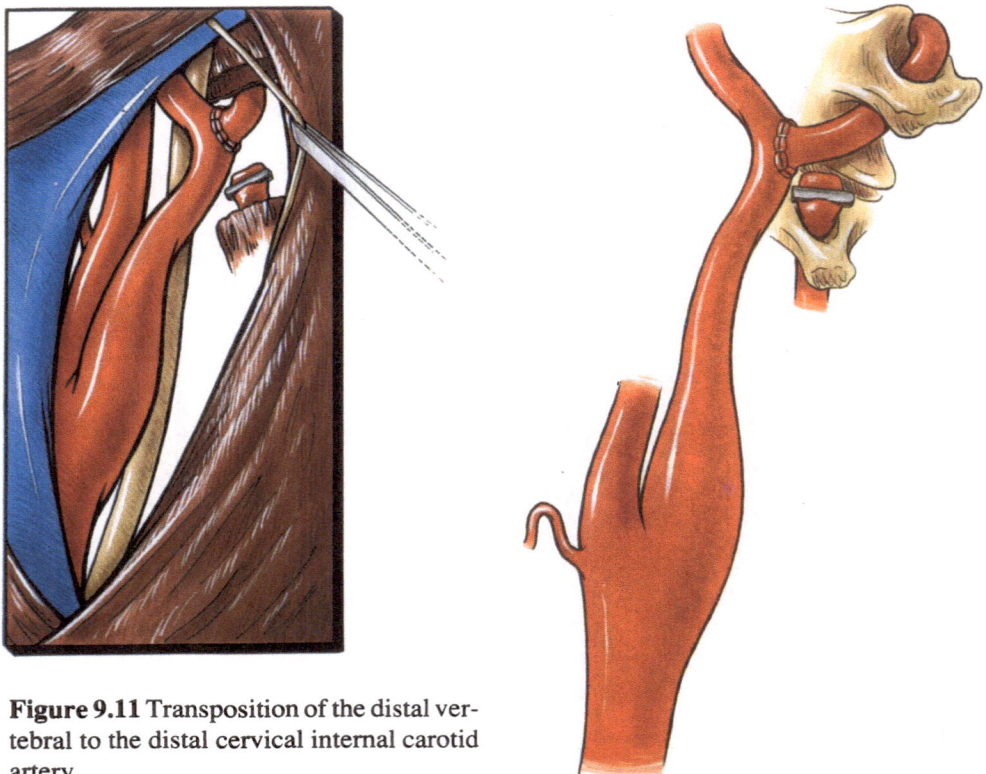

Figure 9.11 Transposition of the distal vertebral to the distal cervical internal carotid artery.

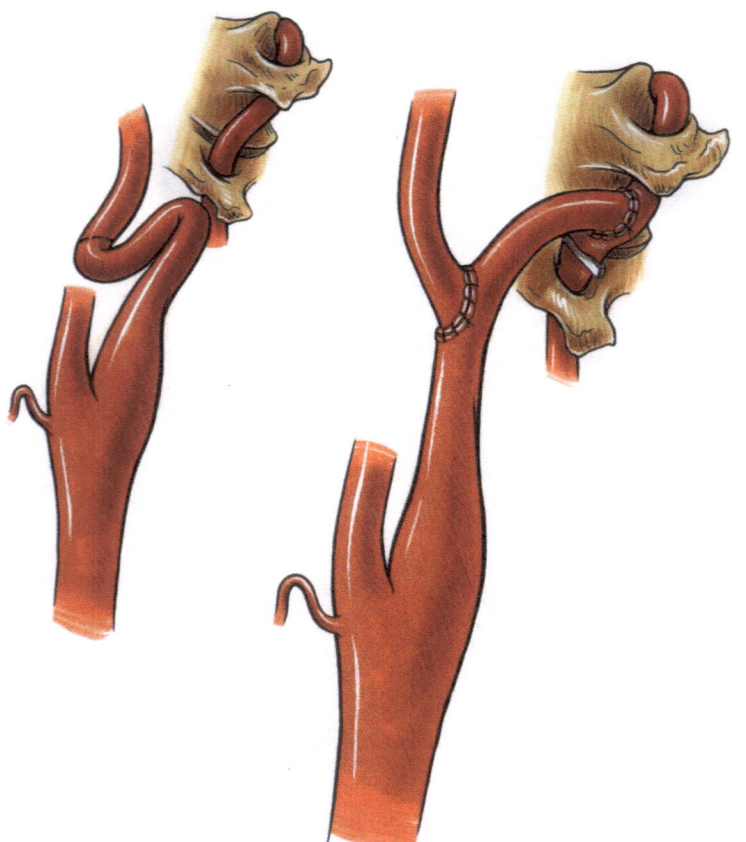

Figure 9.12 Technique for revascularizing the distal vertebral artery when the latter is too short for transposition to a redundant internal carotid artery and no suitable saphenous vein is available.

Figure 9.13 Recently occluded internal carotid artery (**a**) may be used as a bypass conduit to revascularize the distal vertebral artery (**b**) following thromboendarterectomy of the former.

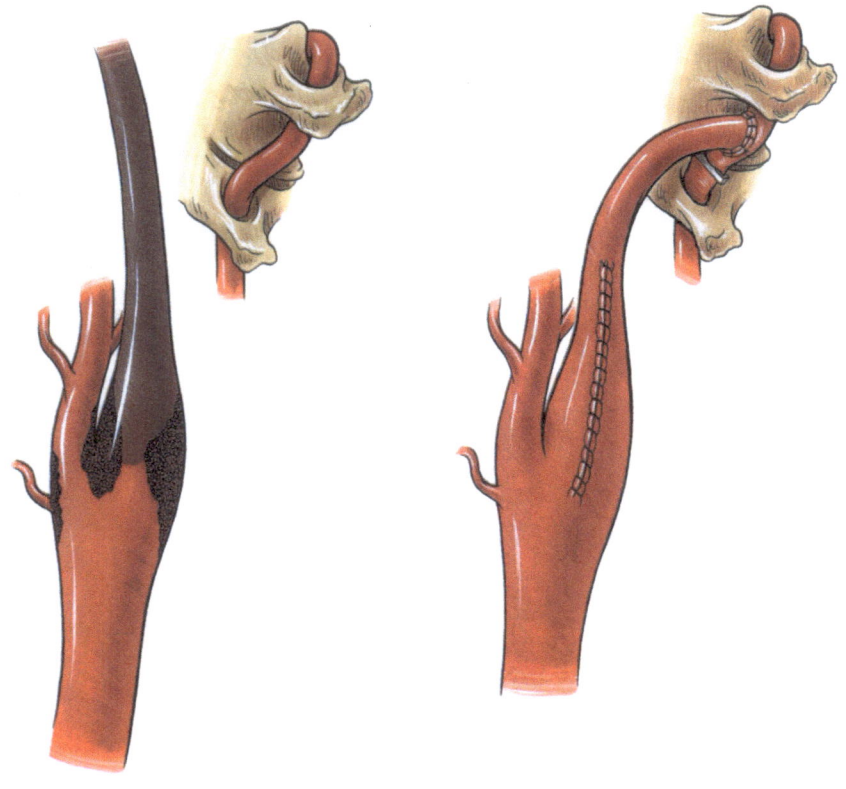

VA (Figure 9.12), transposing the distal ICA to a more proximal site in the cervical ICA and correcting its redundancy. If a suitable vein graft is not available and the ipsilateral ICA is recently occluded, the ECA, which is potentially a valuable collateral pathway, should not be used for a transposition to the distal VA. In this case, the thrombosed ICA is cut high at the level of C1 and a thromboendarterectomy is done through an incision over the carotid bulb. The ICA can then be used as a bypass, transposing its distal end to the VA (Figure 9.13). Finally if the CCA and ICA are thrombosed, the distal VA may be revascularized by a vein graft from the ipsilateral SA (Figure 9.14).

Only rarely does the surgeon need to approach the VA above the transverse process of C1 (Figure 9.15). In such cases the standard incision anterior to the sternomastoid is extended posteriorly by cutting

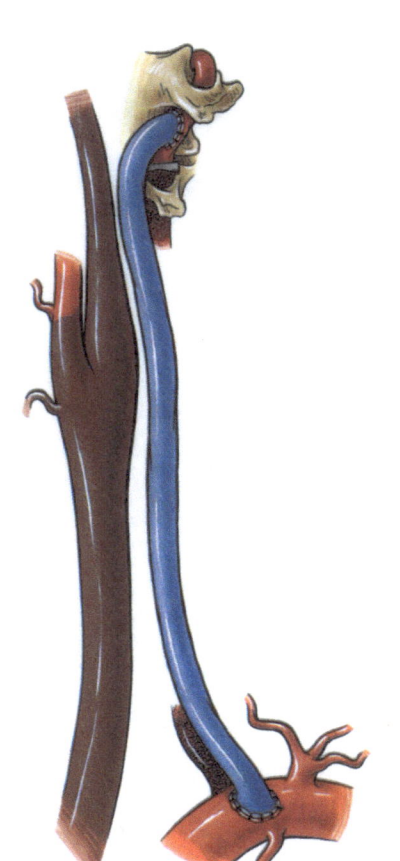

Figure 9.14 Revascularization of the distal vertebral artery by a vein graft from the subclavian artery.

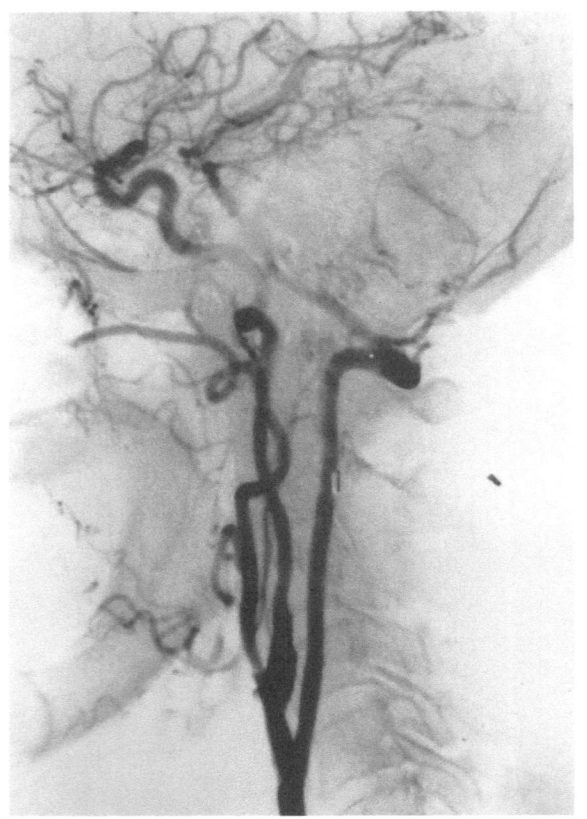

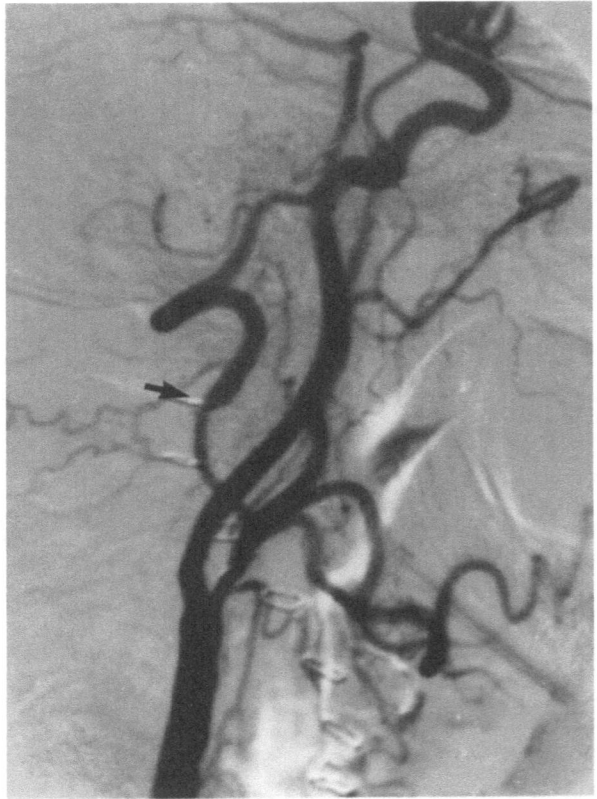

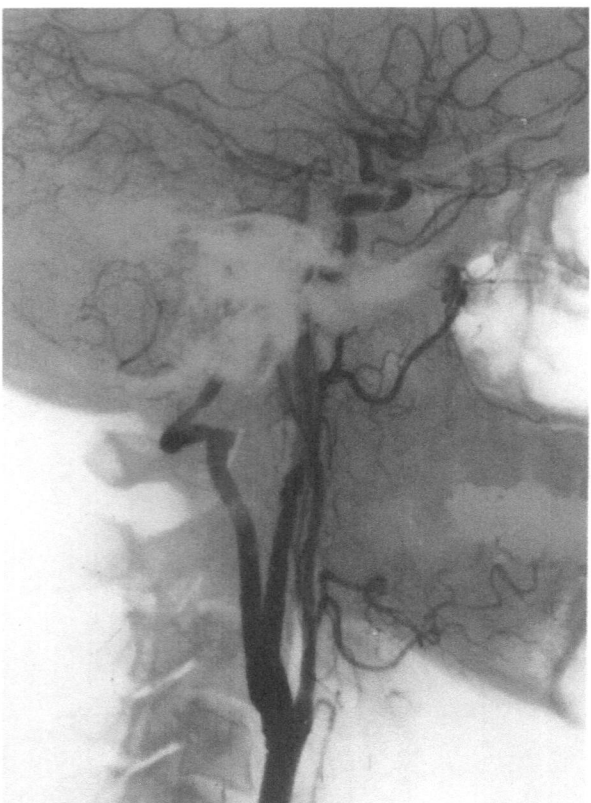

Figure 9.15 Postoperative arteriograms of different types of distal vertebral reconstruction. (**a**) Common carotid to distal vertebral artery vein bypass at the C1–C2 level. (**b**) Transposition of the occipital to the distal vertebral artery at the C1–C2 level (arrow). (**c**) Internal carotid to distal vertebral artery vein bypass above C1.

the upper insertion of the sternomastoid and the splenius capitis muscles. The transverse process of C1 and part of its posterior arch are resected with a rongeur. At this level the VA is surrounded by a rich venous plexus that adheres to the periosteum. The latter tents the veins open and prevents them from collapsing, which may result in troublesome bleeding. In such cases the best solution is to free the VA, looping it to get it out of the way before concentrating on control of venous bleeding by a combination of unipolar coagulation, bone wax, compression, and elevating the head of the table. With this approach the VA may be dissected up to and including the level of the atlantooccipital membrane. For revascularization at this level a saphenous vein bypass from the CCA is the best solution. It is advisable to obtain a complete arteriogram after a distal reconstruction to ensure a good technical result.

10 Complex Repairs

Combined Repair of the Carotid-Vertebral/Subclavian Arteries

Combined operations on the ipsilateral ICA and VA/SA have been considered risky and seldom justified. The traditional approach in patients with vertebrobasilar symptoms has been to operate on the ICA stenosis first and to proceed with the secondary repair of the VA/SA only if the symptoms fail to disappear or they recur. To the contrary, we believe that combined operations of the ICA and VA/SA are usually safe and appropriate in patients with VBI because they avoid a secondary operation in nearly 50% of cases where the carotid operation fails to relieve VBI symptoms. We also advocate combined ICA and VA/SA operations in patients with a carotid lesion that is either critical or causing hemispheric symptoms, who have, in addition, a critical lesion of a large dominant VA on the same side.

The incision for combined operations on the ICA and *proximal VA/SA* depends on the particular anatomy of the patient (Figure 10.1). In patients with long necks, two separate incisions may be done (see Chapters 8 and 9). In patients with short necks a continuous presternomastoid incision gives good exposure for both operations, provided the neck is not placed in excessive hyperextension, which may make

retraction of the sternomastoid difficult. If access to the VA or SA is difficult with the presternomastoid incision, cutting the sternal head of the sternomastoid muscle provides the needed additional exposure. Combined reconstructions are done sequentially starting from the bottom up. The VA, SA, or both are first transposed into the CCA and flow is reestablished into the VA or SA, leaving the distal CCA clamp in place. The ECA and ICA are then clamped to allow performance of standard carotid endarterectomy.

Combined operations of the carotid bifurcation and *distal VA* are done through the same high presternomastoid incision. If a vein graft is to be placed in the distal VA, it is easier to do the more demanding distal anastomosis first. The CCA is then cross-clamped in its midportion, and the proximal part of the vein graft is anastomosed to it, establishing inflow to the distal VA after removal of the proximal clamp (Figure 10.2). The distal CCA clamp, which lies above the takeoff of the distal VA graft, is left in place, and the ICA and ECA are then clamped to preform the endarterectomy of the carotid bifurcation.

If a vein graft is not available, the surgeon may choose to do the ICA endarterectomy and transposition of the distal VA into the ICA at the same time. In this situation the ICA is dissected through the same

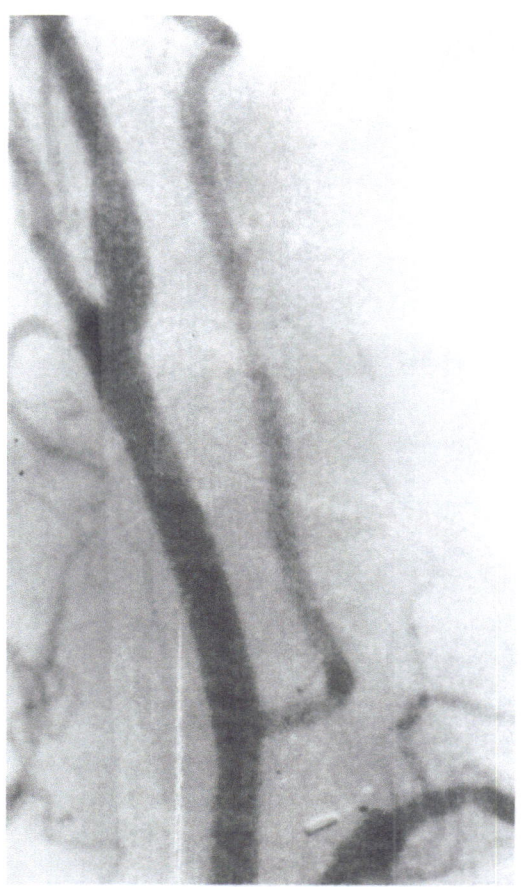

Figure 10.1 Combined transposition of the proximal vertebral and carotid endarterectomy. Some compression of the vertebral artery at C4 with the neck rotated to the right is noted in the postoperative arteriogram.

retrojugular approach, which is standard for exposure of the distal VA. This combination of carotid endarterectomy and distal VA transposition is more difficult in this setting than the vein bypass to the VA and has the disadvantage of prolonged simultaneous clamping of both arteries. The latter is to be avoided if the opposite ICA is diseased or occluded.

With these combined reconstructions, if there is severe contralateral carotid disease or occlusion, even a short period of simultaneous clamping of the ICA and VA is risky. If the VA lesion is in the proximal segment, two alternatives should be considered. For the first a shunt is placed in the proximal CCA and ICA and opened to flow (Figure 10.3). With the ICA perfused by the shunt the proximal VA (or SA) is transposed. Flow is reestablished into the VA (or SA)

by moving the proximal end of the shunt distal to the site of transposition, allowing perfusion through the VA. A standard carotid endarterectomy follows. The second alternative is to reconstruct the VA lesion directly by endarterectomy, SA-to-VA bypass, or transposition of the VA to another SA site and follow, at the same operative session, with a standard carotid endarterectomy with or without shunting.

If the VA needs to be revascularized at its distal level, the shunt is first placed in the carotid and opened to flow (Figure 10.4). Then the distal VA bypass is constructed as described before placing the proximal anastomosis low in the CCA in a segment of the latter excluded by the shunt. The proximal end of the shunt is then moved distally, the VA bypass is opened to flow, and the carotid endarterectomy is

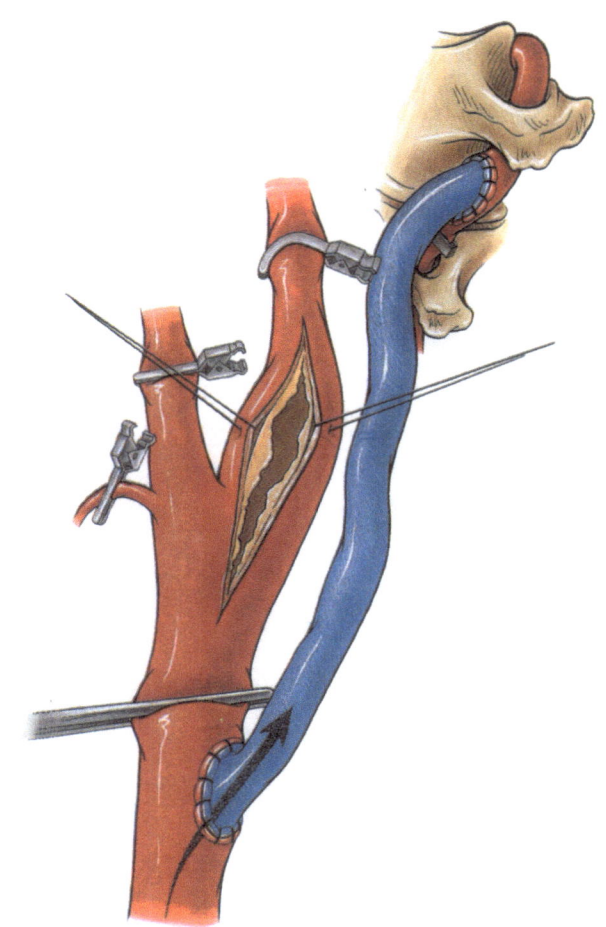

Figure 10.2 Reestablishing flow to the distal vertebral artery before carotid endarterectomy.

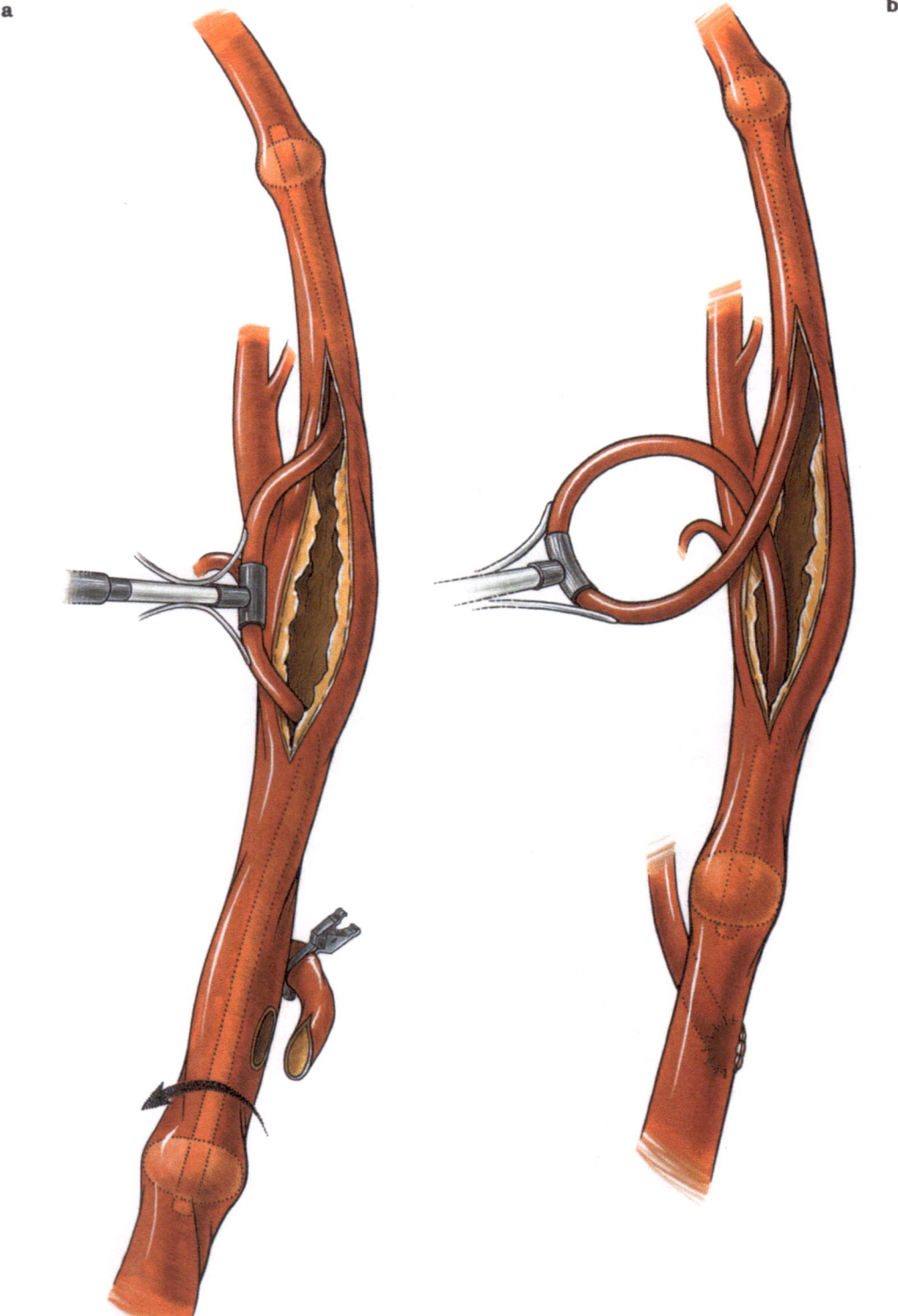

Figure 10.3 Combined internal carotid endarterectomy and proximal vertebral reconstruction in a patient with contralateral internal carotid occlusion. (**a**) Transposition of the vertebral artery is done after ensuring perfusion of the internal carotid artery with a shunt. (**b**) Proximal end of the shunt is moved distal to the site of transposition of the vertebral artery. With the latter open to flow, the carotid endarterectomy is done.

a

b

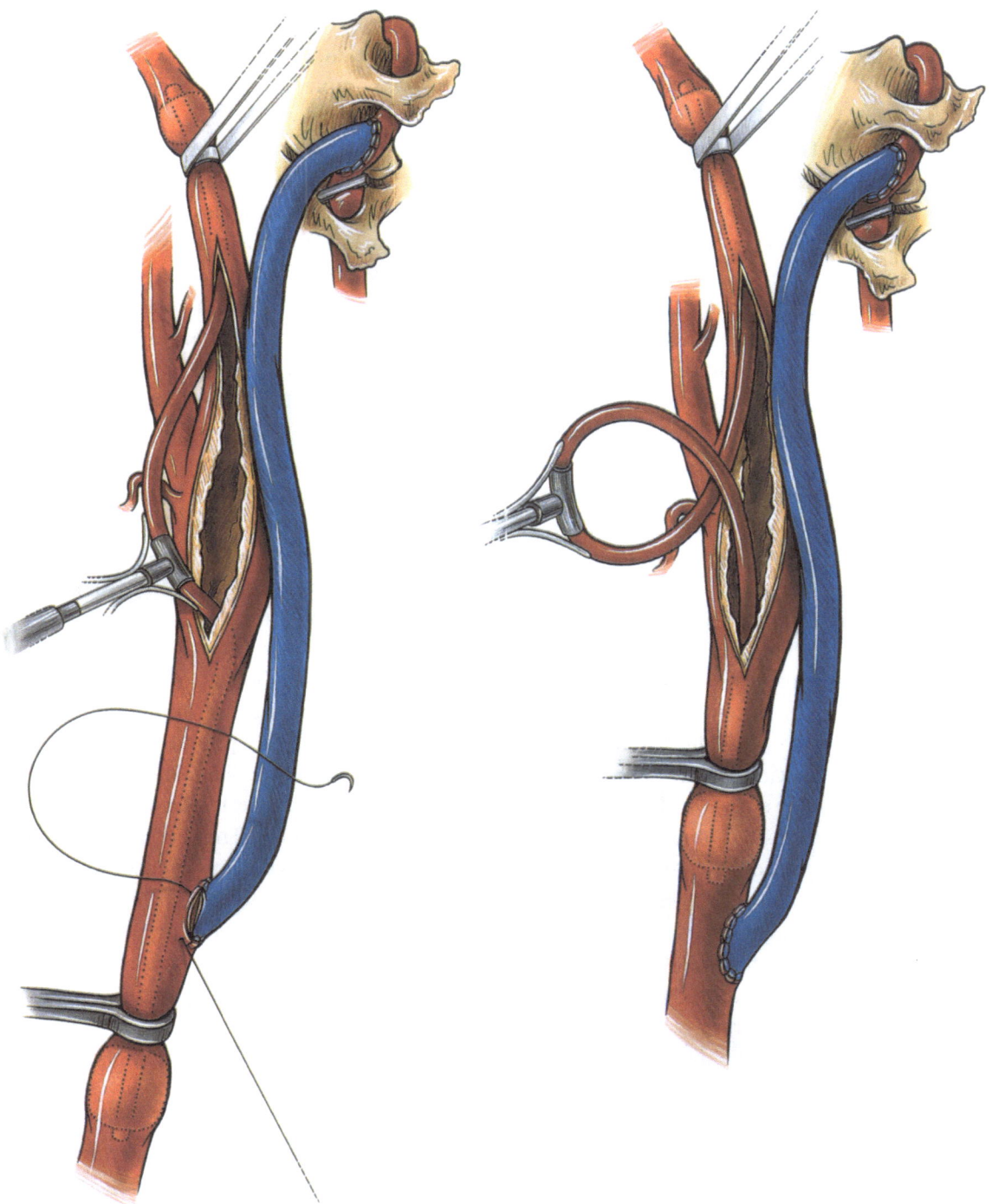

Figure 10.4 Combined carotid endarterectomy and distal vertebral artery reconstruction in the presence of contralateral internal carotid artery occlusion. (**a**) With a shunt placed in the internal carotid artery, the distal vertebral bypass is constructed. (**b**) Proximal end of the shunt is then moved distal to the takeoff of the vertebral artery bypass to allow perfusion of the latter during endarterectomy of the carotid bifurcation.

performed with the protection of the shunt and the functioning VA bypass.

Reconstruction of all Proximal Trunks

Transsternal Reconstruction

For reconstruction of all the branches of the aortic arch, an important strategic decision must be made as to whether a sternotomy incision can be used. In patients in whom a midline sternotomy is feasible, the best repair should also encompass severe lesions of the left SA, even if they are asymptomatic. This maneuver adds little to the complexity of the operation and provides a safe source of inflow for an eventual extrathoracic reconstruction should any of the bypassed trunks occlude in the future. It also provides appropriate inflow for eventual myocardial revascularization using the left internal mammary artery.

Traditionally, access to the left SA from a median sternotomy incision has been thought to be difficult and sometimes impossible. We have found that division of the brachiocephalic vein provides satisfactory exposure of the entire vertical segment of the left SA as well as the SA–VA junction. Other than occasional thrombosis of the left internal jugular or left subclavian veins, division of the brachiocephalic vein has no important consequences. During dissection of the left SA the surgeon should avoid injury to the thoracic duct and to the vagus and phrenic nerves, which are adjacent to the pleura.

In patients with disease involving all the SATs the best alternative is a prosthetic bypass. Three theoretic choices are available: (1) multiple bypasses between the ascending aorta and the individual trunks; (2) a bifurcated bypass inserted in the ascending aorta with one limb to the IA and one to either the left SA or left CCA with the remaining vessel in the left side transposed into the left limb; or (3) sequential bypasses from the ascending aorta to the left- or right-sided arteries, which can take a number of configurations.

Multiple bypasses are impractical. They require separate exclusion clamping of the ascending aorta, and generally there is not enough room in the ascend-

ing aorta to insert all these grafts. In addition, they occupy too much space in the thoracic inlet and may become compressed there or cause tracheal or venous compression.

The configuration of *bifurcated grafts* has the appeal of a ready-to-use prosthesis with a single trunk for the aortic anastomosis and two limbs for the distal anastomoses. Other than this small convenience, their geometry offers mostly disadvantages. Bifurcation tubes are constructed with an area ratio* between the trunk and the limbs that has no counterpart in human anatomy. This ratio is 0.5 for most commercially available bifurcation prostheses. In humans, the normal area ratio in bifurcations of large arteries is always more than 1.0 and continues to increase progressively as the arteries reach the periphery. To achieve anatomic similarity (assuming an area ratio of 1.1, which is common in large arteries) the trunk of a bifurcated prosthesis with limb size 8 should be a size 11 tube rather than the size 16 in which they are manufactured.

In addition, the narrow anterior mediastinum requires an acute angle of implantation lest the trunk of the graft end up pointing forward toward the sternum and kinking. To achieve such an angle, the proximal end of a size 16 prosthetic trunk is beveled in a curved fashion. This cut increases the already large perimeter to be anastomosed by a factor of 1.6 (Figure 10.5). For the aortotomy to accommodate a beveled size 16 tube, it must be approximately 23 mm in length (Figure 10.6), which requires a large bite from the exclusion clamp in the ascending aorta. Such a bite may cause a pressure drop and dangerously increase the left ventricular afterload, and it may not even be feasible in female patients with small ascending aortas.

Another problem with bifurcated prostheses is that their large main trunk, when distended under normal blood pressure, may not fit in the narrow

---

*Area ratio for a bifurcation

$$\beta = \frac{(A_1 + A_2)}{A_0}$$

where A_0, A_1, A_2 are the cross-sectional areas of the trunk and of each branch, respectively.

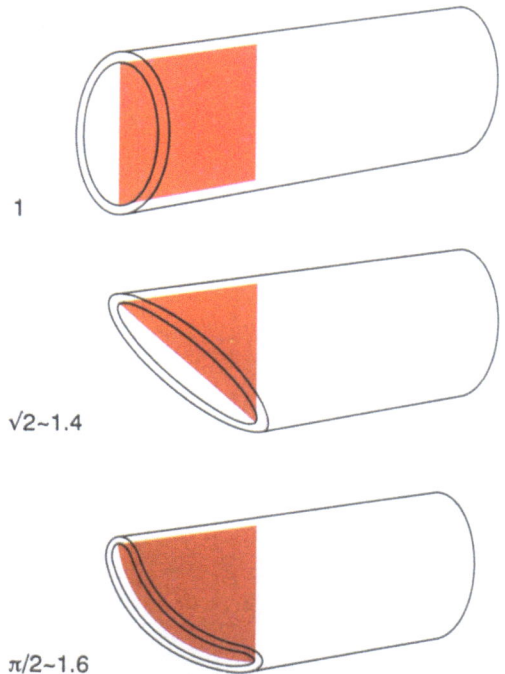

1

√2~1.4

π/2~1.6

Figure 10.5 Change in the length of the cut end of a prosthesis of unit diameter (after a "straight" and, a "curved" beveling).

space between the sternum and the aorta may kink or compress neighboring structures or later become compressed by firbrosis.

Sequential grafting is preferable by far. The main graft is usually from the ascending aorta to the IA or its branches. Our preference is to use a size 10 prosthesis anastomosed proximally to the aorta and distally to the bifurcation of the IA. This configuration requires a smaller arteriotomy in the ascending aorta (and a smaller bite of the exclusion clamp) and does not crowd the anterior mediastinum. The smaller caliber of a size 10 prosthesis also allows use of the thymus as a cover interposed between the prosthesis and the sternum (Figure 10.7). A spatulated size 10 tube is anastomosed so it leaves the ascending aorta at an acute angle, thereby fitting with ease in the substernal space (Figure 10.8). The prosthesis is a polytetrafluorethylene (PTFE) or a knitted Dacron tube that matches the size of the IA distally. To this tube we anastomose a size 8 branch that will replace the left common carotid (Figure 10.9). This arrangement results in an area ratio of 1.6, which is close to the normal anatomic configuration and, in fact, simi-

lar to that found in individuals in whom the left CCA arises as a branch of the IA. The attachment of the size 8 side branch is made within 5 cm of the aortic anastomosis. This placement keeps the takeoff of the side branch low in the mediastinum, mimicking better the course of the left CCA, which it replaces, and lying in the groove between the aortic arch and the trachea just above the stumps of the IA and left CCA. In addition, it does not crowd the retrosternal space. The left SA is then transposed into the conduit that supplies the left carotid system, whether it be a graft (Figure 10.10) or the native CCA.

The branch from the main trunk may also be anastomosed to the left SA, excluding a lesion of the proximal segment of the latter. The left CCA may be transposed to this branch (Figure 10.10). In rare anatomic circumstances a large left SA may receive the prosthesis from the aorta, and the smaller trunks may be anastomosed to it. The length of these side branches to the left-sided arteries must be determined after releasing the sternal retractor to avoid redundancy.

In the rare patient whose plaques are limited to the ostia of the three supraaortic trunks and are contiguous with severe atheroma of the dome of the aortic arch, the repair may be done by *transaortic endarterectomy*, as described by Thevenet.[35] For this procedure cardiopulmonary bypass is instituted between an atrial caval cannula and an ascending aortic or femoral arterial cannula. The patient is cooled to

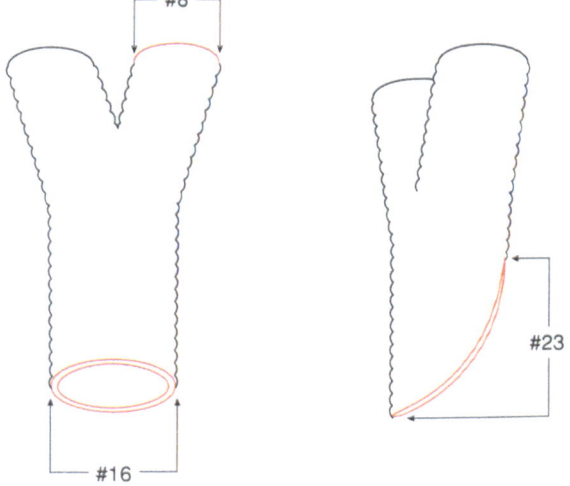

Figure 10.6 Beveling of the prosthesis requires an increase in the size of the aortotomy.

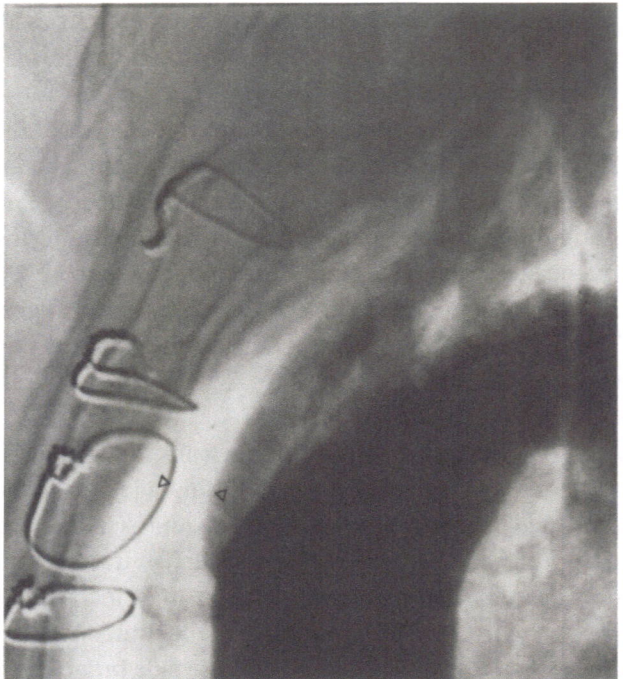

Figure 10.7 Space between the prosthesis and the sternum (between arrowheads) occupied by the thymus.

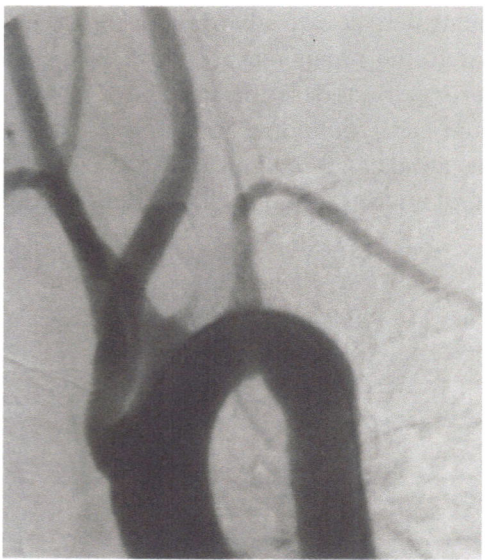

Figure 10.8 Bypass from the ascending aorta to both carotid bifurcations. The graft arises tangentially from the ascending aorta.

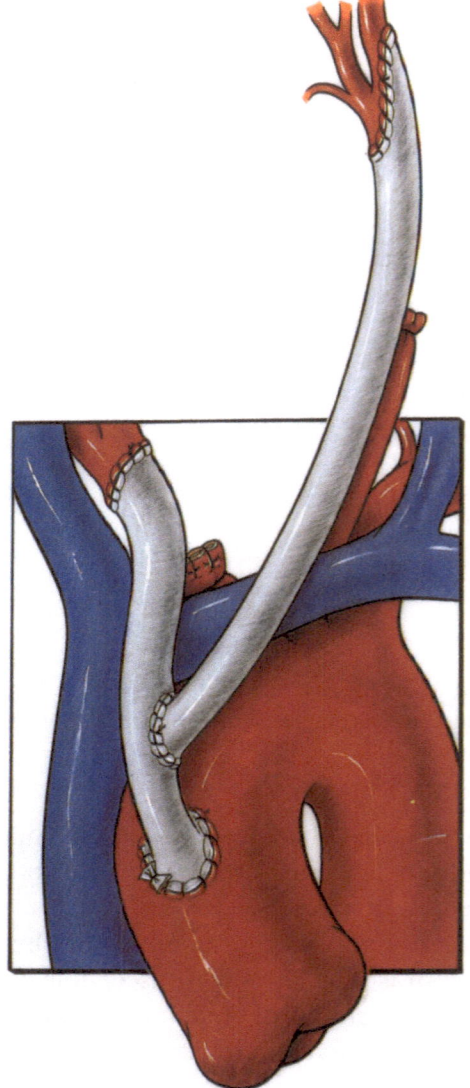

Figure 10.9 Frequent pattern of reconstruction involving the innominate and left common carotid arteries.

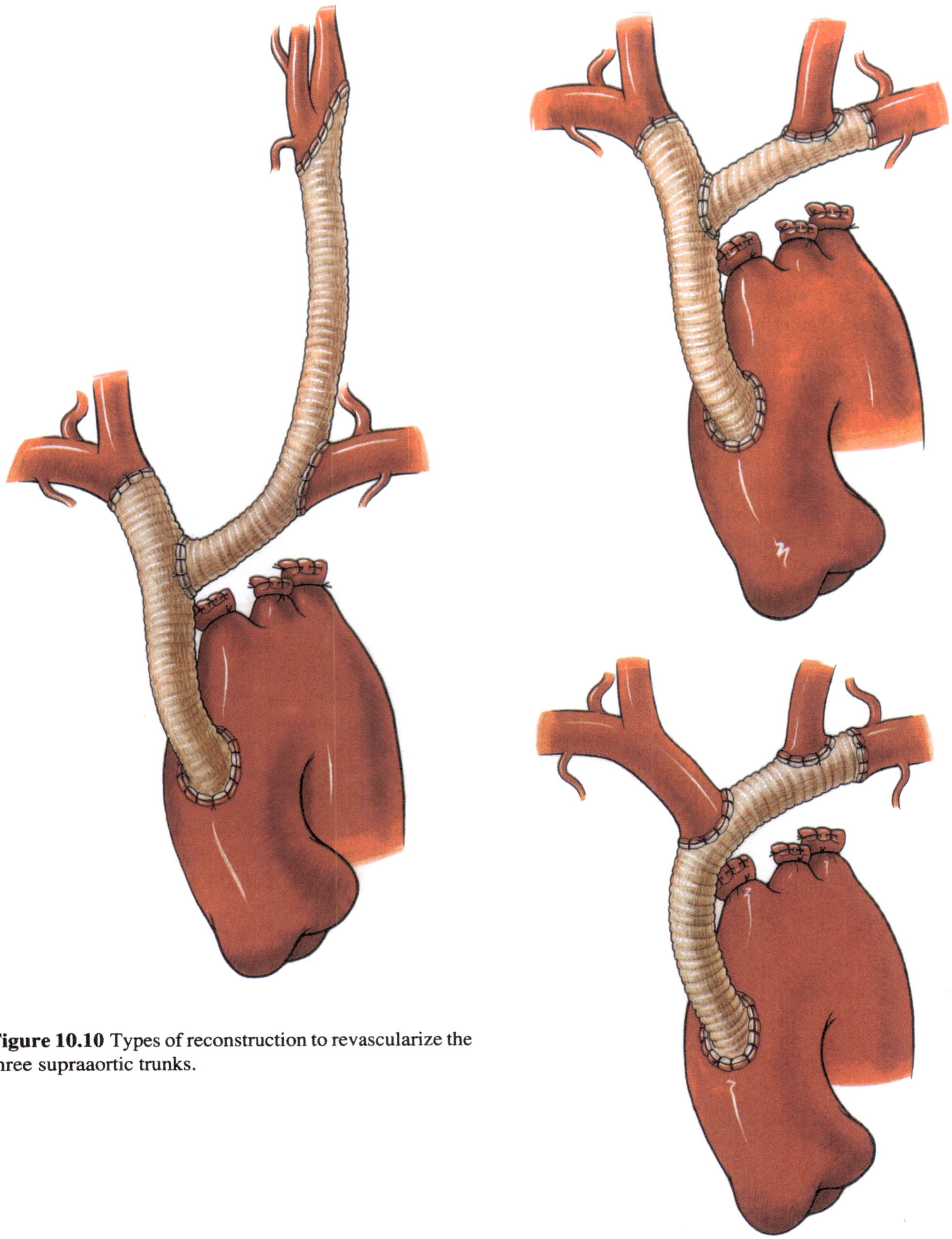

a
b
c

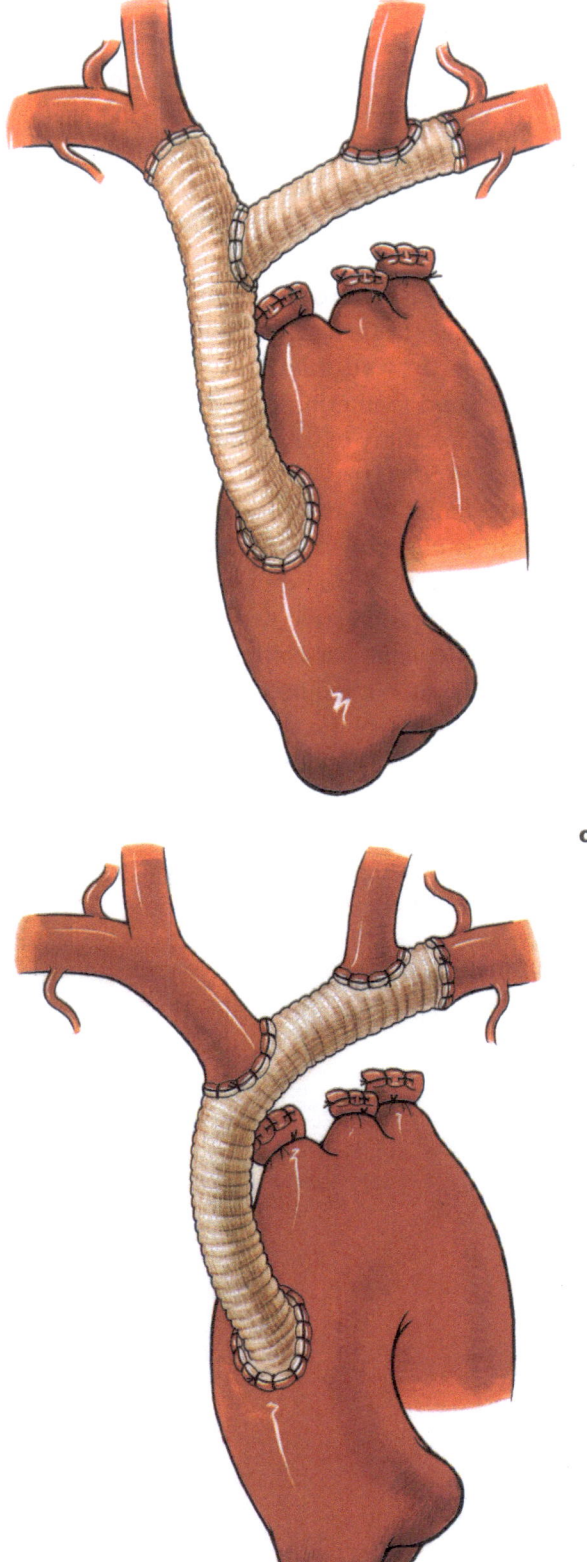

Figure 10.10 Types of reconstruction to revascularize the three supraaortic trunks.

15° to 18°C and then placed in the head-down position under circulatory arrest or low flow circulation (<100 ml/min). The brachiocephalic vein is retracted upward. A curvilinear incision is made in the anterior wall of the aortic arch near the origins of its branches. The endarterectomy is performed first in the arch, then in each branch, using the eversion technique to clear the end of the plaque in each ostium (Figure 10.11). The deep plane of endarterectomy at the level of the external elastic lamina should be avoided, as it leaves an aortic wall that is too thin and does not provide a good feathering off when doing the eversion endarterectomy of the branches of the arch. The aortic intimal edges may have to be tacked using interrupted or more conveniently, running suture. The aortotomy is closed with a running suture, and air is evacuated from the aortic arch with resumption of the circulation and progressive rewarming. Although this elegant technique allows complete repair of all supraaortic trunks without requirement of a graft, it is indicated only in the specific anatomic circumstances described above, and it requires special technical support.

Patients who undergo simultaneous reconstruction of all the supraaortic trunks are at risk of developing the "revascularization syndrome" (see Chapter 11) and should have their blood pressure closely monitored during the postoperative period. Postoperative anticoagulants should be avoided. We use prophylactic steroids, although we recognize that

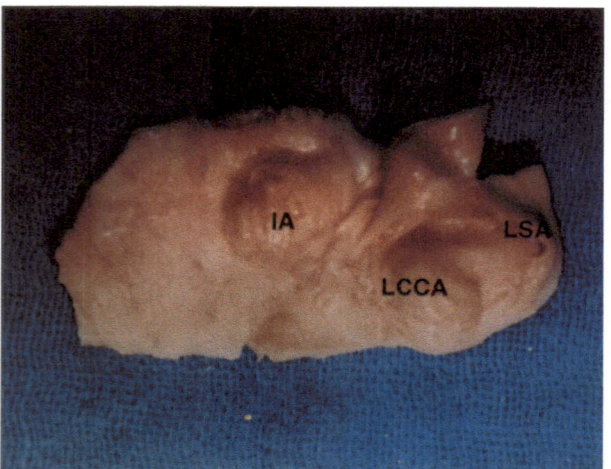

Figure 10.11 Specimen obtained by transaortic endarterectomy. IA = innominate artery; LCCA = left common carotid artery; LSA = left subclavian artery.

evidence for their beneficial effect in preventing this complication is lacking.

Remote Reconstructions

In a few patients with multiple proximal lesions of the SATs, a sternotomy incision may be contraindicated owing to poor cardiopulmonary reserve, previous operations on the ascending aorta (usually an aortocoronary bypass graft), previous sternal infection, or previous irradiation of the mediastinum. In such cases, an alternative is a remote reconstruction using femoroaxillary, femorosubclavian, or femorocarotid bypasses combined with various types of crossover cervical extension. This technique, however, is reserved for the rare elderly and debilitated patient who does not have concomitant aortoiliac occlusive disease. Our technique of choice for good risk patients with an inaccessible ascending aorta is a bypass *originating from the descending thoracic aorta*. It can be done using one of the following techniques.

1. The descending thoracic aorta may be approached *from the left side* (Figure 10.12). The patient is placed in the right lateral position with his neck, left arm, and left hemithorax in the field. An L-shaped cervical incision combines a presternomastoid and a supraclavicular approach, transecting the sternomastoid muscle. The descending thoracic aorta is isolated through the left fourth intercostal space. A 10 mm graft is first anastomosed end-to-side to the descending thoracic aorta and then tunneled through the pleural apex to the supraclavicular fossa, where it passes between the SA and the subclavian vein. In the neck the graft is anastomosed first side-to-side to the distal SA and then end-to-end to the carotid bifurcation. With the chest wound closed, the patient is placed supine; and revascularization of the arteries on the right side of the neck is done by a crossover cervical bypass either in front of or behind the tracheoesophageal column.

2. The descending aorta may also be approached *from the right side* (Figure 10.13). The right chest is slightly elevated, and the descending aorta is isolated low in the thorax between the esophagus and the vertebral bodies through an anterolateral thoracotomy in the right fifth intercostal space. Care should be taken not to open the left pleural space. After anastomosing a 10 mm graft end-to-side to the aorta, the graft is

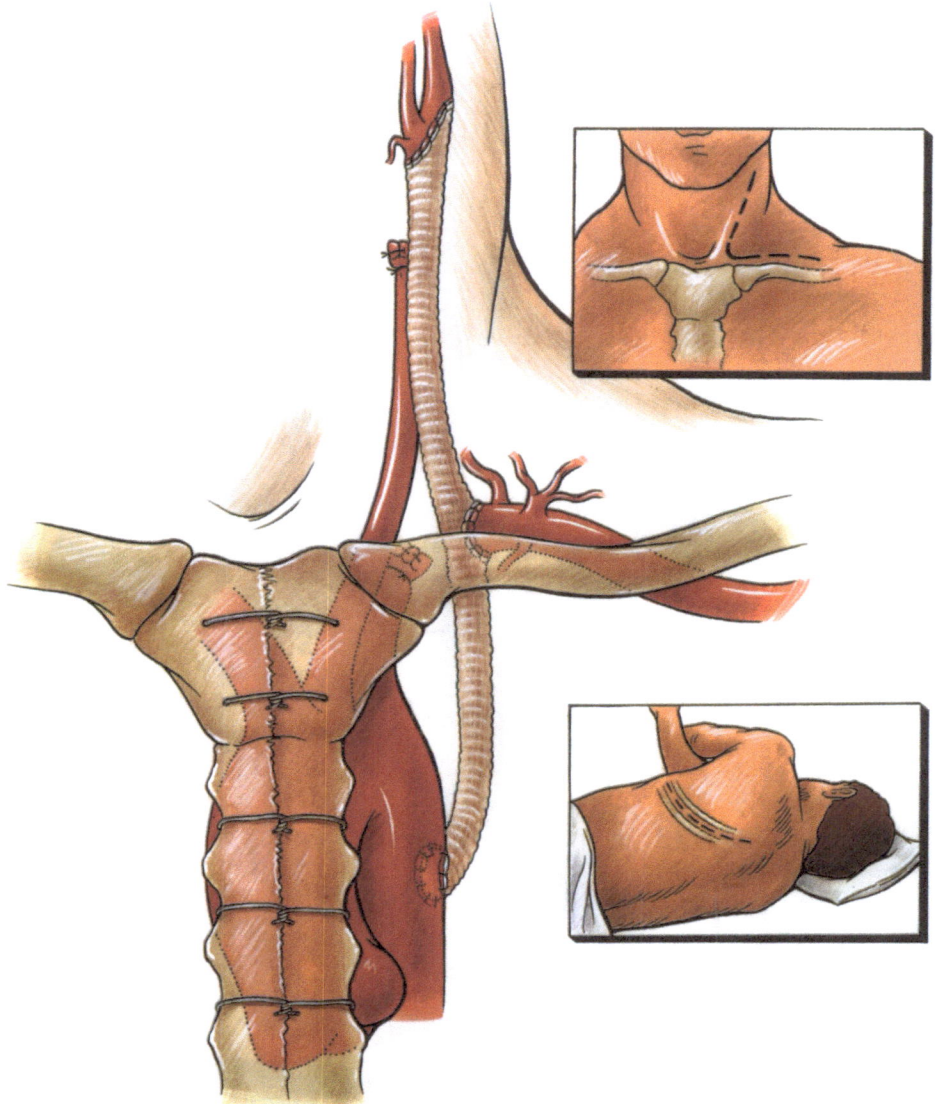

Figure 10.12 Left-sided approach to revascularization of the supraaortic trunks from the descending thoracic aorta.

tunneled in the right hemithorax along the mediastinum and behind the pulmonary pedicle to the right side of the neck, where it can be anastomosed sequentially to the right SA and then to the right carotid bifurcation. With this right-sided approach, it is possible to do the crossover graft to the left side of the neck without having to change the patient's position.

    3. The third option for bringing a bypass to the neck when the ascending aorta cannot be used is to expose the *supraceliac aorta* through an upper median or chevron laparotomy by dividing the crus of the diaphragm. After end-to-side anastomosis to the supraceliac aorta, the graft is tunneled to the right or left side of the neck through an intra- or extrathoracic pathway to perform the distal anastomosis there to the appropriate vessels.

Combined Intrathoracic and Cervical Operations

A carotid stenosis may be associated with proximal lesions of the IA or CCA. Although it may be impossible to ascertain which of the two lesions is responsible for the symptoms, we believe that both should be

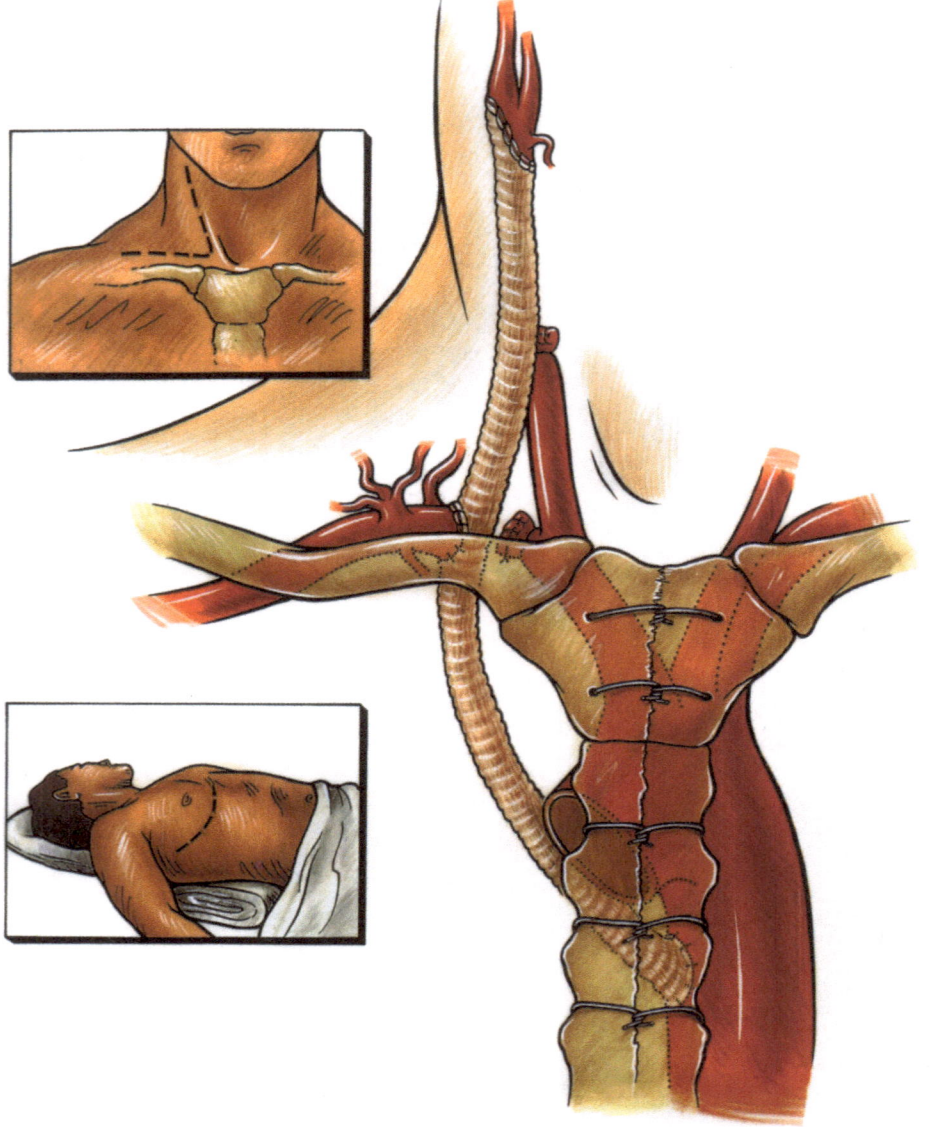

Figure 10.13 Right-sided approach to revascularization of the supraaortic trunks from the descending thoracic aorta.

corrected at the same operation to avoid the consequences of disregarding one of them. The carotid endarterectomy can be done as a separate procedure following proximal reconstruction or when the carotid bulb is prepared for the distal anastomosis of the aortocarotid bypass (see Chapter 7).

We have never seen a case where the simultaneous reconstruction of the proximal supraaortic trunks and distal VA were indicated in the same operation. Should it occur, we would proceed first with the proximal reconstruction and then with the distal VA using a vein graft implanted into the carotid bifurcation supplied by the aortocarotid graft.

Reconstruction of the proximal VA in combination with intrathoracic lesions can be done under the following circumstances: (1) As a part of the endarterectomy of the proximal SA before it is transposed to the left CCA or to a prosthetic limb substituting for it. The endarterectomy of the VA in these circumstances is made easy by an eversion maneuver (see Figure 7.20). (2) If revascularization of the SA is deemed unnecessary or impossible, the VA itself may be transposed into the left CCA or into the bypass substituting for it. (3) On a few occasions we have placed separate venous bypasses from the left side of the ascending aorta to the proximal left VA.

Combined Cerebrovascular and Coronary Artery Reconstruction

Supraaortic Trunks

Previously inserted multiple vein bypasses to the coronary arteries may pose a problem finding a good site to insert a bypass in the ascending aorta, now crowded with the vein grafts. Under these circumstances and unless an endarterectomy of the IA is feasible, alternative sources of inflow as described above must be sought or the graft may have to be anastomosed to the right side of the ascending aorta.

Because of the frequent coexistence of coronary artery disease we advocate routine coronary arteriography for atherosclerotic patients in whom an intrathoracic reconstruction of the SAT is planned. If both diseases are present, they should be corrected at the same operation (Figure 10.14). This practice avoids the difficulty of having to do a later myocardial revascularization through a secondary transsternal approach.

When a patient has severe occlusive disease of all SAT, the risk for stroke during cardiopulmonary bypass is increased. If the SAT disease involves *only the IA* and can be corrected by endarterectomy, it is done first to ensure the best blood supply to the brain during cardiopulmonary bypass. If the IA lesion is to be corrected by means of a bypass but the other trunks are patent, myocardial revascularization is done first. The proximal anastomosis of the bypass to the ascending aorta is done in the usual place after the proximal anastomoses of the vein grafts are completed.

In patients with severe disease of *all trunks* and of the coronary arteries, one must ensure at least one major avenue of brain inflow before starting cardiopulmonary bypass. If the anatomic setup permits, the main prosthetic graft (usually to the IA or right CCA bifurcation) is anastomosed higher than usual in the aorta, allowing room to cross-clamp later the ascending aorta below it during cardiopulmonary bypass. After the proximal aortic anastomosis is completed, a left-sided branch is sewn onto the main graft, the distal anastomosis to the IA or right carotid bifurcation is completed, and the bypass is open to flow. The

a 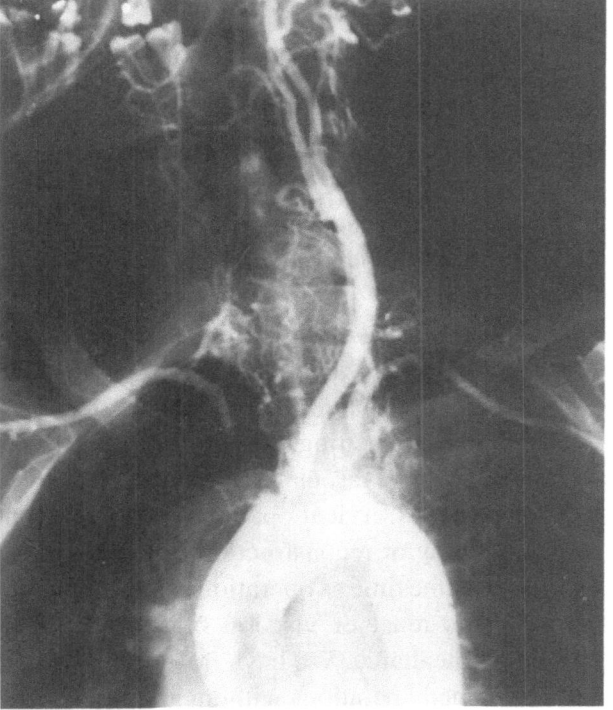 b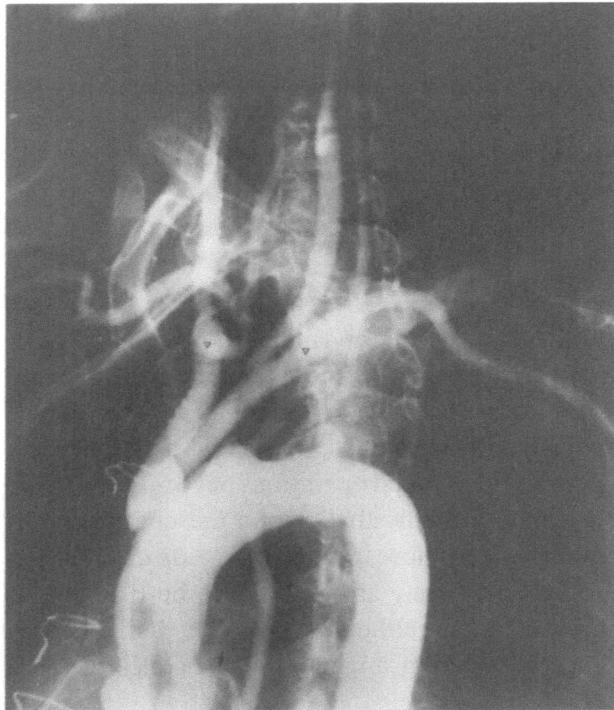

Figure 10.14 (a) This patient had proximal atherosclerosis of all supraaortic trunks together with left main coronary artery disease. **(b)** Postoperative arteriogram shows multiple reconstructions and a vein bypass graft to the left anterior descending artery.

coronary arteries are then revascularized, with the proximal anastomosis being done to the remaining ascending aorta or to lateral aspect of the prosthetic tube, or else anastomosing two or more veins as branches, leaving only a single proximal vein anastomosis to do. While the patient is being rewarmed, the left-sided SATs are revascularized by completing the distal anastomosis of the branch extension(s) previously sewn onto the main graft.

Patients who are candidates for coronary artery bypass may have atheromatous disease in the ostia of the SAT contiguous with extensive disease in the dome of the aorta. This anatomic setup is a good one for the technique of transaortic endarterectomy under hypothermia and circulatory arrest. The distal anastomoses of the coronary bypasses are done first while the patient is being cooled to 15° to 18°C. After circulatory arrest and transaortic endarterectomy, cardiopulmonary bypass is resumed; and the proximal coronary graft anastomoses are completed while the patient is being rewarmed.

Patients scheduled for coronary revascularization using one or both internal mammary arteries may have disease of the SA. If the latter is isolated, transposition of the SA into the undiseased left CCA is the first step in the operation. If severe lesions of the other branches of the arch are present, they are reconstructed before the coronary revascularization, as already described.

Carotid Artery

Much has been written and more has been said regarding the management of concomitant coronary and carotid artery disease. It appears to us that the evidence at hand does not support a dogmatic policy in this matter. Combined operations have the advantage of avoiding two anesthetics and the complications from the lesion whose treatment is being delayed. On the other hand, they are reported to be riskier than staged operations, although we wonder if differences in patient selection might be responsible for these results.

In general, our choice is to do a combined operation when there is a severe unilateral carotid lesion. Patients with severe bilateral carotid lesions present a special problem, as simultaneous bilateral carotid endarterectomy is probably to be avoided. If the coronary artery disease is stable, we prefer to operate first on the more diseased carotid artery and then do the coronaries together with the second carotid endarterectomy a few days later. If the coronary disease is unstable, we do first a simultaneous repair of the most critically diseased ICA and of the coronaries, with the second carotid dealt with a few weeks later.

The combined technique does not present any serious problem. The carotid bifurcation is dissected during harvesting of the saphenous vein. In stable patients the carotid endarterectomy is done first, followed by median sternotomy and myocardial revascularization. In patients with unstable coronary artery disease this sequence is reversed, with the carotid endarterectomy being done after opening the chest, during bypass, or after rewarming. If a carotid patch angioplasty is necessary, one should avoid a prosthetic patch because of its potential for bleeding under the full heparinization required for cardiopulmonary bypass. A small segment of the harvested saphenous vein is usually available for patching.

Combined Cerebrovascular and Aortic/Peripheral Vascular Reconstruction

Combined transthoracic and transabdominal operations pose hazards mainly from respiratory complications and should be done only in young patients who are good surgical risks. In these patients reconstruction of the SAT and repair of abdominal aortic disease, either atherosclerotic or inflammatory, can be done in the same setting. Combining transthoracic operations with revascularization of the legs adds little morbidity. Cervical operations such as carotid endarterectomy or reconstruction of the VA can be done at the same time as operations on the abdominal aorta and its renal or visceral branches or in the femoropopliteal area. We have done more than 100 such combined operations without additional neurologic morbidity, while sparing each of these patients and the health care system the trauma and costs of an additional operation.

11

Special Surgical Problems

Trauma

Trauma to the arteries supplying the head may result from upper thoracic or neck injuries. Blunt or, more often, penetrating trauma causing acute, external, intrapleural, mediastinal or cervical hemorrhage is an obvious indication for emergency surgery. Some patients, however, have contained hemorrhage with formation of false aneurysm, occlusion of the artery, or an arteriovenous fistula. Such cases require further diagnostic evaluation, which is different for penetrating and blunt trauma.

Penetrating injuries to the neck are traditionally divided into three zones (Figure 11.1), according to the site of injury: zone 1, below the clavicle; zone 2, from the clavicle to the angle of the jaw; and zone 3, above the angle of the jaw. This rough, topographic description corresponds generally to three types of arterial injury requiring specific management steps. We say "generally" because it is obvious that the trajectory of a missile is not defined by its point of entrance.

Injuries to zone 1 are often associated with trauma to the supraaortic trunks. After obtaining airway control and ensuring that the patient is hemodynamically stable, an arteriogram is obtained to assess the presence and to define the location and

extent of the injuries to the SAT. With injuries to zone 2 we do not use arteriography because surgical exploration is a straightforward procedure. Those who advocate arteriography in a stable patient with wounds in zone 2 have shown that in selective instances an exploration can be averted provided injuries to other vital structures (pharynx, esophagus, larynx, or trachea) are excluded by appropriate studies. On the other hand, patients may also deteriorate

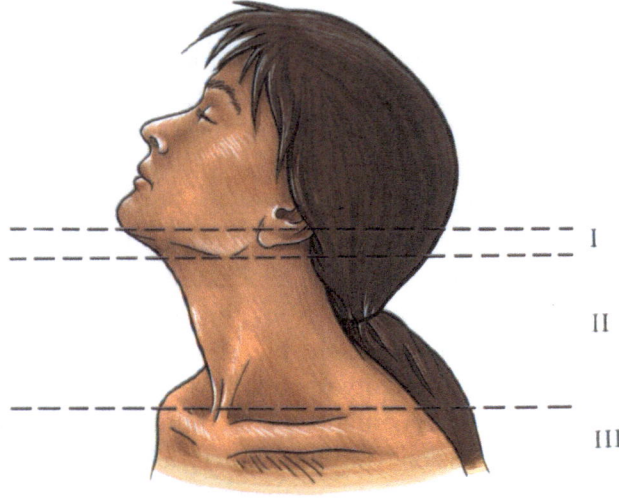

Figure 11.1 Penetrating trauma to the neck may be classified into three zones of injury.

rapidly during arteriography, which, with midneck injuries is unlikely to provide unexpected or new positive findings. For zone 3 injuries, once airway control is obtained and if the patient has no neurologic symptoms and is stable, we recommend evaluation by arteriography to define the accessibility of the injured artery. Patients with intact neurologic status, no evidence of bleeding, and moderate-sized hematomas are best watched if the arteriogram is negative. Exploration of the skull base is more complex and risky than of the midneck.

The indications for arteriography in stable patients with *blunt trauma* to the neck or upper chest are based on the presence of various findings, including a history of deceleration trauma, cervical hematoma, mediastinal widening suggesting hemomediastinum, central neurologic deficit, brachial plexus palsy, and loss of pulses in the neck or upper extremity with or without evidence of ischemia. Isolated first rib or sternal fractures are no longer indications for arteriography.

Management of Trauma to the Supraaortic Trunks

For acute intrathoracic bleeding due to injury to the SAT, if a preoperative arteriogram is not feasible the choice of approach may be life-saving. The patient is draped, exposing the entire neck and chest (Figure 11.2). An arterial line is inserted in the radial artery contralateral to the injury or in the femoral artery. Both thighs are prepared for harvesting saphenous vein grafts if a concomitant injury of the carotid or vertebral artery is suspected. In most patients a median sternotomy is preferable. In combination with a small cervical incision, it allows rapid exposure of the IA and its branches and of the left CCA. Control of hemorrhage from the left SA can be difficult even through a median sternotomy, particularly if the injury involves the proximal portion of the SA. In the latter situation, one should extend the midsternal incision with an anterolateral thoracotomy. The upper mediastinum can then be compressed from within the pleural cavity to obtain control of the proximal left SA, being careful of the vagus and

phrenic nerves, which run close to it. In stable patients with isolated blunt trauma to the proximal left SA, demonstrated by preoperative arteriography, the incision of choice is a left posterolateral thoracotomy.

Once control has been obtained, repair of the lesions in the SAT does not pose any special difficulty. Penetrating injuries can often be handled by lateral repair or end-to-end anastomosis. With more destructive lesions a venous or prosthetic interposition graft or a transposition may be needed.

The most frequent lesion following blunt trauma to the SAT is subadventitial disruption of the IA at its origin from the aortic arch (Figure 11.3). It presents as a hematoma around the origin of the artery. The best solution is to use the proximal ascending aorta to insert a prosthetic bypass to the distal IA. This procedure should be carried out before entering the hematoma that surrounds the origin of the IA. Once the bypass is open to flow, the origin of the IA is isolated by lateral exclusion-clamping of the aortic arch and is obliterated with sutures using a Teflon felt strip reinforcing both sides. Cardiopulmonary bypass is not needed unless there is an associated rupture of the aortic arch.

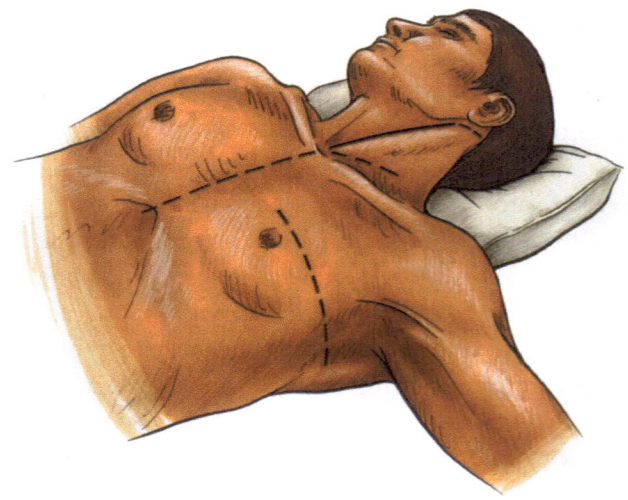

Figure 11.2 Incisions used after penetrating trauma of the vessels of the chest and neck. Prolongation of the midsternotomy into the neck (shown here on the left) can be made into either side.

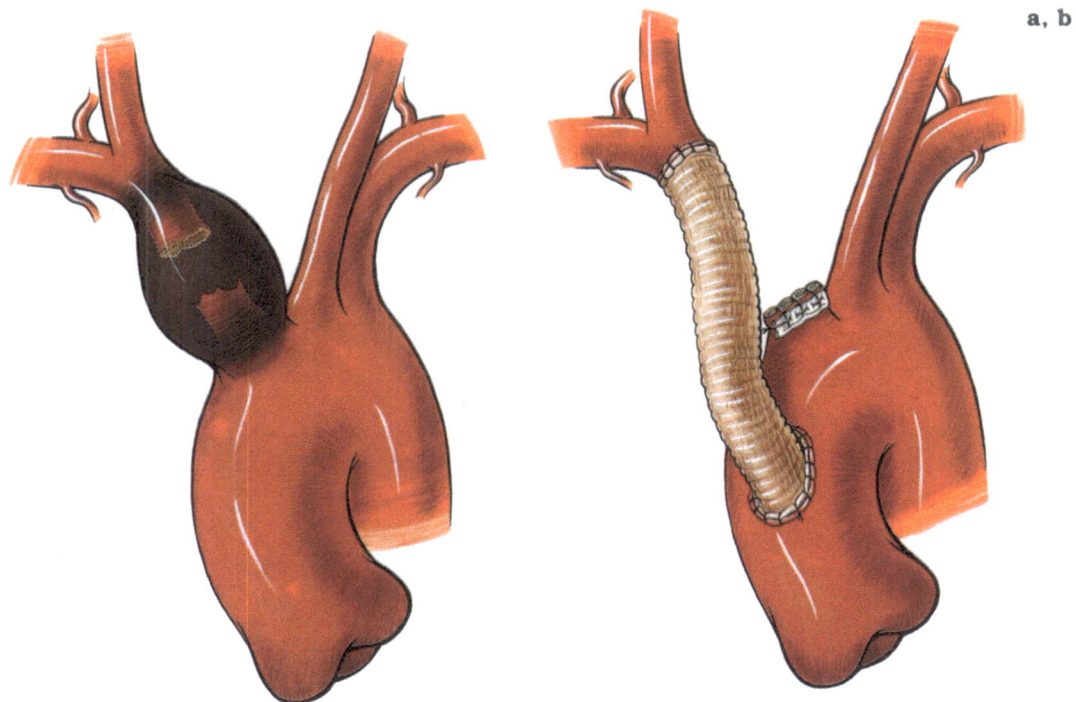

Figure 11.3 Repair of a subadventitial disruption of the innominate artery (**a**). Construction of an aorto-innominate bypass before entering the hematoma to close the aortic defect (**b**).

Management of Trauma to the Carotid Artery

Patients with suspected injuries to the carotid artery require immediate control of the airway and hemodynamic stability. If there is active bleeding from the neck wound, the latter can be controlled by manual pressure while the endotracheal intubation is performed. A minimal neurologic assessment should be made, stating the level of consciousness and if the patient can move the extremities and facial muscles. It is important to remember that the neurologic deficits present may be due not only to carotid embolization or thrombosis but also to associated injuries to the brachial plexus, brain, spinal cord, or cranial nerves.

Two large-bore intravenous lines are started, with one usually placed in the femoral vein. Subclavian lines are not to be used on the side or in the path of injury. Patients who are stable and neurologically intact and do not have tense, expanding hematomas or bleeding should undergo esophagoscopy if the trajectory of the missile suggests coexistence of an esophageal injury.

In patients with zone 3 injuries where the arteriogram indicates a high-lying carotid injury, it is preferable to do an nasotracheal intubation, which allows further anterior displacement of the jaw during exploration of the high cervical ICA (Figure 11.4).

With the exception of patients who are in a coma, those with a neurologic deficit who have a patent ICA artery are best managed by reconstruction if the latter is technically feasible. We have found no convincing evidence, either in the literature or in our own experience, that carotid reconstruction should be avoided in patients with acute carotid trauma even if they present with gross neurologic deficits (except coma). Sometimes the severity of the neurologic deficit is difficult to ascertain because of high blood alcohol levels or shock.

The handling of *injuries to the CCA, carotid bifurcation, and proximal ICA* (up to the digastric muscle) is straightforward (Figure 11.5). If the bleeding injury to the CCA is low in the neck and one anticipates difficulty obtaining proximal control, the neck incision is prolonged with a median sternotomy. Small injuries of the CCA, such as those caused by a knife wound, may be repaired by lateral arteriorrhaphy or by resection and anastomosis. Freeing of a mildly tortuous CCA by dissecting above and below the

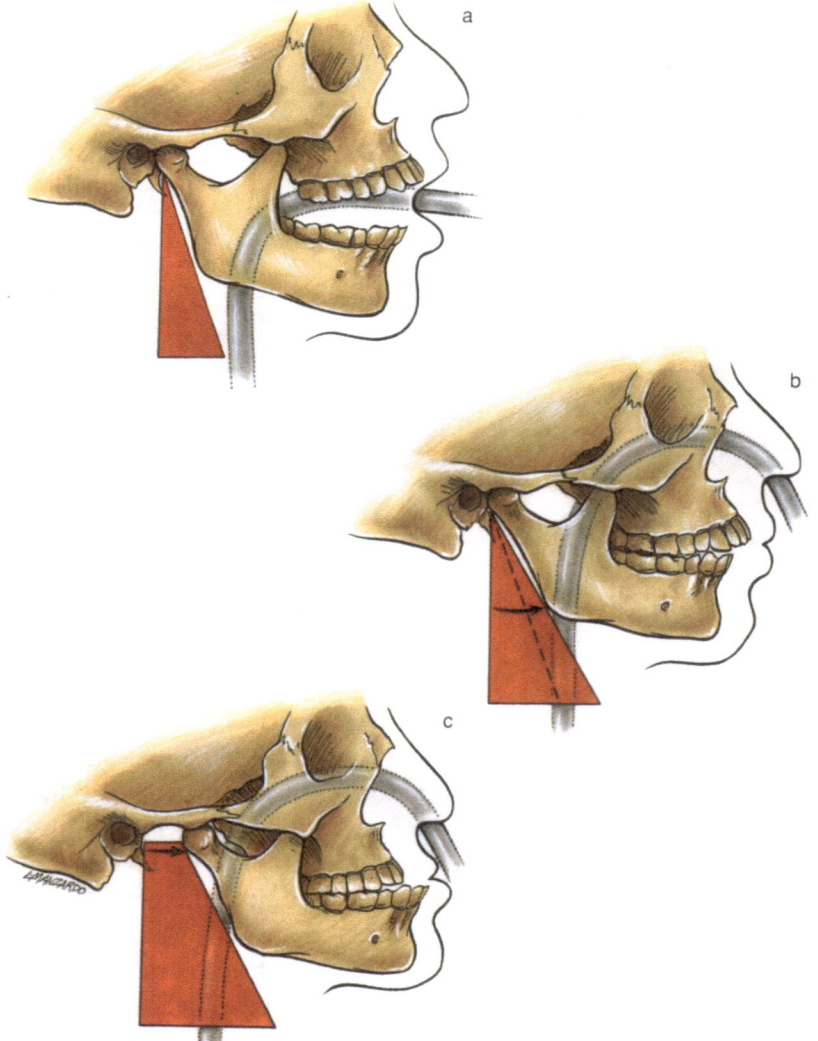

Figure 11.4 Nasotracheal intubation improves the approach to the high cervical ICA. The switch from oral (**a**) to nasotracheal (**b**) intubation results in anterior displacement of the angle of the jaw (more so in edentulous people). Anterior subluxation (**c**) provides additional access to the high cervical carotid.

cross-clamped area may permit a direct anastomosis to bridge a short defect. If there is any tension on the anastomosis or if the defect is too long to be repaired in this manner, the CCA is replaced with a saphenous vein graft. When there is a substantial mismatch in size between the CCA and the vein graft, the repair can be made by closing both ends of the CCA and bridging the defect with the vein graft anastomosed end-to-side to the CCA stumps. The repair can be made with a PTFE prosthesis if the CCA injury is extensive, provided there is no associated tracheal or esophageal injury, and the wound is not contaminated. If there has been contamination, the gap in the CCA can be bridged with a segment of superficial

femoral artery and the latter is replaced with a segment of polytetrafluorethylene (PTFE). The surgical field and instruments used to retrieve the femoral artery graft and to replace it with PTFE should be separate from the neck field which presumably is contaminated. Alternatively, a low CCA injury near its origin can be repaired by ligating the proximal stump of the CCA and anastomosing the distal portion of the CCA to the neighboring SA.

Injuries to the carotid bifurcation or to the proximal cervical ICA are repaired by lateral arteriorraphy or venous bypass grafting. Control of bleeding from the ICA below the digastric muscle is usually straightforward. Digital pressure over the bleeding site may permit dissection above and below to loop the vessel prior to clamping. Back-bleeding from the ICA may also be controlled by compressing the artery against the transverse process of C1.

If at the time of exploration the carotid artery is thrombosed at the site of injury but after removing a thrombus plug at the site of injury there is brisk anterograde and retrograde bleeding, the artery is reconstructed. No effort should be made to obtain retrograde flow by manipulation of balloon catheters

into the distal ICA. If spontaneous, brisk back-bleeding does not occur after removing a thrombus plug, ligation is the most sensible way to handle the thrombosed ICA. In patients who have an associated pharyngeal or esophageal injury of some duration, where contamination of the neck is likely, the ICA may be ligated or grafted with autogenous vein (saphenous) or artery (superficial femoral). Patients in whom the ICA is ligated are placed on intravenous heparin for 5 days (if the concomitant injuries permit)

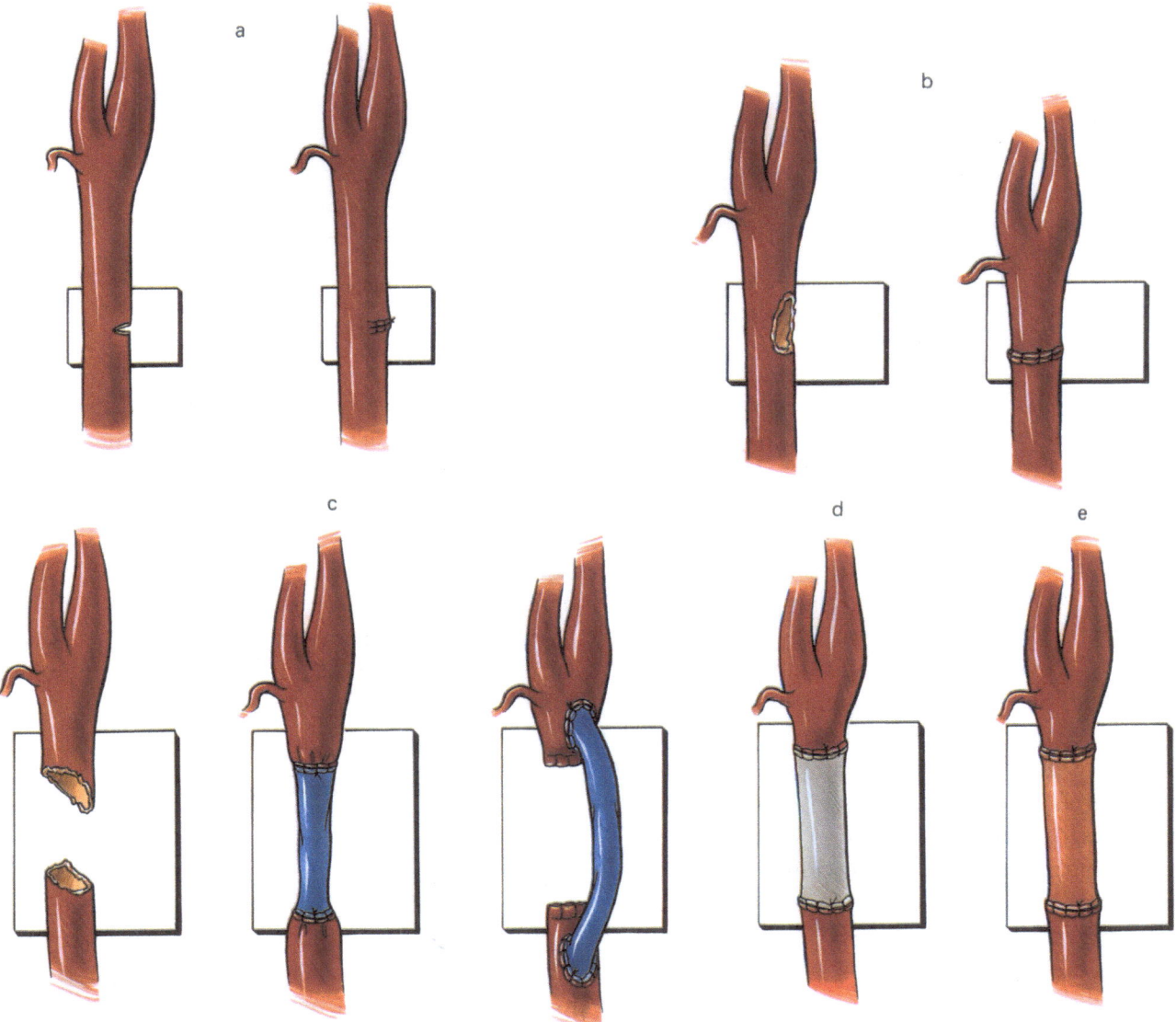

Figure 11.5 Alternatives for repair of common carotid artery injuries (**a**) Lateral repair. (**b**) End-to-end anastomosis. (**c**) Interposition and bypass vein graft. (**d**) Prosthetic replacement. (**e**) Autograft of superficial femoral artery. (The latter is replaced with a PTFE prosthesis.)

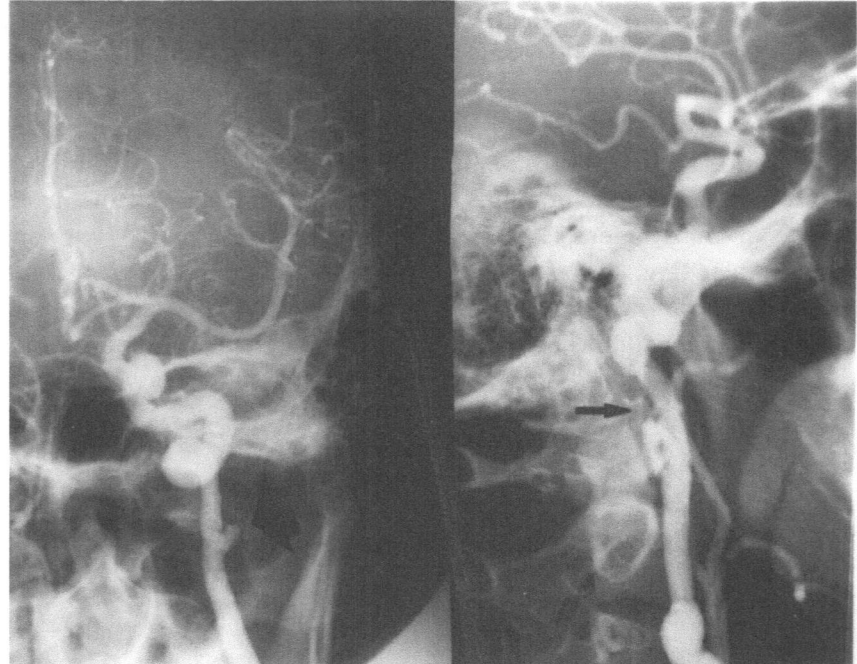

Figure 11.6 **(a)** Injury to the internal carotid artery above the digastric muscle. **(b)** This injured segment was replaced with a vein graft that extends to the upper level of C1 (arrow).

to minimize the possibility of progression of the thrombus into the intracranial branches of the ICA. Patients with gross neurologic deficits should not be given heparin treatment even if the carotid is ligated.

Injuries to the distal cervical ICA (above the digastric muscle) are difficult to control. Proximal CCA or ICA control is obtained by clamping the corresponding vessel. Digital pressure of the distal cervical ICA over C1 may provide temporary distal control. The digastric muscle is divided. The occipital artery, which crosses the ICA path below the posterior edge of the digastric, is also divided. In high-lying injuries of the ICA (Figure 11.6), when the intention is to reconstruct the vessel, it may be easier to do so from behind rather than in front of the internal jugular vein (see Chapter 8). In high-lying carotid injuries where it is impossible to obtain distal control, suture ligation is advisable.

If a distal segment of normal ICA is accessible through the neck, the carotid is repaired by resection and grafting, preferably using a saphenous vein. The ICA is approached from behind the jugular vein and is opened at C1 through a longitudinal arteriotomy.

Thrombus is cleared by a short Fogarty catheter that must never reach the intracavernous carotid. If brisk back-bleeding is obtained after the thrombus is cleared and if the intima of the distal cervical ICA is intact, plans are made for a CCA-to-distal cervical ICA saphenous vein bypass graft. The ICA is ligated immediately below the distal anastomosis of the graft. A completion arteriogram of the ICA is a good way to ensure that these difficult reconstructions are technically satisfactory.

Management of Trauma to the Vertebral Artery

With the exception of the V1 segment, where active bleeding is the usual presentation, penetrating VA injuries have a tendency toward spontaneous hemostasis and formation of a false aneurysm or, more often, an arteriovenous fistula. These abnormalities can appear either early or after an interval following trauma. The management of arteriovenous fistulas is outlined later in this chapter.

Patients presenting with *penetrating injuries*

with active bleeding are best explored immediately through a generous sternomastoid incision. It is only at this point that the surgeon can determine if the VA is the bleeding source and whether the injury involves the first or second segment.

Injuries to the first segment of the VA (Figure 11.7) may also involve the neighboring vertebral vein, and their control is straightforward. The sympathetics may have been damaged before or may be damaged during the operation with a resulting Horner syndrome. The injured artery is ligated if it is small and has a good back-flow. Care must be taken with the proximal ligature if it is made near the vertebral origin. The SA wall is particularly thin and may be torn. We prefer to close the proximal end of the VA with fine, 6-0 polypropylene suture. After control of the vertebral vein and other associated lesions, the field is checked for a lymphatic leak. If found, usually on the left side, the thoracic duct is doubly ligated. If a patient has a large VA, we recom-mend its reconstruction using a saphenous vein graft from the SA or CCA or transposing it to the latter should there be enough length of VA available.

If the injury to the VA involves its second segment, the artery is approached by mobilization of the carotid medially and exposure of the transverse processes covered by the insertions of the anterior scalene muscle. The artery is difficult to isolate directly at the bleeding point, and placing large, occluding suture bites at this level risks injury to the neighboring brachial plex-us or creation of an arterio-venous fistula. It is more prac-tical to control bleeding with direct pressure while the transverse processes above and below the point of bleeding are unroofed to electively ligate the artery above and below the point of injury. Tamponade, unipolar cautery, bone wax, and elevating the head are all helpful in controlling venous bleeding from the transverse process and from vertebral veins around the artery. We prefer to reconstruct the distal VA at the

Figure 11.7 Repair of proximal vertebral artery injuries (**a**) by ligation (**b**) or grafting (**c**) from the adjacent subclavian or carotid artery.

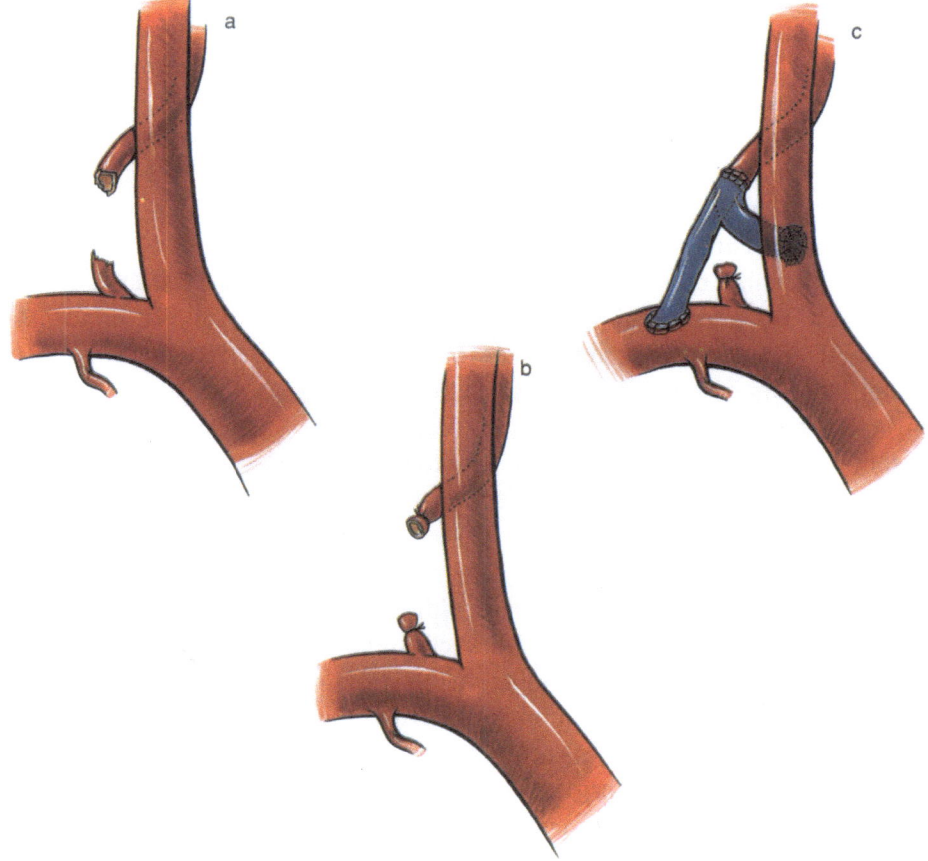

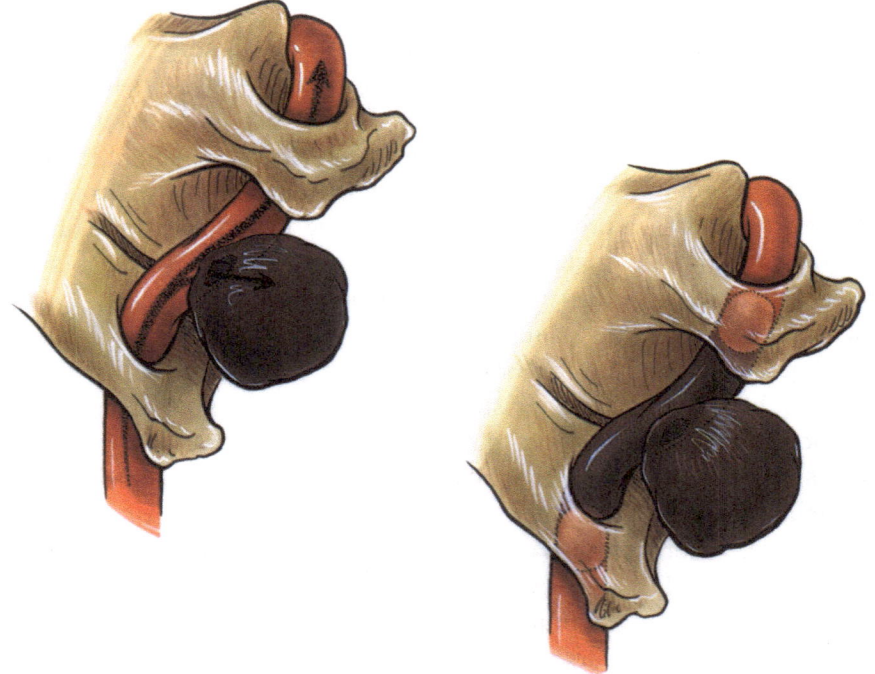

Figure 11.8 False aneurysm of the vertebral artery occluded with the double balloon technique.

C1–C2 level in patients who have injured a large dominant artery.

In patients with penetrating injuries and a stable or slowly expanding hematoma without active bleeding from the first or second segment of the VA, we do an arteriogram. It identifies the site of injury, ensures the adequacy of the opposite VA, and, at the same time, allows an attempt to occlude the injured artery with a detachable balloon. This technique, however, is not always successful in the VA, where after proximal occlusion brisk retrograde bleeding may occur from its distal end. If possible, a balloon is passed distal to the bleeding point first (Figure 11.8). A second, more proximal balloon, should then stop the bleeding. If it fails to do so, direct exploration is mandatory.

Blunt trauma to the VA in any segment usually results in intramural dissection with or without occlusion of the artery. The diagnosis of dissection is often made during the workup of a vertebrobasilar stroke or TIA caused by embolization into the posterior circulation. In these patients arteriography permits assessment of the feasibility of surgical correction. Reconstruction, however, is often contraindicated either because the patient has a severe neurologic deficit or because it is technically impossible owing to the intracranial extension of the dissection or occlusion of the VA. In lesions below C2, a distal bypass of the VA with exclusion of the proximal artery has worked well in some cases.

Aneurysmal Disease

Aneurysms of the Supraaortic Trunks

Resection of *aneurysms of the first portion of the left SA* requires a left thoracotomy (Figure 11.9). The usual technique includes partial exclusion clamping of the aorta around the origin of the left SA, lateral aortorraphy between two Teflon felt strips, and an aortosubclavian bypass.

For large aneurysms extending to the base of the neck, it may be wise to dissect the first and second portion of the SA through a supraclavicular approach first. If the VA originates low or within the aneurysm (Figure 11.10), the artery is transposed to the CCA. Preliminary transposition of the left SA to the CCA is

Figure 11.9 Repair of aneurysms of the left subclavian artery (**a**) limited to the prevertebral segment using aorta to left subclavian artery bypass followed by closure of the aneurysmal neck (**b & c**).

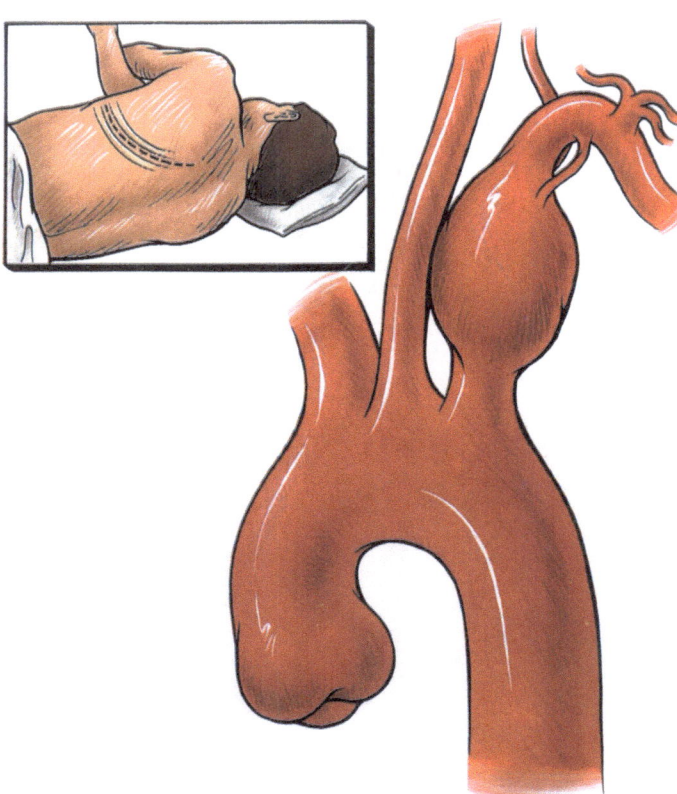

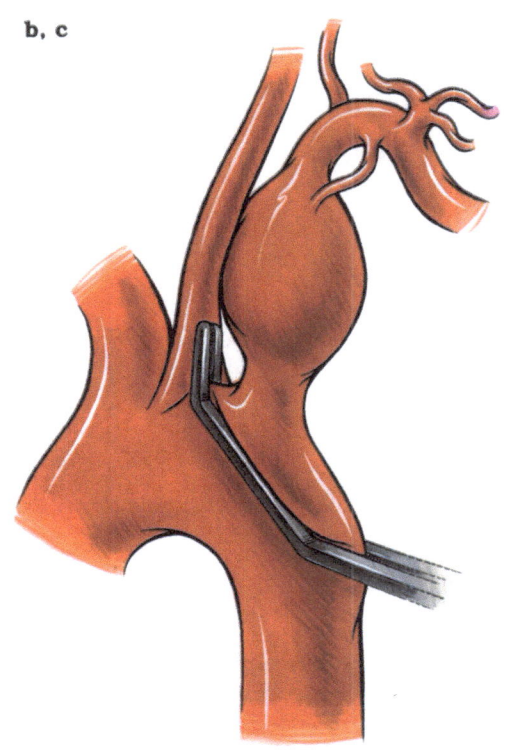

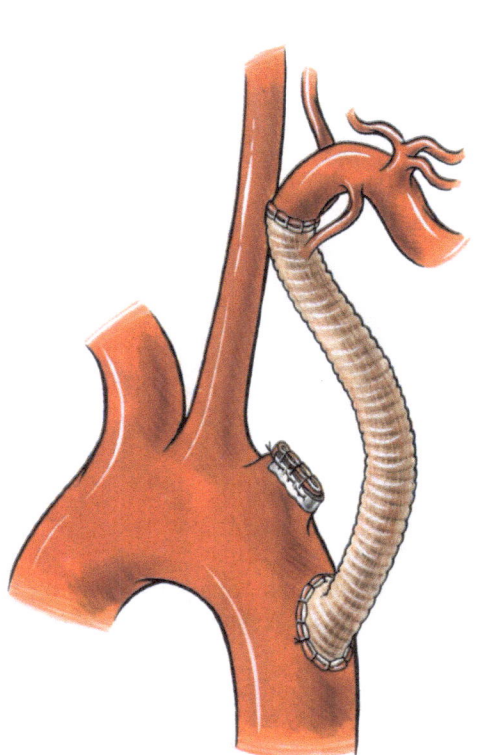

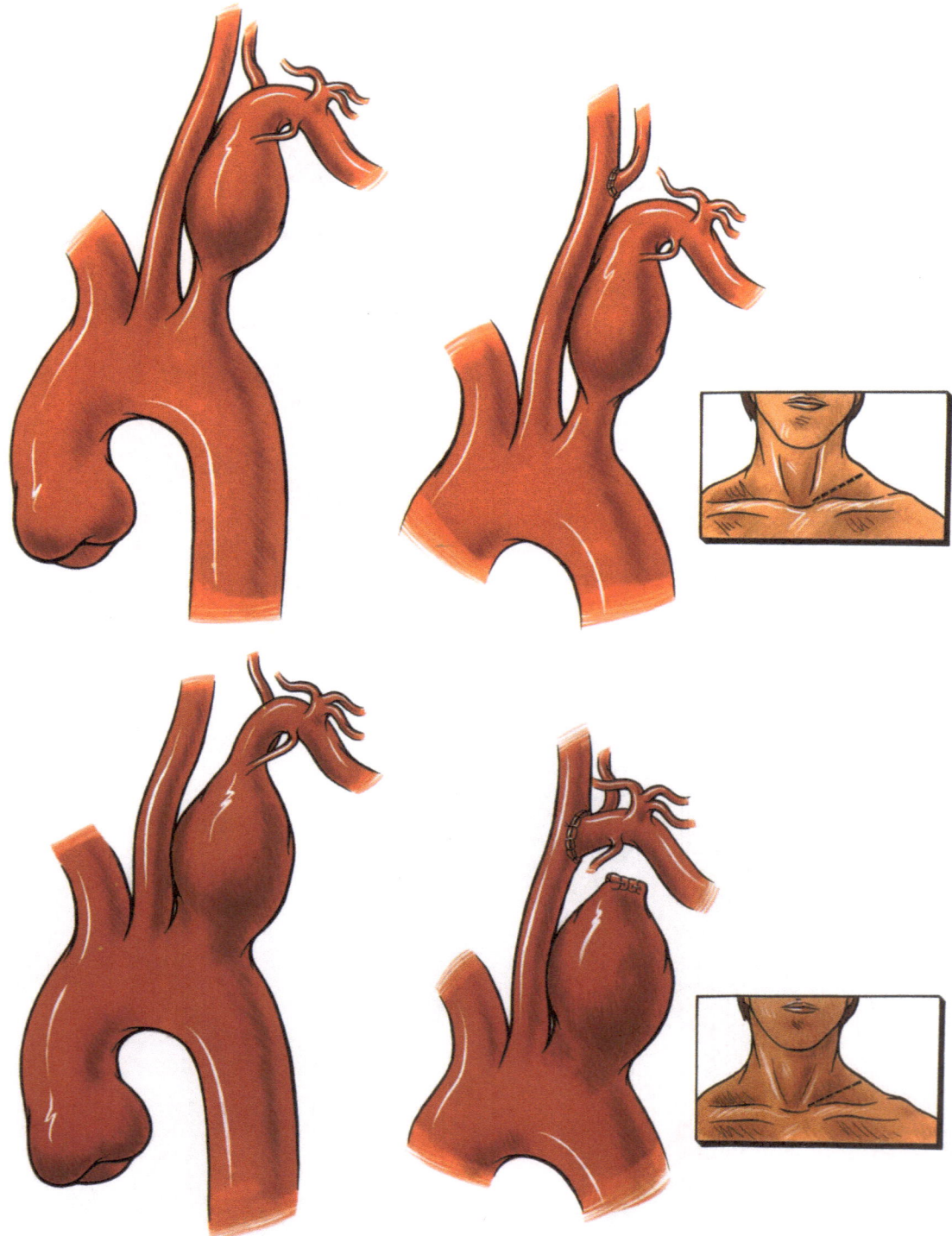

Figure 11.10 Repair of aneurysms of the intrathoracic left subclavian artery extending into the neck is facilitated by previous transposition of the left vertebral or, rarely, the left subclavian artery.

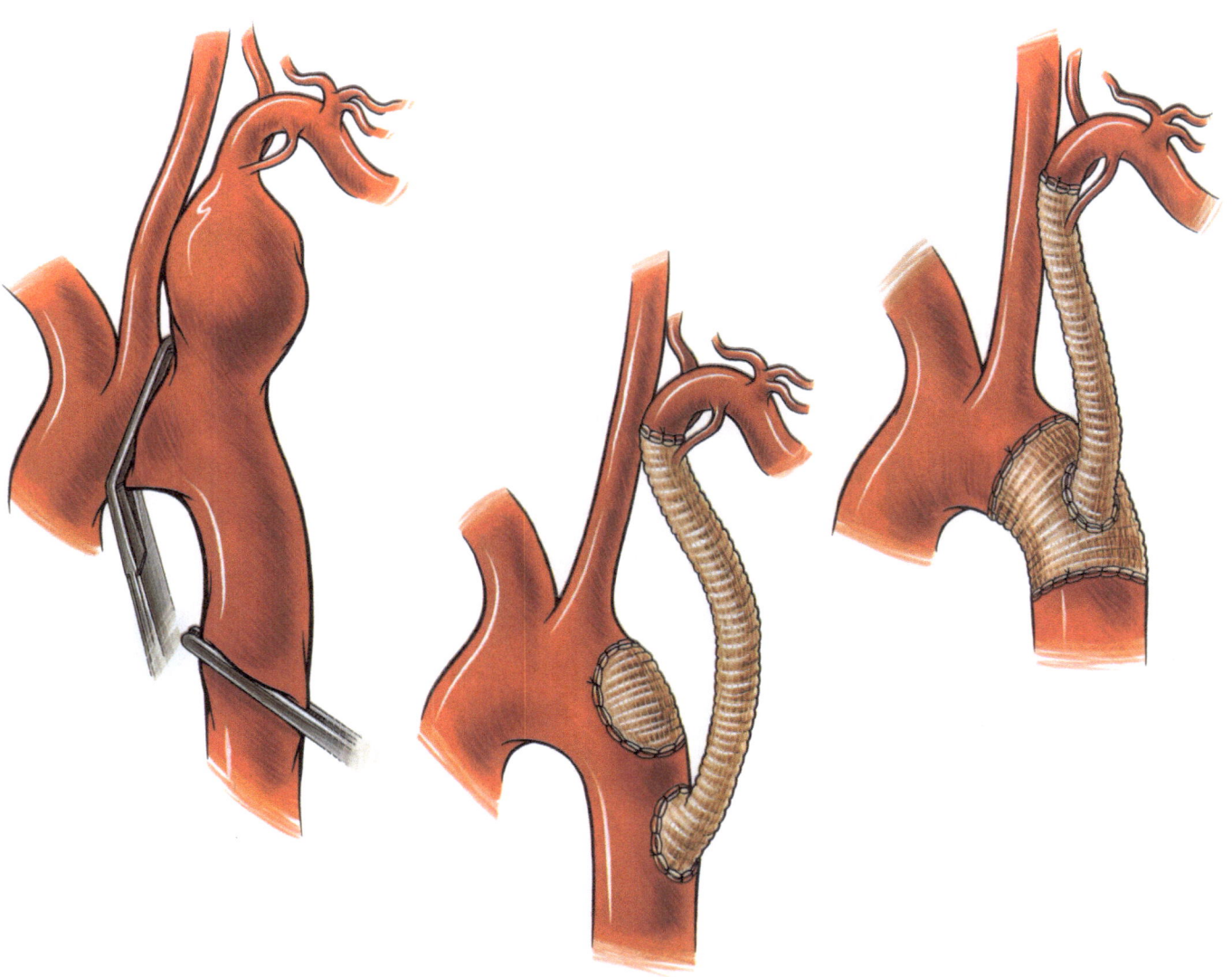

Figure 11.11 Repair of aneurysms of the intrathoracic left subclavian with a wide base of implantation on the aorta calls for aortic cross-clamping and patch repair or tube replacement of the diseased aorta. A bypass graft is used to revascularize the left subclavian artery.

less appealing, as it usually entails a potentially risky supraclavicular dissection of the distal part of the aneurysm. In both cases the rest of the operation is done through a thoracotomy. The distal anastomosis is greatly facilitated by the previous supraclavicular dissection of the second portion of the SA.

If the aneurysm has a wide base of implantation in the aorta (Figure 11.11) closure of its proximal end may not be safely done by exclusion-clamping of the aorta and may require cross-clamping and closure with a patch or segmental aortic replacement. These procedures may be done by cross-clamping under pharmacologic control of proximal hypertension or by using a left atriofemoral bypass or partial femorofemoral cardiopulmonary bypass.

All *other aneurysms of the SAT*, including those of the proximal right SA, require an anterior approach, usually a median sternotomy. With large aneurysms the CT scan may suggest attachment to the sternum, and in such cases it is wise to avoid the midsternotomy approach. Proximal control can be obtained through bilateral anterolateral thoracotomies, usually through the right second and left third or fourth intercostal spaces, and an oblique sternotomy.

a

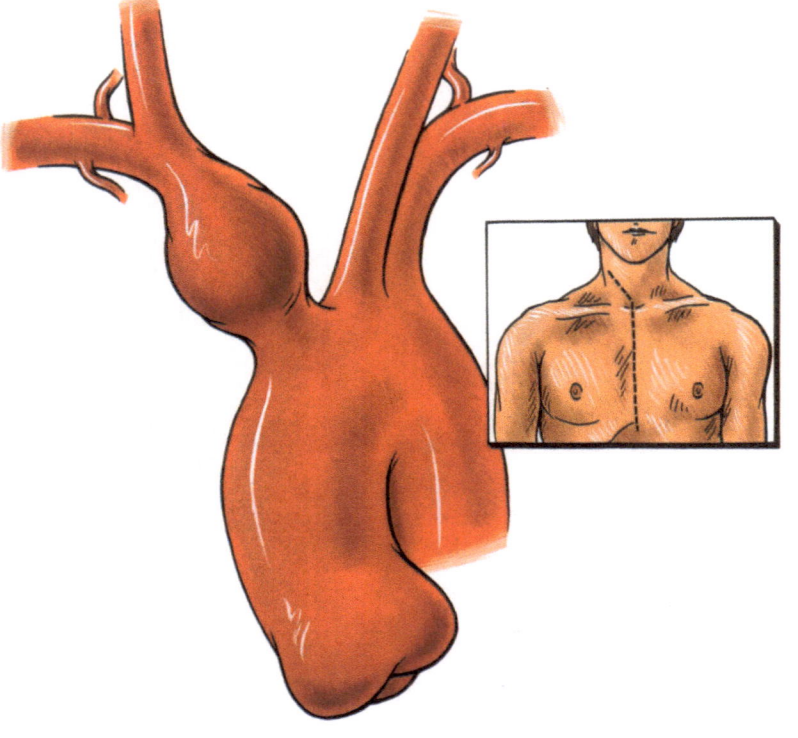

Figure 11.12 Repair of an innominate artery aneurysm (**a**) using interposition grafting (**b**)

b

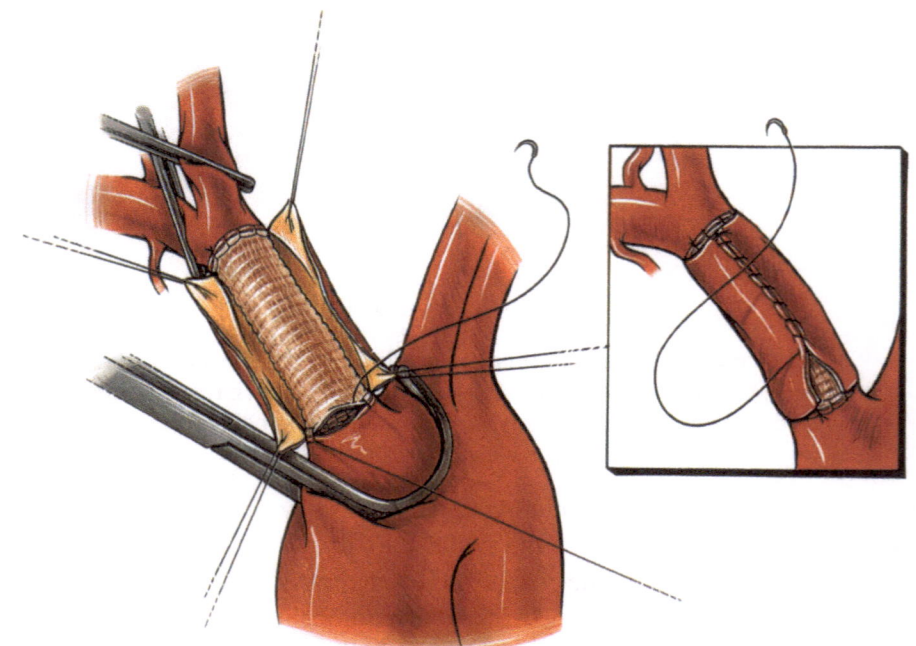

c

or bypass grafting from the
ascending aorta followed by
lateral closure of the origin of
the innominate artery (c).

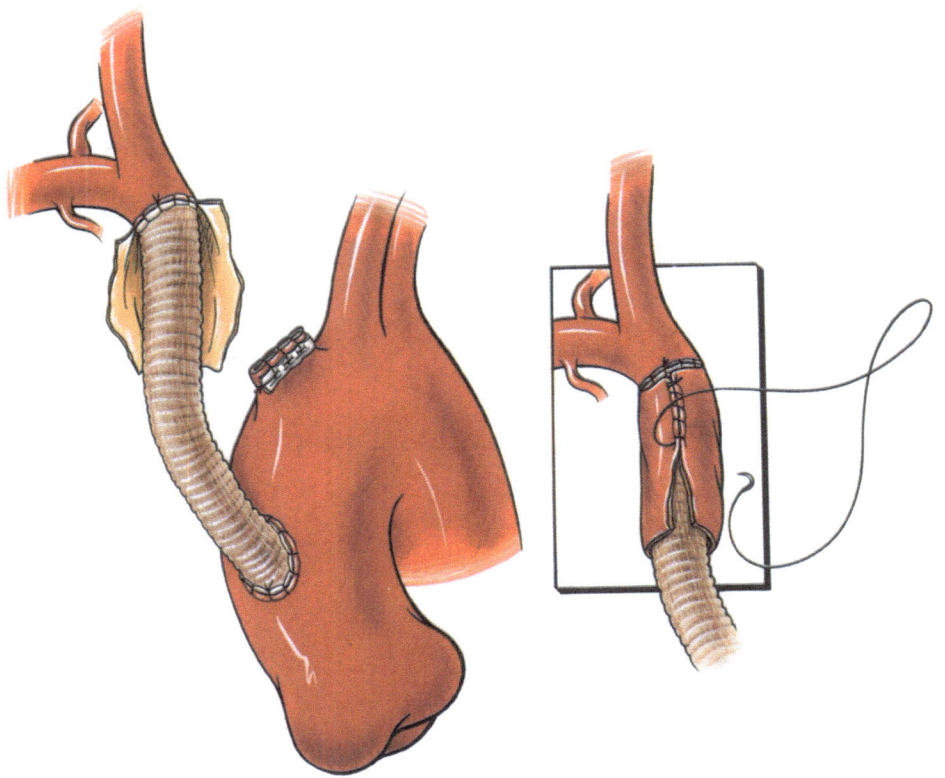

After proximal control is secured, distal arterial control is obtained in the neck through a separate incision. Once the aneurysm is isolated between clamps, the two incisions can be joined, with the upper half of the sternum being split longitudinally to gain direct access to the aneurysmal sac. A better solution to this unusual problem is femorofemoral cardiopulmonary bypass to induce deep hypothermia and circulatory arrest before opening the sternum through the midline. As soon as proximal control of the aneurysm is obtained, circulation and rewarming may be resumed rapidly unless there is some associated repair that needs to be done in the aorta itself.

Once proximal control of the trunk bearing the aneurysm has been obtained, either by clamping the artery itself or by exclusion-clamping of the aortic arch, the treatment is usually an interposition graft or a bypass graft from the neighboring aorta (Figure 11.12). Thrombus and debris are removed from within, and the wall is left in place to avoid injury to adjacent structures, e.g., the brachiocephalic vein, trachea, and esophagus. The graft suture is done from the inside, and the wall of the aneurysm is wrapped over the graft after flow is resumed. An alternative technique includes preliminary ascending aorta to distal IA bypass followed by partial exclusion clamping of the aorta around the origin of the IA and pledgetted closure of the latter.

Some aneurysms of the IA originate from large openings in the aortic arch that preclude exclusion-clamping of the aorta (Figure 11.13). They may be best managed by median sternotomy, deep hypothermia, and circulatory arrest, replacing the mouth of the aneurysm on the aortic arch using a prosthetic patch to which an interposition graft has been attached. Alternatively, a bypass to the distal IA or both IA and left CCA may be implanted first in the proximal ascending aorta and the aortic arch repaired using partial cardiopulmonary bypass or even single aortic cross-clamping.

a

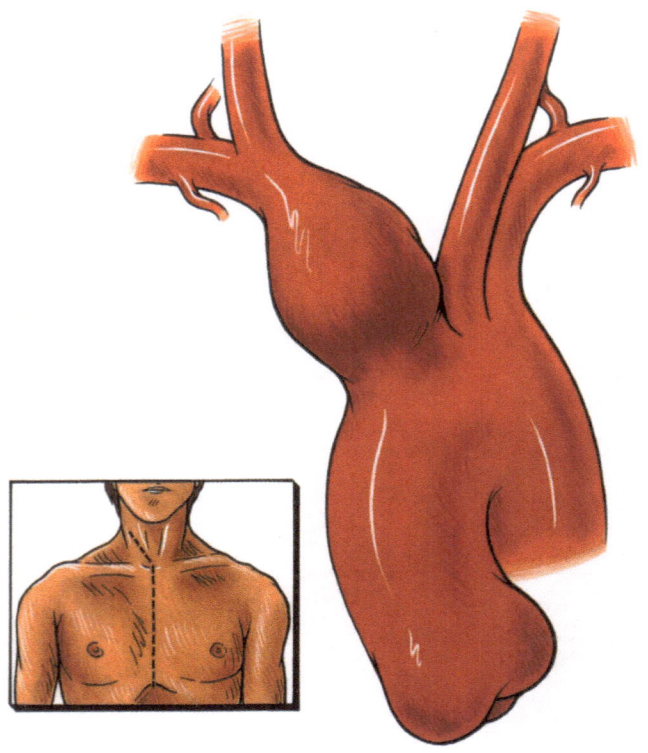

Figure 11.13 Repair of aneurysms of the innominate artery that involve the arch of the aorta (**a**) requires either patch closure or an interposition graft. The distal innominate artery is revascularized by a bypass graft from the proximal aorta (**b&d**)

b, c

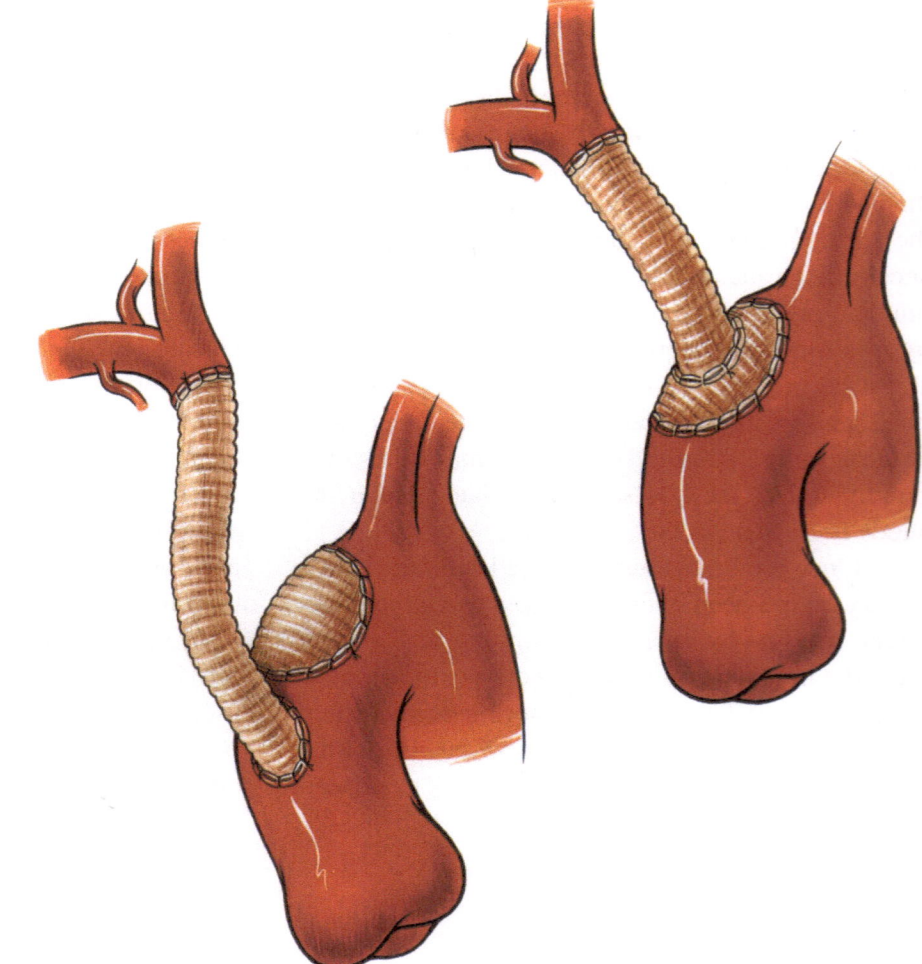

d, e

or from the patch (**c**) or tube graft
(**e**) used to repair the aorta.

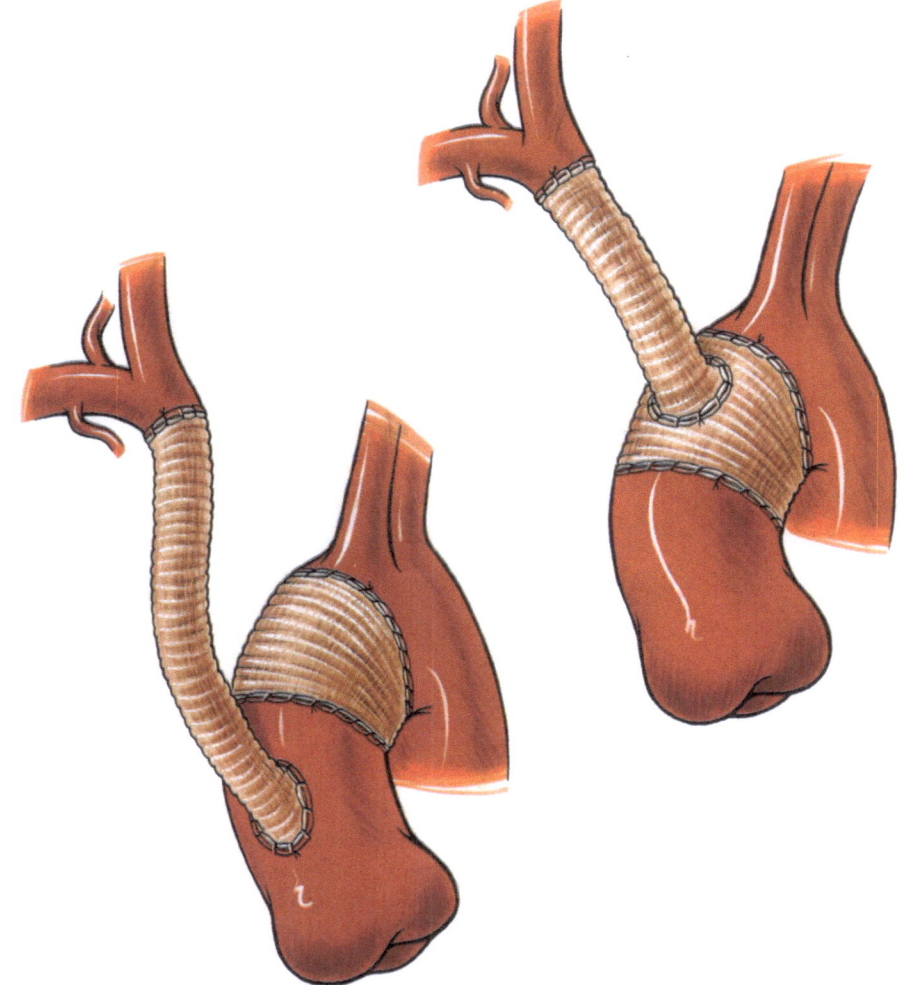

Carotid Aneurysms

Most carotid aneurysms can be handled through a
neck incision. Occasionally, a median sternotomy is
needed to gain proximal control of aneurysms of the
proximal left CCA and even the right CCA. Aneurysms of the CCA are treated with interposition
grafts, usually a prosthesis. Aneurysms that involve
the carotid bifurcation pose the secondary problem of
preserving the continuity of the ECA (Figure 11.14).
It can be done by constructing a venous bifurcated
graft or by reimplanting the external carotid artery
(ECA) into the interposition graft that links the CCA
to the ICA. Aneurysms of the proximal cervical ICA
(below the digastric muscle) are repaired with an
interposition or bypass vein graft (Figure 11.15).

Rarely, an elongated ICA permits excision of the
aneurysm-bearing segment and direct end-to-end
reanastomosis (Figure 11.16).

Aneurysms of the distal cervical ICA (above
the digastric muscle) are a different story. The approach to the base of the skull requires complex
maneuvers (see Chapter 8), which may result in
injury to the seventh, ninth, tenth, and twelfth cranial
nerves and to the upper sympathetic ganglion. The
distal cervical ICA is usually controlled by a balloon
catheter that has been passed through the vein graft
intended for reconstruction. The graft is anastomosed to the distal ICA with interrupted 7-0
monofilament sutures; after checking the back-flow
and testing the anastomosis, the balloon catheter is
removed. The proximal anastomosis is constructed

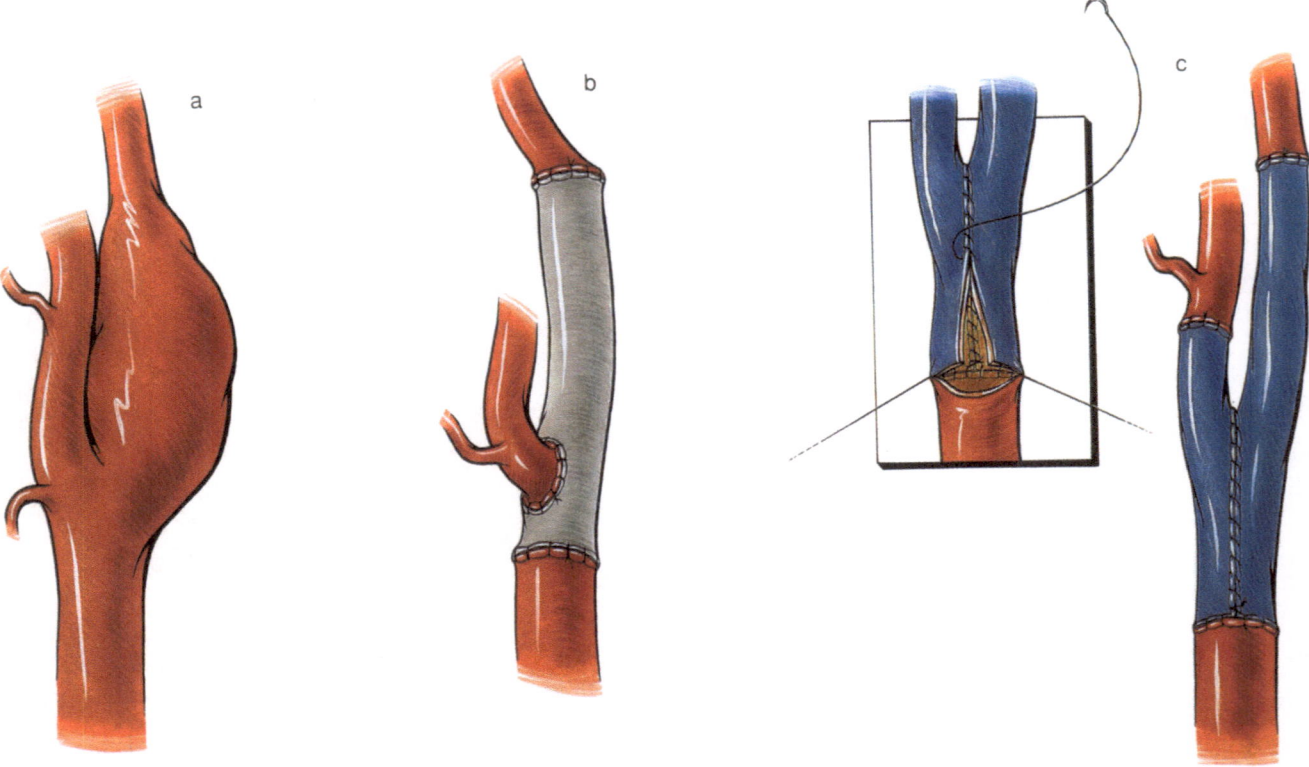

Figure 11.14 Resection and grafting of a carotid aneurysm (**a**) that involves the bifurcation, by (**b**) an interposition PTFE graft placed between the common and internal carotid arteries with reimplantation of the external carotid artery, or by (**c**) construction of an interpositon bifurcated venous graft.

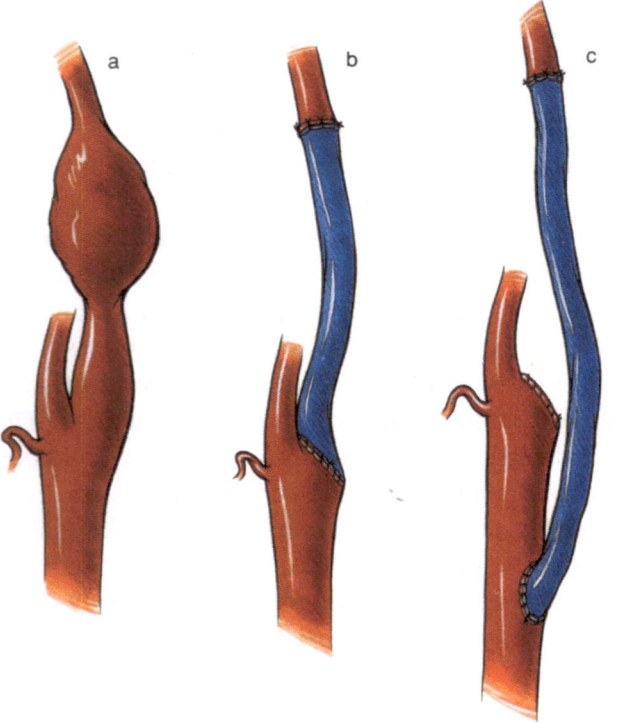

Figure 11.15 Repair of an aneurysm (**a**) of the proximal internal carotid (below the digastric) by interposition (**b**) or bypass grafting (**c**).

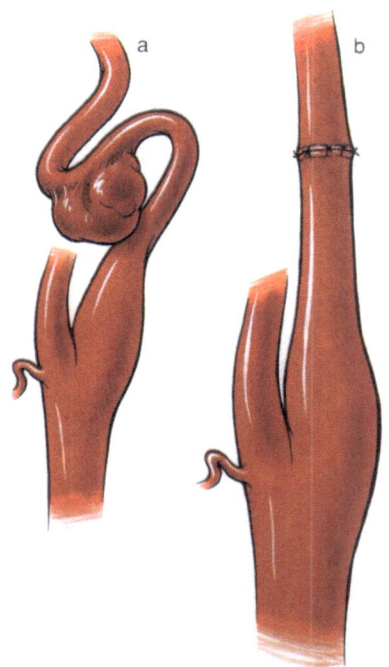

Figure 11.16 Redundancy of the internal carotid artery (**a**) allows resection of the aneurysm and end-to-end anastomosis (**b**).

end-to-end to the proximal ICA or to the carotid bifurcation.

In patients with truly juxtacranial (infratemporal) aneurysms this technique does not provide safe access to the distal ICA. In a few cases and in conjunction with an otolaryngologic surgeon, we have used a technique described by Fisch.[77] It consists in a transtemporal approach with petrosectomy and temporary transposition of the intrapetrosal portion of the facial nerve. This technique allows control of the vertical part of the intrapetrosal ICA. Although it facilitates reconstruction of the distal cervical ICA, it has the major drawback of creating loss of hearing on the operated side and a prolonged facial palsy that does not always recede completely. Today we would restrict its use to patients who have either symmetric contralateral carotid disease or a previous contralateral carotid ligation where one must ensure, by all means, a safe and patent carotid reconstruction on one side. We are currently evaluating the technique described by Pech and Mercier[78], a variant of the approach of Purdue[79], in which the middle ear is pre-

served but access to the intrapetrosal course of the ICA is less satisfactory.

For other patients, proximal ligation or balloon occlusion of the ICA using the safety criteria indicated in Chapter 5 are reasonable alternatives. In these patients the tolerance to carotid occlusion is tested by temporary balloon occlusion in the arteriographic suite. The patient is fully heparinized, and the blood pressure is monitored through an arterial line. A second catheter is advanced into the origin of the opposite CCA. The proximal ICA in the site of the aneurysm is occluded by inflating the balloon, and the neurologic status is monitored. Injection of the opposite ICA demonstrates if there is good cross-filling. The systemic arterial pressure is lowered approximately 20 mm Hg to ascertain the adequacy of collateral supply within the range of systolic blood pressures that may occur during the postoperative period. If the patient fails to pass the carotid occlusion test, prophylactic superficial temporal-middle cerebral artery anastomosis should be considered before occlusion of the ICA.

Vertebral Artery Aneurysms

Vertebral artery aneurysms are rare. Aneurysms in the first segment of the VA (Figure 11.17) are repaired using a vein graft originating either in the adjacent CCA, the SA, or the uninvolved VA. Aneurysms in the second segment or the initial portion of the third segment of the VA (Figure 11.18) are treated by either an interposition vein graft or exclusion and distal bypass (Figure 11.19) to the C1 level or above it.

Takayasu's Arteritis

Takayasu's arteritis is sometimes confined to the subclavian-axillary artery with isolated chronic upper extremity ischemia. More frequently, this disease involves the proximal IA, CCA, or SA. It may cause no symptoms in young patients with good cervical and intracranial collateral circulation. When the disease extends to both CCAs, patients usually develop chronic ischemic symptoms of the brain and eyes and

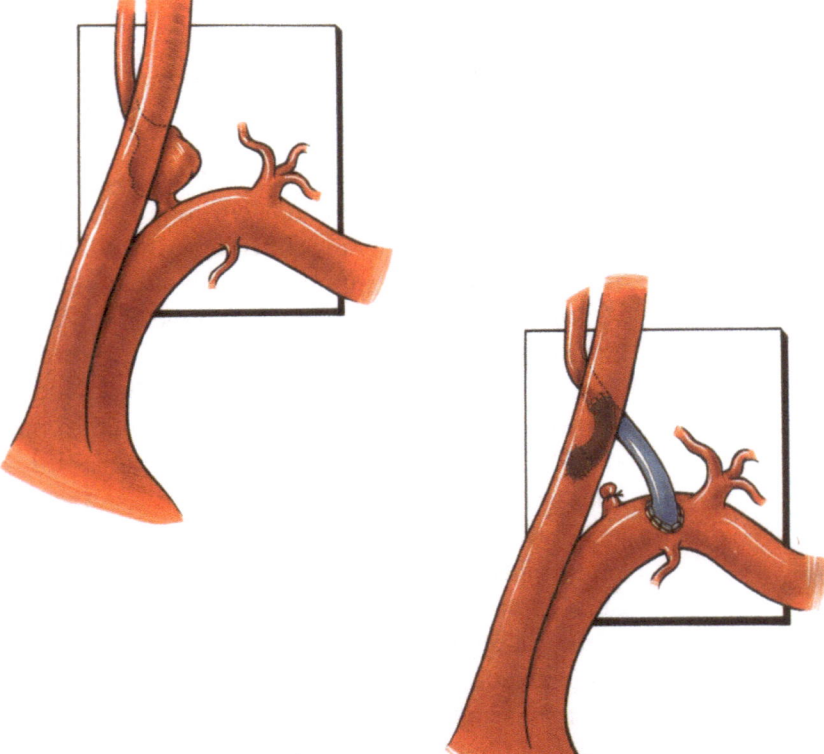

Figure 11.17 Repair of a proximal vertebral artery aneurysm by resection and a vein graft from the subclavian or common carotid arteries.

a, b

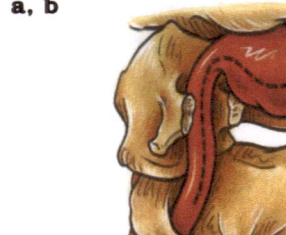

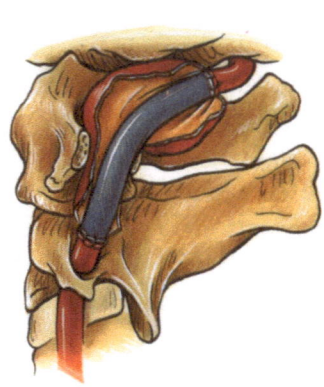

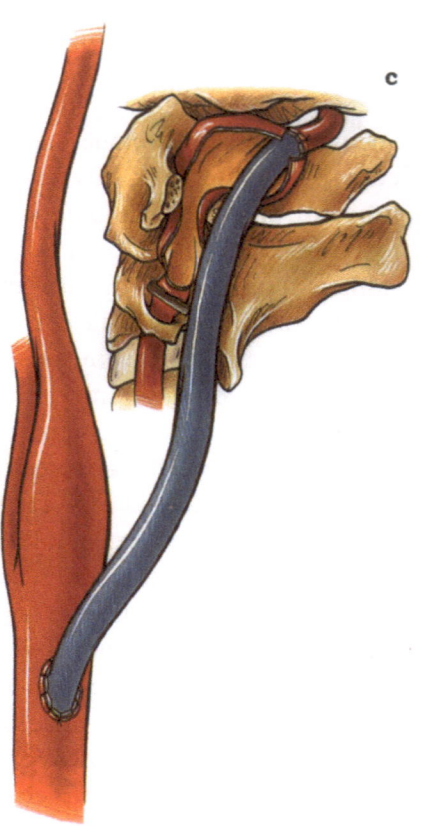

c

Figure 11.18 Repair of a distal vertebral artery aneurysm at the level of C1 (**a**) requires unroofing the transverse process and dissection of the sub-occipital course of the vertebral artery. It may repaired by (**b**) endo-aneurysmorraphy interposition grafting or (**c**) bypass grafting from the common carotid artery.

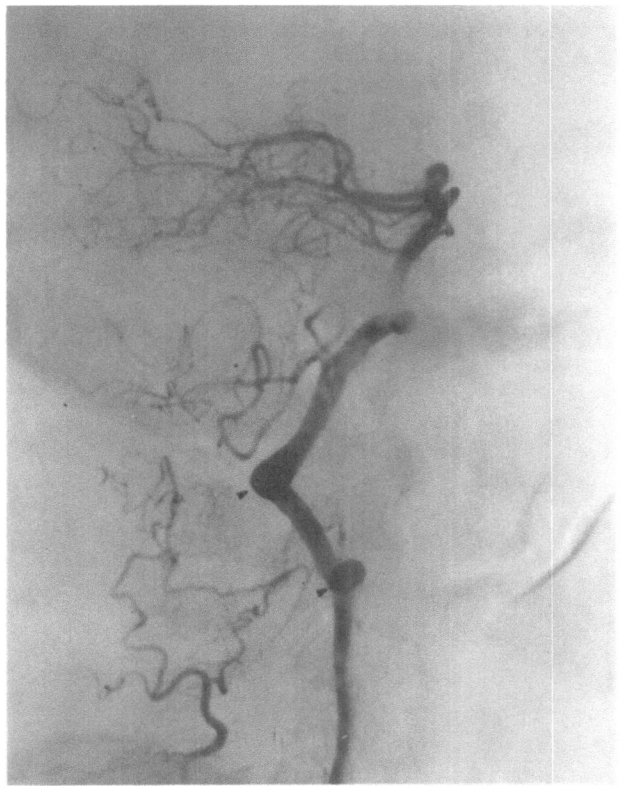

Figure 11.19 Aneurysm of the distal vertebral artery repaired by a vein graft extending up to the horizontal segment of the vertebral artery above C1.

even the face. Hemispheric strokes may occur in patients with Takayasu's arteritis after CCA occlusion.

Most patients who are seen with extensive involvement of their SAT by Takayasu's disease have at least one large VA, sometimes originating from a diseased SA, and a good circle of Willis that has prevented their death by stroke. Vertebrobasilar insufficiency is a common clinical feature in these patients and is explainable by either a deficit in total blood inflow or an intracranial vertebral-to-carotid steal through the circle of Willis. In patients with extensive involvement of the SAT, the hemispheric values of regional blood flow (measured by xenon 131) are usually below normal limits. They also show loss of autoregulation and maximal vasodilation of the cerebral arteries. This confluence of circumstances

accounts for the cerebral edema and even the hemorrhage that may follow revascularization.

Isolated occlusive disease of the SA (Figure 11.20) is best treated with a transcervical carotid to axillary (or brachial) venous bypass, although wall involvement of the CCA (which should be ruled out preoperatively on duplex examination) may preclude its use as a good site for the proximal anastomosis. In such cases we have used an anterolateral thoracotomy to obtain a source of inflow from the descending aorta, the IA, or the left proximal SA.

When there is *proximal involvement of several SAT*, the best solution is a prosthetic bypass from the ascending aorta to both carotid bifurcations, where the disease stops abruptly unless distal extensive thrombosis has taken place (Figure 11.21). Every effort should be made to keep the ECA patent. A venous bypass may be attached to any CCA graft in order to revascularize an ischemic upper extremity, if only to allow monitoring of the blood pressure in patients who have bilateral SA disease. Any large existing VA should be revascularized by either transposition to the posterior wall of the carotid graft or indirectly through a separate autogenous vein graft. A surgeon managing these complex cases should be ready to use a wide array of technical solutions.

Rarely, the ascending aorta is not suitable for the proximal anastomosis of a bypass. In such cases one can use a remote bypass from the descending thoracic aorta, supraceliac aorta, or iliac or femoral arteries (see Chapter 13).

Patients with Takayasu's disease of the branches of the aortic arch commonly have associated lesions *of the thoracoabdominal aorta and its branches*. In the young, low-risk patient they can be repaired at the same operation (Figure 11.22). This combined approach is particularly convenient when there is a thoracoabdominal aortic lesion that has to be repaired by an ascending aorta-to-abdominal aorta bypass. This bypass is inserted first by using a median sternolaparotomy. From the proximal part of the aortic bypass one can tend additional branches to the supraaortic trunks in need of revascularization.

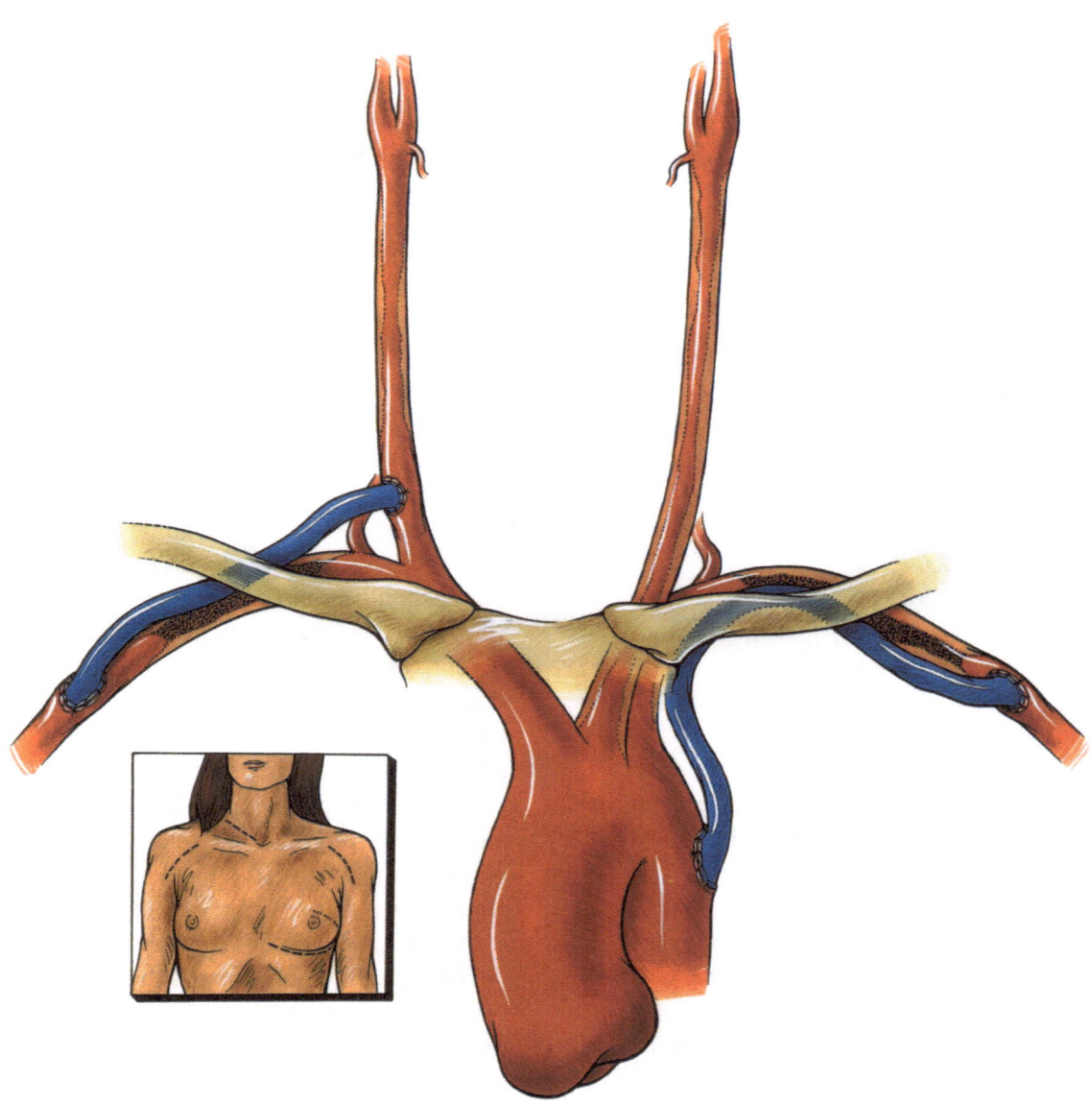

Figure 11.20 Revascularization of ischemic upper extremities in a patient with Takayasu's arteritis by carotid-axillary vein bypass and aortoaxillary vein bypass.

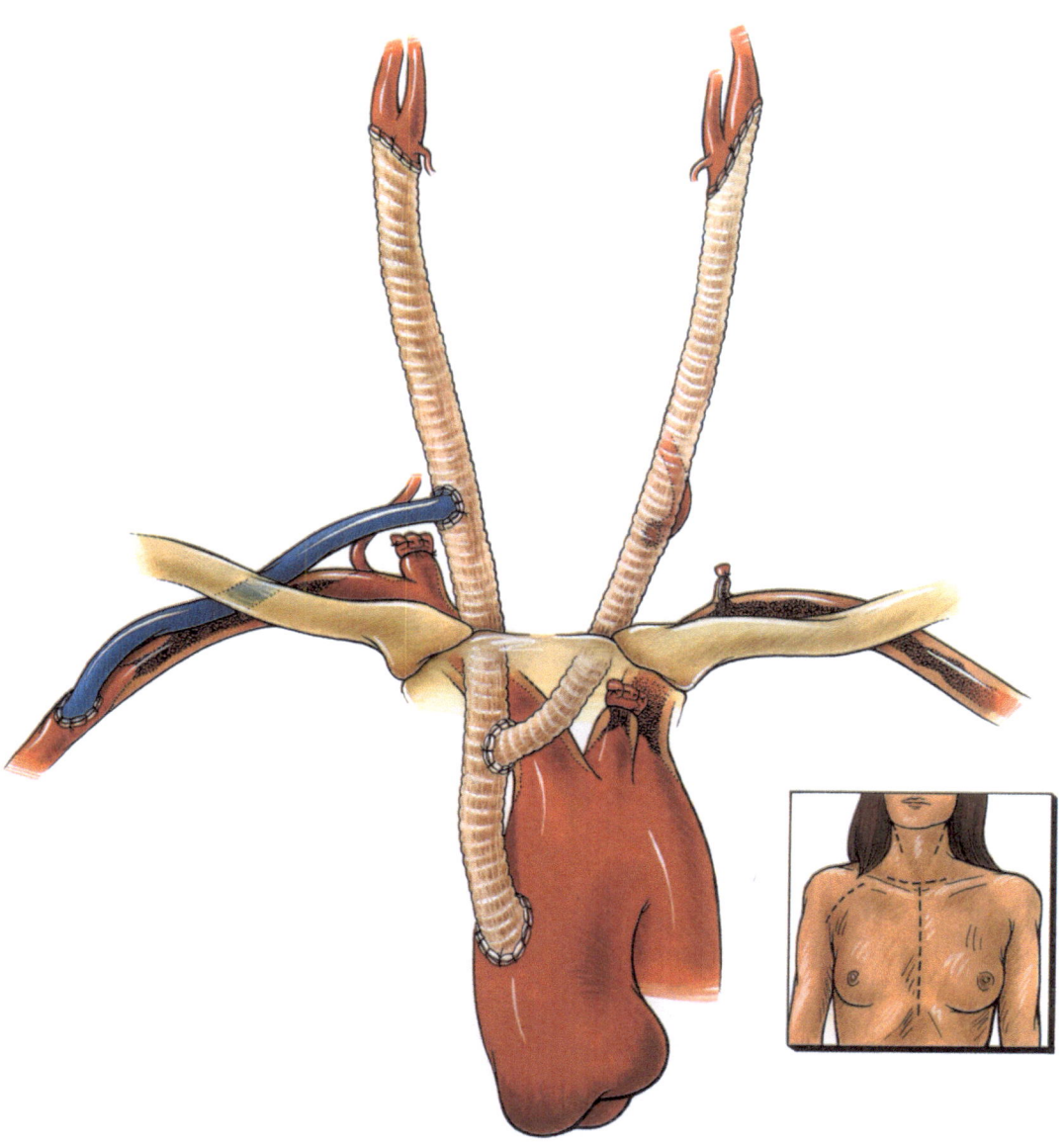

Figure 11.21 Multiple bypasses from the ascending aorta in a patient with Takayasu's arteritis.

a

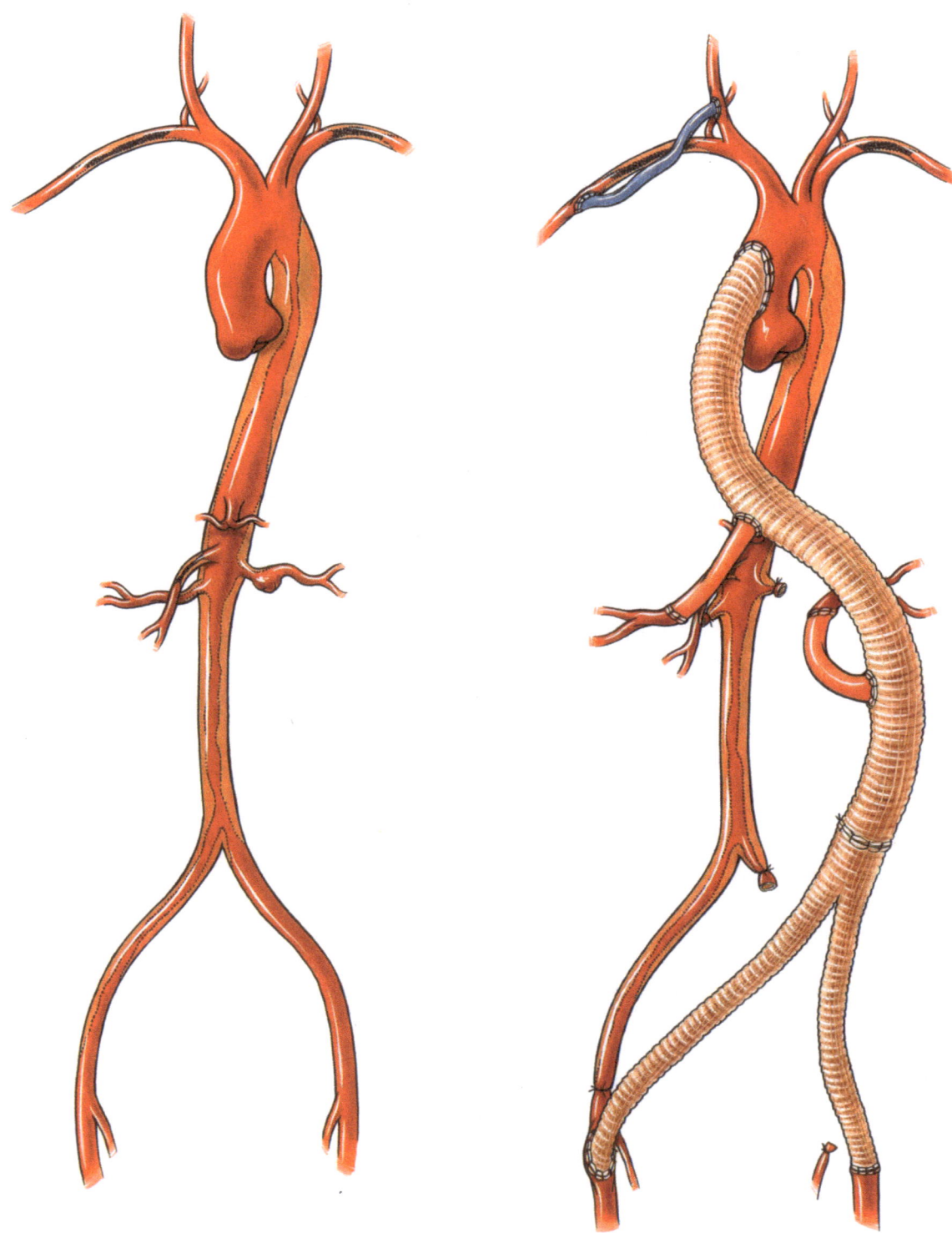

Figure 11.22 Two types (**a,b**) of combined revascularization of the branches of the arch and thoracoabdominal aorta for patients with Takayasu's arteritis. In (**a**) the left iliac artery was used as a free autograft to the left renal artery.

b

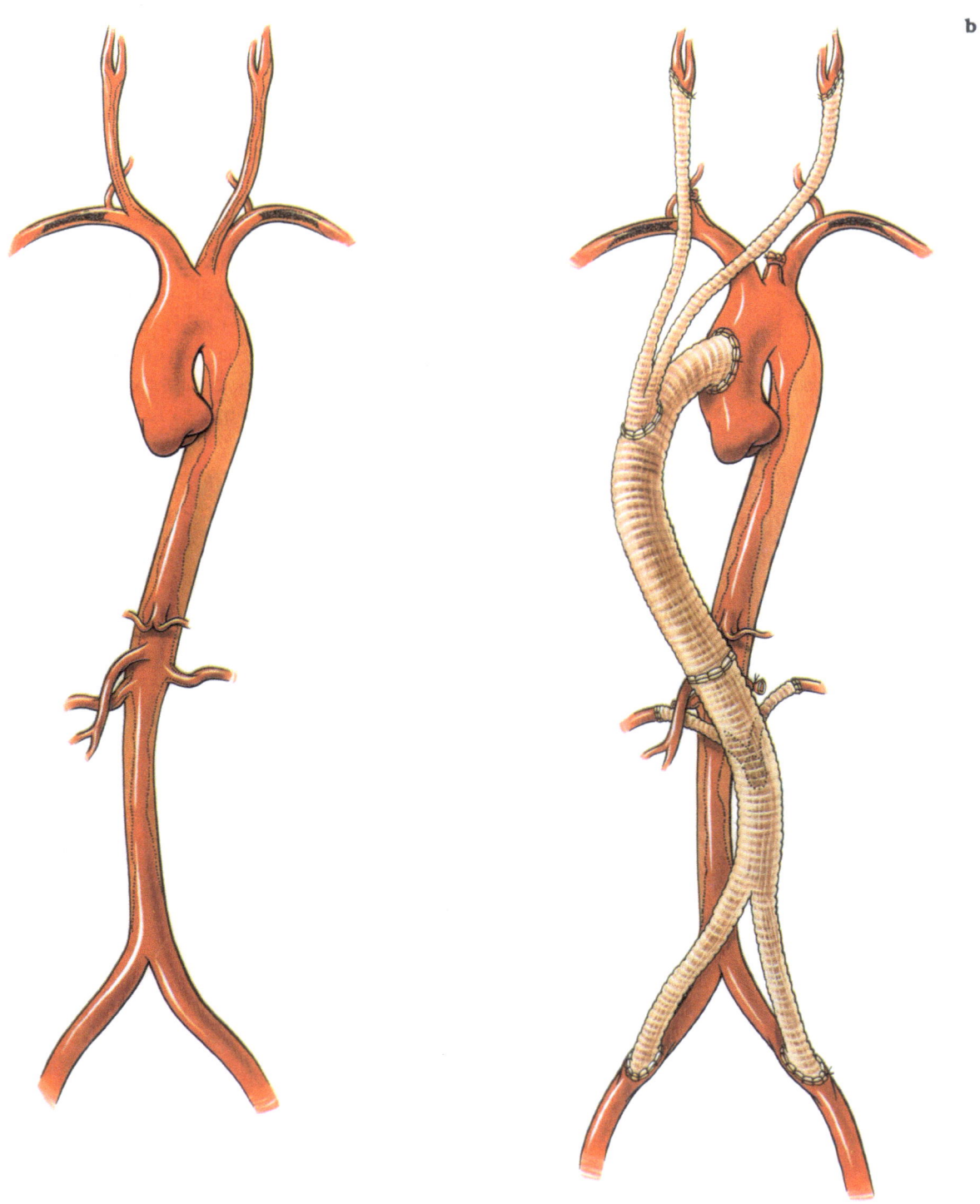

In **(b)** both renal arteries are supplied by a small bifurcated prosthesis attached to the main graft.

The Retroesophageal Subclavian Artery

Most RSA are incidental and asymptomatic and require no treatment. Surgical repair of an RSA is, however, indicated in four circumstances: the presence of dysphagia lusoria, occlusive disease, aneurysmal disease, or associated aortic disease.

Dysphagia Lusoria

Dysphagia lusoria is seen either in young children, often associated with respiratory problems, or in middle-aged adults where it manifests as isolated

swallowing difficulty (Figure 11.23). The traditional approach to this condition has been to relieve the esophageal compression by transection and ligature of the anomalous artery at its origin from the aortic arch followed by mobilization of the posterior aspect of the esophagus as far as the left thoracotomy allows. Unfortunately, ischemia of the right upper extremity or VBI may result from this procedure.

Today the accepted surgical approach includes transposition of the distal portion of the RSA into the right CCA (Figure 11.24). It is done through a supraclavicular approach in combination with any of several techniques designed to handle the abnormal origin of the artery (Figure 11.25). The most common

a 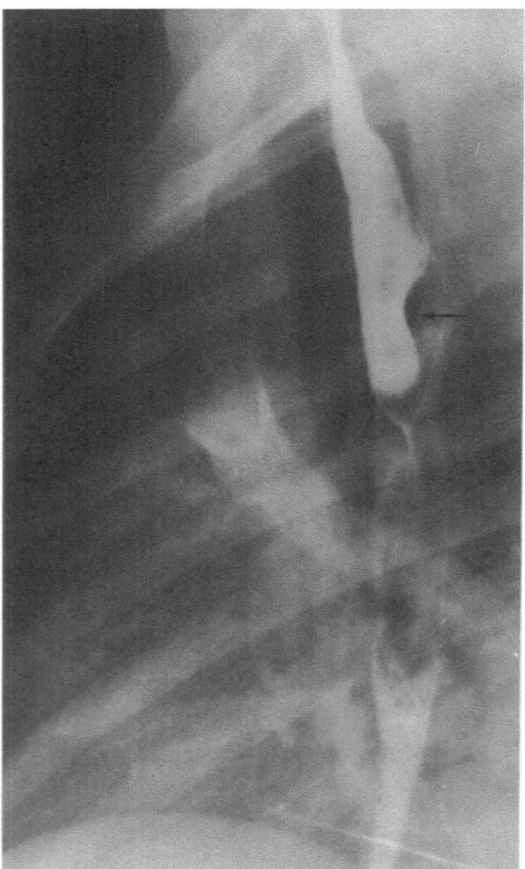 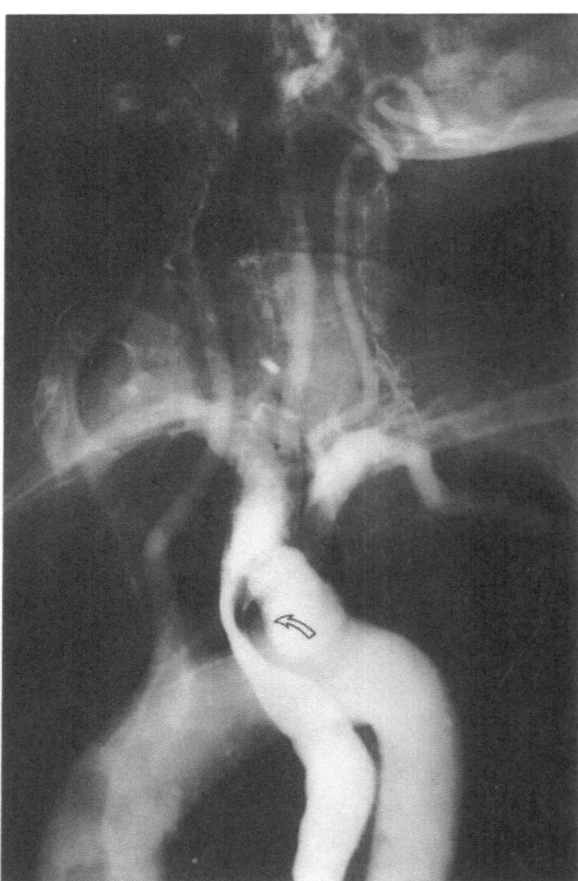 b

Figure 11.23 A retroesophageal subclavian artery as a cause of dysphagia. **(a)** Impression of a retroesophageal right subclavian artery on the esophagogram. **(b)** Combined esophagogram and arteriogram showing a retroesophageal right subclavian artery with an aneurysmal dilatation compressing (arrow) the esophagus.

a, b

Figure 11.24 Retroesophageal right subclavian artery (**a**) transposed to the right common carotid artery (arrow) (**b**).

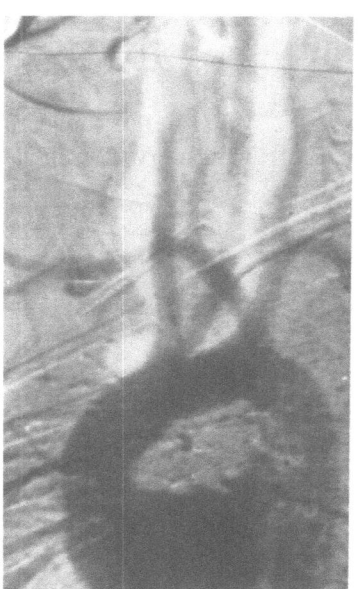
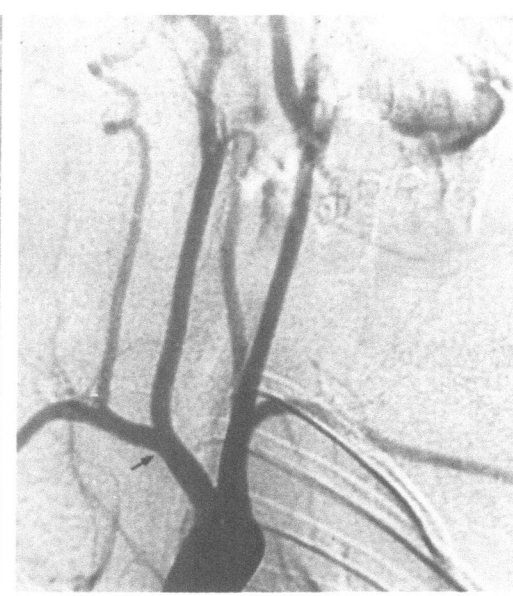

and probably the safest technique is to obliterate the origin of the RSA through a left posterolateral thoracotomy. A small inconvenience with this approach is that it requires changing the position of the patient. Otherwise the ligature of the origin of the RSA may be done through a median sternotomy (dividing the brachiocephalic vein) or through a transverse neck incision by cutting both sternomastoid muscles. The latter approach works only in patients with a large thoracic inlet and a high-lying aortic arch. Both anterior approaches to the proximal RSA require ample mobilization of the tracheoesophageal column in order to dissect the RSA completely and obliterate its origin with sutures. (Transposition of the distal RSA to the right CCA is done first through the same incision.) If the median sternotomy approach has been chosen, the RSA may also be transposed to the distal ascending aorta, a convenient alternative if the right CCA is unsuitable as a source vessel because of disease or small size. A short interposition prosthetic graft may be needed to reach the ascending aorta easily.

Occlusive Disease

Atherosclerotic or Takayasu's disease of the RSA may cause VBI or right arm ischemia. In patients with isolated occlusive disease of the RSA, revascularization is done through a right neck incision by transposing the RSA into the right CCA or, occasionally, by doing a carotid-subclavian bypass. In patients who have occlusive disease of the RSA associated with disease of other SATs, the approach should be through a median sternotomy with insertion of a bypass from the ascending aorta to the right SA and to any other trunk needing repair.

a

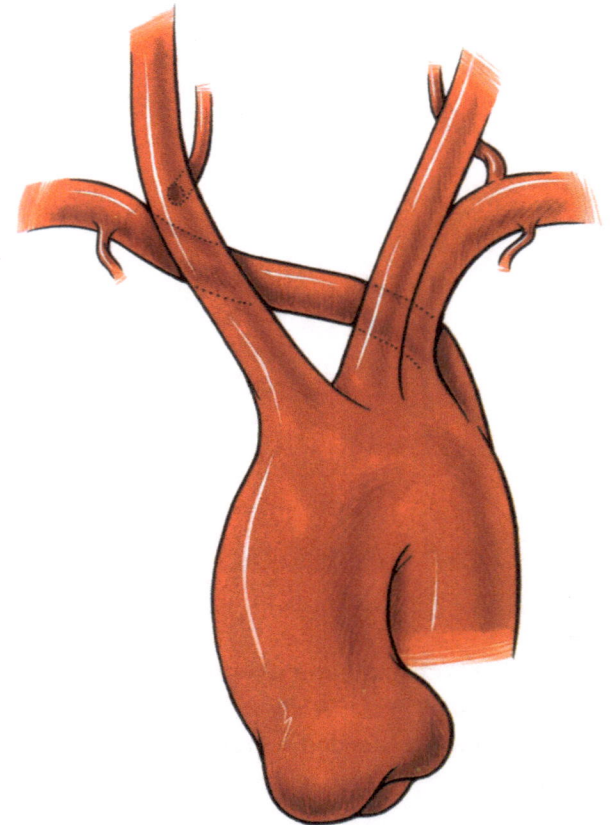

Figure 11.25 Repair of a symptomatic retroesophageal subclavian artery (**a**) using cervical (**b**),

b

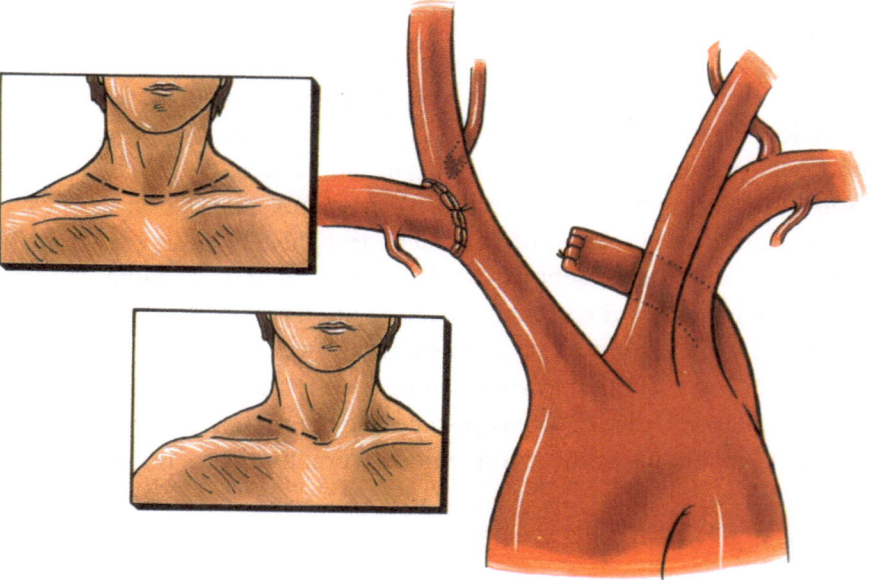

combined cervical, and left thoracic (**c**), or transsternal
(**d**) approach.

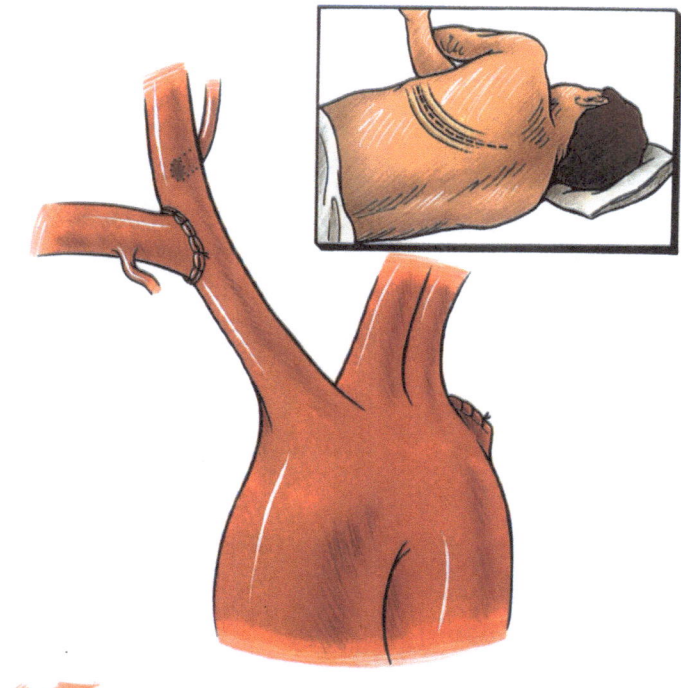

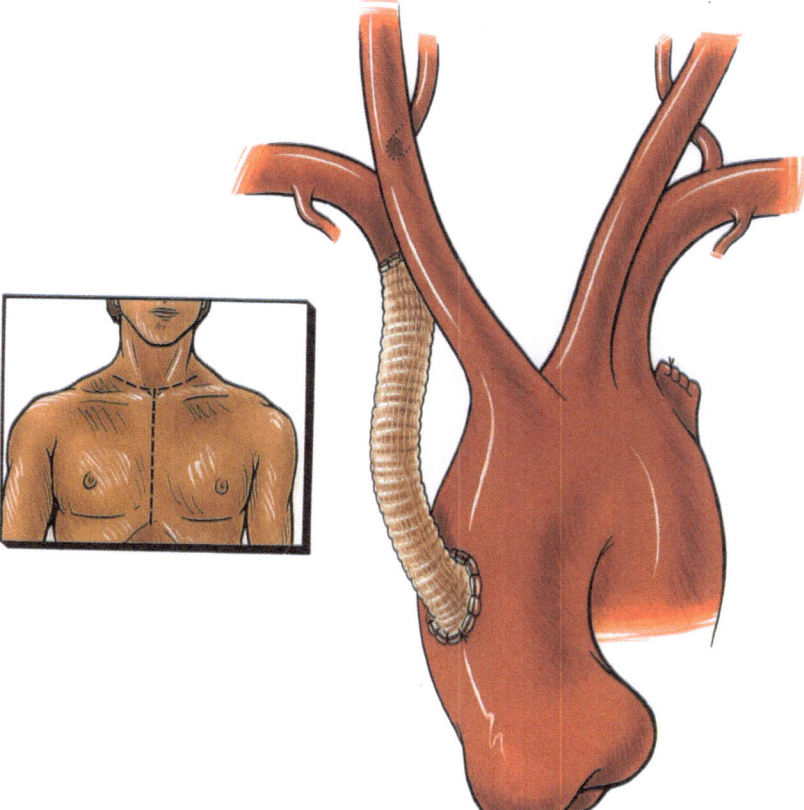

a

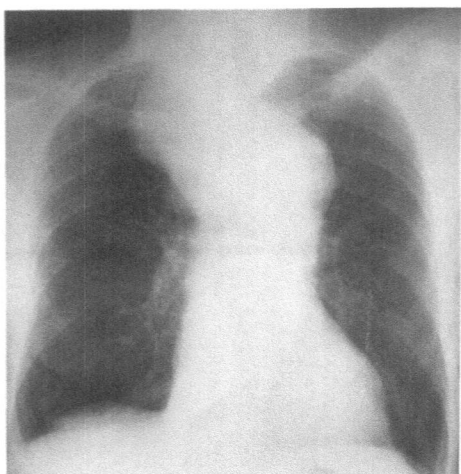
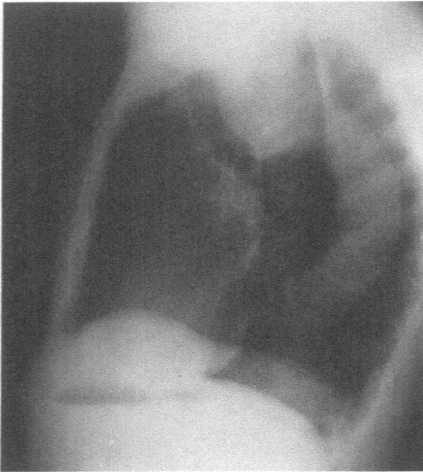

Figure 11.26 (**a**) Posteroanterior and lateral chest roentgenographic views of a patient with a large aneurysm of a retroesophageal subclavian artery. (**b**) CT scan of the chest showing the aneurysmal cavity largely filled with thrombus. (**c**) Arteriogram in the same patient.

b

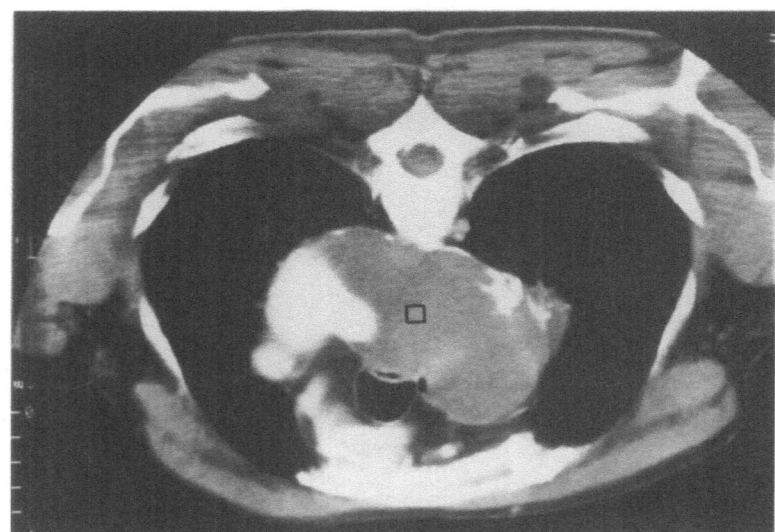

c

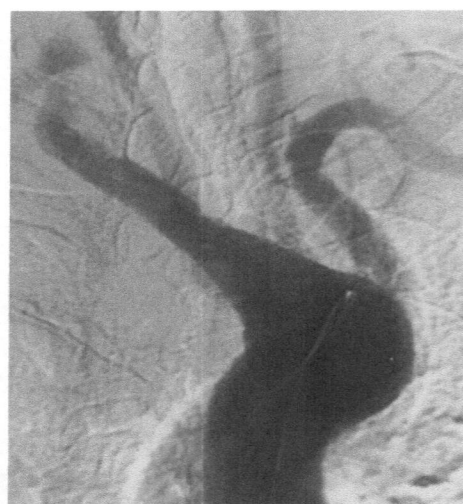

Aneurysmal Disease

The RSA may become aneurysmal owing to atherosclerotic disease (Figure 11.26). In these rare cases it may cause dysphagia or distal emboli, or it may rupture into the mediastinum, esophagus, or either pleural cavity. Aneurysms of an RSA are usually located at its origin and probably develop from the congenital outpouching known as Kommerel's diverticulum. Aneurysms of the midportion of the RSA are rare, and some may be traumatic in origin.

Aneurysms of the RSA usually have a broad implantation on the medial part of the distal aortic arch (Figure 11.27) and involvement of the adjacent aorta by atheromatous or aneurysmal disease. These features obviously require the use of a left thoracotomy to obtain control of the aorta. The operation, however, starts first with a right neck incision in a supine patient, transposing the distal RSA to the right CCA. Having ensured perfusion of the right distal SA, the patient is moved to a right lateral position. A left thoracotomy permits clamping of the aorta between the left CCA and left SA proximally and below the RSA distally. A separate clamp is required for the proximal left SA. If the adjacent aorta appears normal, the ostium of the RSA can be isolated by aortic cross-clamping. Lateral clamping is generally difficult and risky because of the posterior origin of the RSA. Once the aorta is cross-clamped, its lateral wall is opened and the origin of the RSA is closed from within the aorta, using a prosthetic patch sewn from inside; the anterior aortotomy is then closed with a running suture. In cases where the aorta is diseased, it is best handled by segmental resection and graft replacement.

Associated Aortic Disease

An RSA may be found in association with coarctation, trauma, aneurysm, and dissection of the aorta. Its presence places the patient at great risk of perioperative vertebrobasilar stroke because it is usually necessary to interrupt flow to both SAs for surgical repair of the aortic disease. In elective cases this threat should be anticipated and treated by an initial operation that transposes the RSA into the right CCA. Under emergency conditions it may be best to deal with this situation by using deep hypothermia and circulatory arrest.

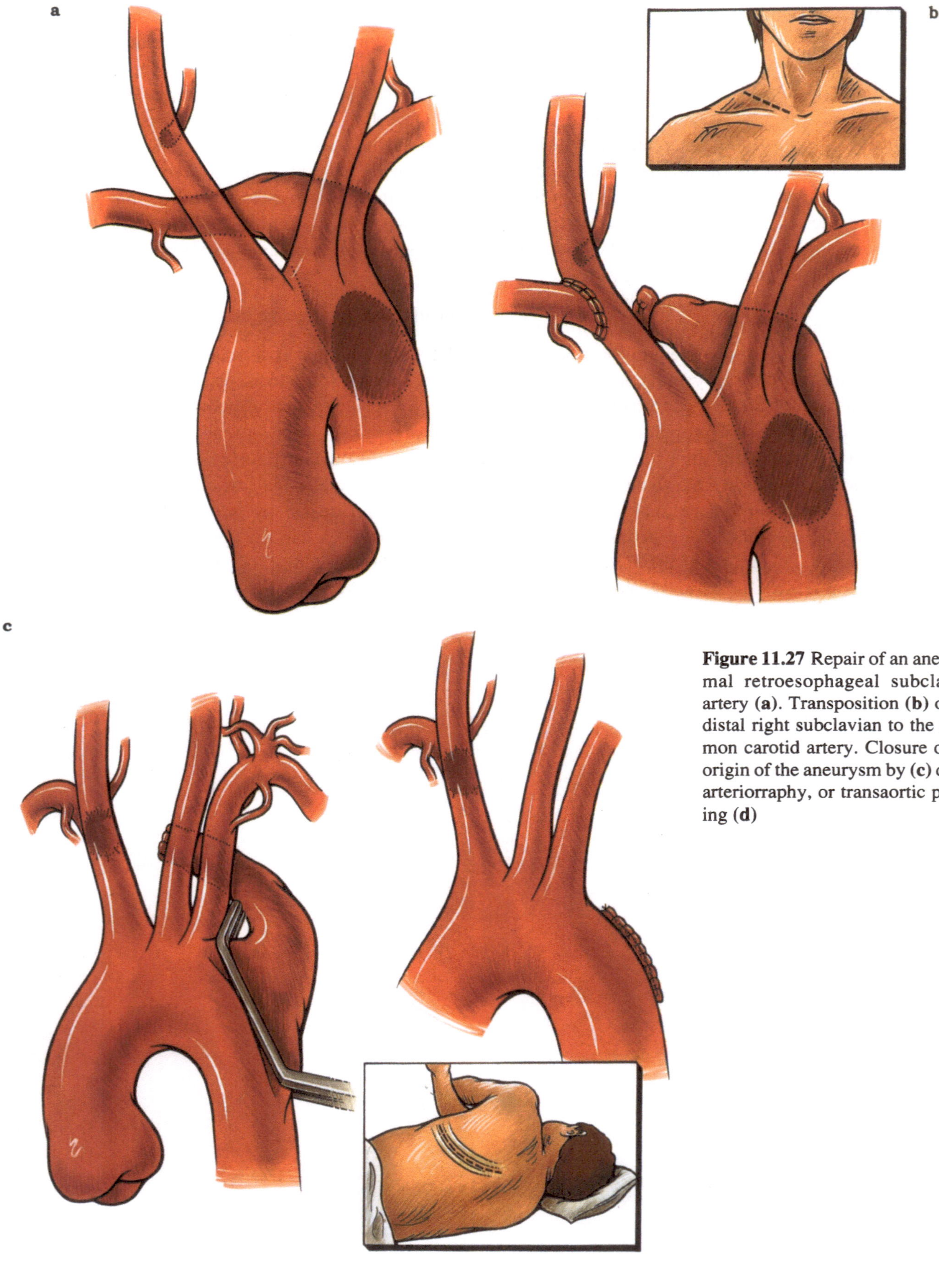

a

b

c

Figure 11.27 Repair of an aneurysmal retroesophageal subclavian artery (**a**). Transposition (**b**) of the distal right subclavian to the common carotid artery. Closure of the origin of the aneurysm by (**c**) direct arteriorraphy, or transaortic patching (**d**)

d

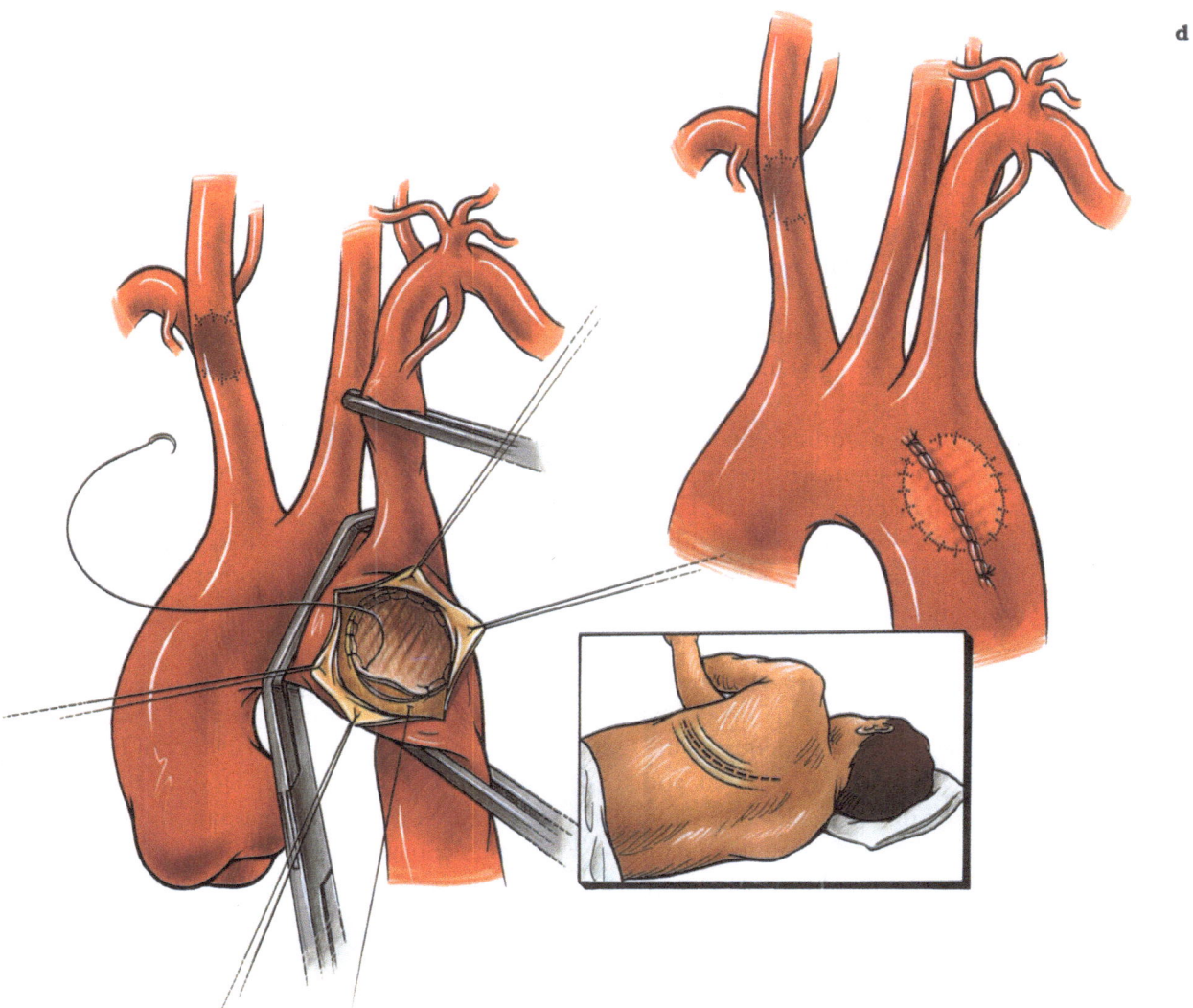

Fibromuscular Dysplasia

An uncommon disease of the SAT, fibromuscular dysplasia primarily affects the cervical segment of the ICA and VA; it occurs more frequently in women. Patients with fibromuscular dysplasia of the ICA are at risk for TIAs and stroke. The most likely mechanism of brain symptoms and damage is thromboembolic (platelet plugs) rather than hemodynamic.

In cases where an intervention is indicated, the type of correction done depends on the arteriographic findings. In a few patients there is minimal elongation and redundancy of the ICA and no associated atheromatous disease of the bulb, proximal to the lesion. In this group of patients the lesion is treated by percutaneous dilatation in the arteriography suite.

Patients with redundancy of the ICA or with associated disease of the ICA bulb are treated surgically. In cases where severe atheroma of the bulb is not present and where the fibromuscular dysplasia is corrected surgically, the cervical ICA is dissected to straighten its course. Graded dilators are preshaped and introduced through a small transverse incision in the bulb up to the temporal bone (which may be felt at the end of the dilator through the ICA wall). The artery is generally dilated to 3.5 to 4.0 mm diameter. It may be necessary to relieve the spasm of the ICA with topical papaverine. Prior to reestablishing flow, the ICA is back-bled to avoid embolization from intimal fragments.

If there is gross redundancy after dilatation, the artery is cut at the origin of the bulb, shortened, and reanastomosed. If gross redundancy is noted while dissecting the artery, it is best handled by cutting its origin, dilating the artery with dilators while it is in a straightened position, and finally transposing it to the bulb, after shortening, or to a CCA site. If there are associated atheromas of the ICA bulb, they should be dealt with in the usual fashion by endarterectomy, with the fibromuscular dysplastic lesions corrected by intraluminal dilatation. Intraoperative arteriograms or angioscopy shows the shaggy intima that remains after the diaphragm-like lesions are forcibly dilated and torn. After a few weeks the intima smooths out and recovers a normal appearance, as shown by follow-up arteriograms. Restenosis is rare and may be related to an incompletely dilated lesion.

The most common complication of dilatation for fibromuscular dysplasia is intimal dissection. In our experience it occurs much more frequently when the dilatation is done percutaneously than when it is done as an intraoperative procedure. For this reason we prefer intraoperative to percutaneous dilatation. This different outcome probably depends on the fact that, intraoperatively, the carotid is freed and the dilatation is done under direct vision with the kinks being corrected as the artery is fed around the dilator with the fingers: the axis of the dilator is the same as the axis of the artery.

Fibrodysplastic arteries are vulnerable to spontaneous dissection, which may result in occlusion of the artery or in the formation of an aneurysm. Rarely and only in the VA, an arteriovenous fistula may be the consequence of a rupture of the aneurysm.

Spontaneous Dissections

Supraaortic Trunks

Dissection of the SAT is usually the extension of a type A aortic dissection. It may be completely asymptomatic or induce diffuse or focal central neurologic symptoms, e.g., obtundation, or localized ischemic symptoms of the upper limb. Except in comatose patients, the presence of neurologic symptoms is not contraindicative to operation because a type A dissection is a severe threat to the patient's life.

The classic treatment is the prosthetic replacement of the ascending aorta with bypasses to the SAT, as indicated. More and more frequently, the preferred operation is replacement of the ascending aorta and aortic arch with simultaneous reconstruction of the SAT using intima-affixing sutures (with or without surgical glue) or separate bypasses.

Isolated dissections of the SAT (without type A aortic dissection) are rare. When present, they are usually seen in patients who have congenital diseases of the arterial media such as Marfan or Ehlers-Danlos syndrome. The treatment of these isolated dissections is an interposition graft or a bypass from the ascending aorta, depending on the proximal extent of the dissection. In those cases where the ascending aorta, although not involved by the intramural dissection, still appears to the surgeon to be particularly fragile, it may be best to use another SAT as a source of inflow.

Dissections of the Internal Carotid Artery

There is no indication for surgery of ICA dissections during the acute period. Despite the fact that the dissection is usually a hematoma, the accepted therapy is intravenous heparin administration to prevent the thromboembolic complications or final occlusion that may occur. These patients are followed with repeat arteriograms. A few go on to chronic occlusion, but most recanalize the ICA.

There are some secondary surgical indications in cases of spontaneous ICA dissection, such as a residual stenosis or aneurysm. The latter is usually located at the C1 level and may be surgically accessible from the neck, in which case it is treated with an interposition graft. If it is not directly accessible, three options remain: ligation, ligation with superficial temporal to middle cerebral artery anastomosis; and, rarely, a direct approach through the petrous bone (see Chapter 9).

Dissections of the Vertebral Artery

In general, management of VA dissections is similar to that for ICA dissection. Intravenous heparin is the therapeutic choice. Repeat angiograms during follow-up may disclose some of the indications for surgical treatment: a severe proximal stenosis in a dominant VA, an aneurysm, and an identifiable and persistent mechanical compression despite satisfactory recanalization. If an operation is advisable during the follow-up, it is important to determine precisely, with an arteriogram, that the dissection does not extend up to the level of C1. If the dissection goes above this level, reconstruction is contraindicated. If this fact is discovered after opening the artery, the artery should be ligated and closed and the patient placed on heparin for 5 days. On the other hand, if the segment of the vertebral artery entering C1 is intact (undissected), usually the reconstruction can be done with a vein graft from the CCA and, occasionally, by transposition of the ECA into the VA (see Chapter 9).

Radiation Arteritis

By virtue of its location, the carotid artery (CCA and ICA) is the vessel most frequently involved after radiotherapy for head and neck cancer. We have seen, however, radiation arteritis in all of the SAT. These patients are usually a decade or two younger than those presenting with lesions of purely atherosclerotic origin.

The indications for operating on these lesions are similar to those used for atherosclerosis, although three caveats must be considered: (1) The staging of the cancer for which the radiation was given should be taken into account to estimate life expectancy when planning an operation on asymptomatic patients with advanced occlusive disease. (2) The possibility of local recurrence of the malignancy must be excluded. (3) If the patient has had a disease-free interval suggesting that the cancer is cured, the artery bearing a severe plaque should be seen as a rapidly progressing lesion in a young patient whose life expectancy is normal.

The state of the vocal cords should be ascertained before any repair of the neck arteries. An unsuspected inferior laryngeal nerve palsy (due to irradiation or surgery) could turn into a major problem should the opposite recurrent laryngeal nerve be damaged during dissection of a fibrosed CCA or bifurcation of the IA. If such palsy should be present, the mandatory tracheostomy poses a serious risk of contamination to any neighboring graft.

The surgical approach is through atrophic skin and subcutaneous tissue. Dissection of the fibrosed carotid artery may be further complicated by a previous cancer operation: The usual landmarks are missing, the nerves are in abnormal position, and the carotid is in a subcutaneous location. If the disease is limited to the bifurcation, an endarterectomy and patch suffice. If the lesions are extensive, a prosthetic bypass from the CCA to the bifurcation is preferable (see Chapter 8).

When the arterial repair is done through the sternum, the usual prolongation of the midsternotomy incision to the right should avoid the suprasternal notch (which may have been the site of a tracheostomy); rather, it should follow a more horizontal curve to imitate the shape of an "apron" incision. The location of previous neck incisions should also be borne in mind to avoid necrosis of a skin flap. If both sides of the neck need to be exposed to carry the repair to each carotid bifurcation, a bridge of skin should be left intact on the left side to avoid a three-cornered junction, which may become devascularized and contaminate an underlying prosthesis.

Another approach in patients with heavy postirradiation changes in the lower neck is to access the ascending aorta through a third right anterolateral thoracotomy with or without concomitant transverse sternotomy. After anastomosing the graft to the aorta, the former is tunneled through the right pleura between the SA and the subclavian vein to emerge into the supraclavicular incision. From there it should travel behind the sternomastoid, if the latter is present, to the right carotid bifurcation. Crossover cervical bypass (see Chapter 7) may be added as indicated.

The repair of SAT involved with radiation arteritis should aim to bypass, in one setting, all the involved length of artery. If the mediastinal trunks are involved, it usually means a bypass from the ascending aorta to the bifurcation of one or both carotid arteries. The geometry of the bypass should be such that the branch to the left CCA takes off just above the origin of the trunk and is safely tucked to the left side of the trachea, well below the suprasternal notch, and then tunneled under the strap muscles of the left side of the neck. The distal anastomoses are usually carried to the carotid bifurcation.

In necks with severe scarring and contraction

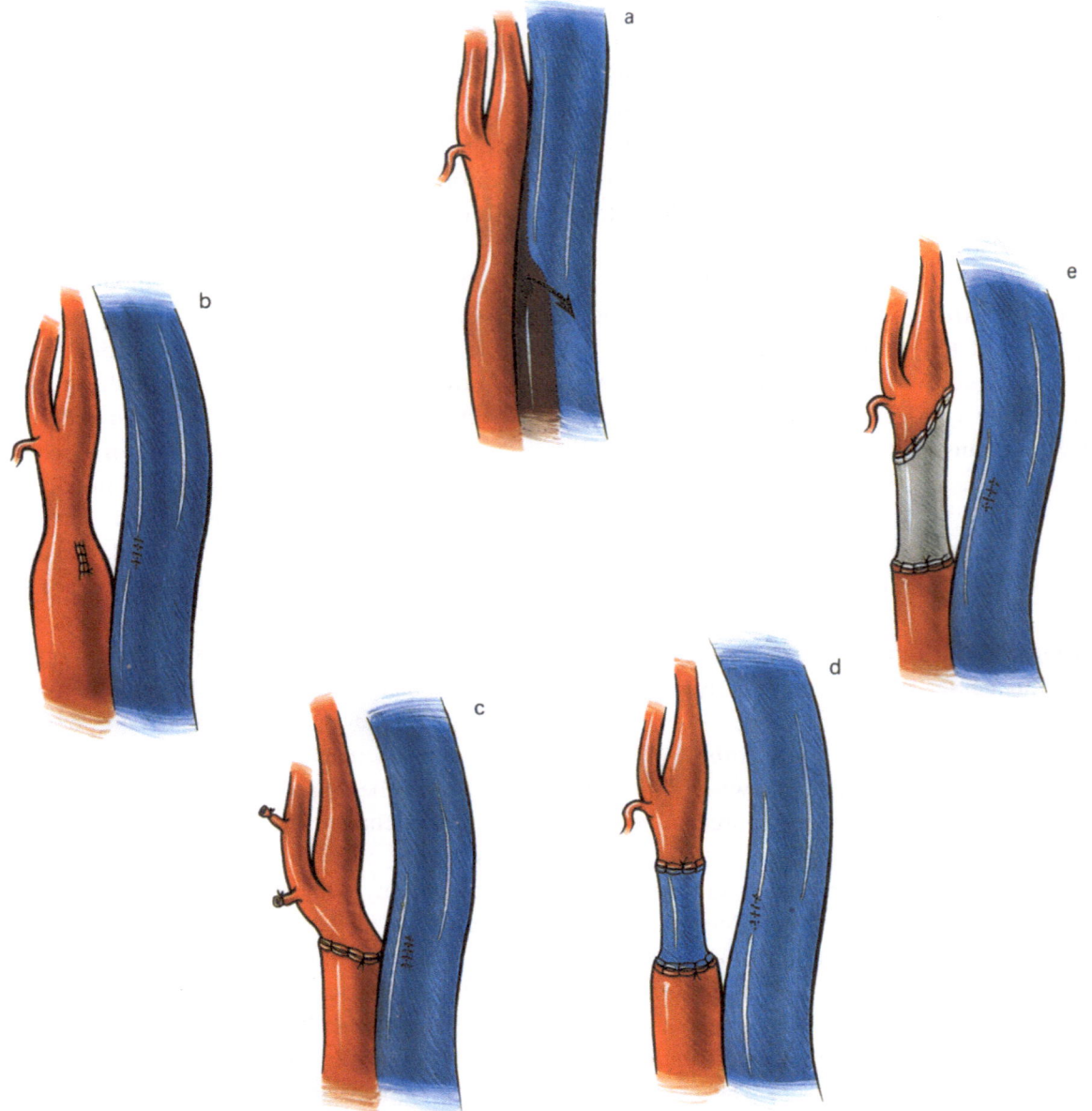

Figure 11.28 Repair of a carotid-jugular fistula (**a**) by lateral suture (**b**) of both vessels; (**c**) end-to-end repair, or (**d,e**) interposition grafting of the common carotid artery with lateral suture of the jugular vein.

after a previous radical cancer operation and irradiation, placement of the left limb of the bypass that substitutes for the CCA may require excision of the native, diseased CCA to make room for the prosthesis and to avoid its bulging under the atrophic skin. The usual method of covering the mediastinal prosthesis with thymus and strap muscles may not be possible owing to atrophy of these structures. There are two alternatives to provide soft tissue coverage for

the graft: One is to prepare an omental flap that can be drawn up to provide retrosternal and supraclavicular cover; the other is to close the neck incision with a deltopectoral musculocutaneous flap covering the prosthesis. If the patient has had necrosis of the sternum due to irradiation, consideration should be given to the use of a remote bypass from the descending thoracic aorta, supraceliac aorta, or iliac or femoral artery (see description in Chapter 14).

Arteriovenous Fistula

Traumatic fistulas of the mediastinal portion of the SAT are approached through a median sternotomy. Cardiopulmonary bypass with hypothermic circulatory arrest may be necessary to manage large arteriovenous fistulas involving the proximal SAT. A small fistulization of the SA and subclavian vein due to needle or catheter injury is best handled by controlled balloon embolization of the fistulous tract.

For fistulas in the cervical portion of the CCA our preference is direct surgical repair. Carotid-jugular fistulas (Figure 11.28) are short in length and large in diameter, and they have high flow rates. The short fistulous tract makes the balloon occlusion unstable and risky. A dislodged balloon may occlude the ICA or cause pulmonary embolization by escaping into the jugular vein. For such fistulas we advise direct repair, which can usually be accomplished preserving the patency of the carotid and internal jugular vein by lateral suture. Fistulas of the ECA territory should never be treated by proximal ligation of the artery. The management by balloon embolization is discussed in Chapter 6.

Arteriovenous fistulas of the VA are handled preferentially by catheter balloon occlusion. It is often possible to "parachute" the balloon into the venous site of the fistulous tract, occluding it, while preserving the integrity of the VA. A full arteriographic study should precede any embolization attempt to determine if the VA can be occluded with a balloon to control the fistula should the need arise. If there is no evidence of a good contralateral VA supply, a distal VA bypass should be constructed before obliterating the fistula.

Carotid Body Tumors and Other Paragangliomas

Infrequent carotid body tumors (also called paragangliomas) develop from the carotid body, a small corpuscle that lies behind the bifurcation near the ECA origin, from which it derives its blood supply (Figure 11.29). Only a few carotid body tumors have a familial incidence, and they are often bilateral, have a high incidence of malignancy, and may be associated with other tumors derived from the neural crest e.g., glomus jugulare or glomus tympanicum. The typical carotid body tumor is single, nonfamilial in origin, and appears in a mature or older woman as an asymptomatic, firm, slow-growing mass in the anterior triangle of the neck. Occasionally the tumor grows inward and causes a visible protrusion within the oropharynx (Figure 11.30). Symptoms are present only with long-standing tumors and are related to compression of the neighboring nerves or the pharynx (dysphagia).

Not all the vascular paragangliomas found in the bifurcation derive from the carotid body. Tumors derived from the vagus or glossopharyngeal nerve also grow in the carotid bifurcation and have a similar clinical and arteriographic appearance. Their blood supply, however, may be derived from higher branches of the ECA, a matter that makes dissection of the carotid bifurcation easier.

Paragangliomas should be excised to avoid the

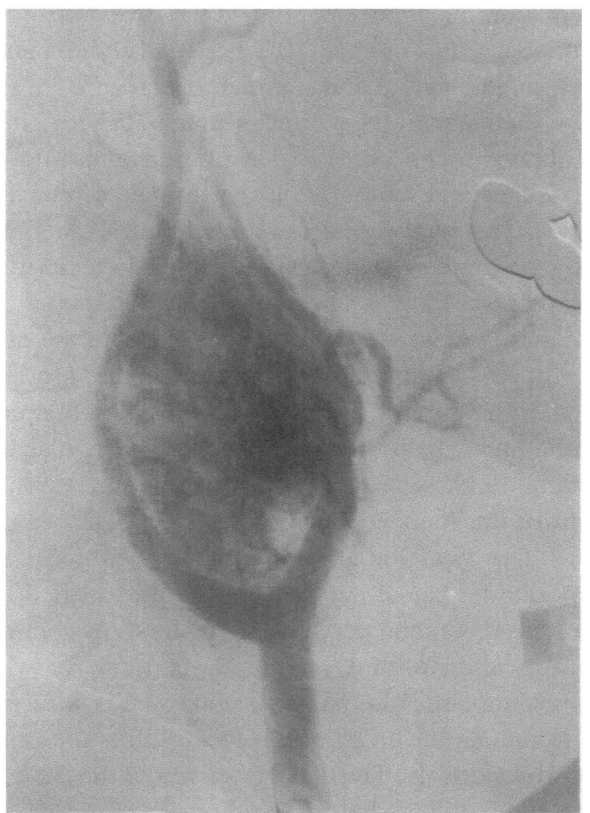

Figure 11.29 Characteristic arteriographic appearance of a carotid body tumor.

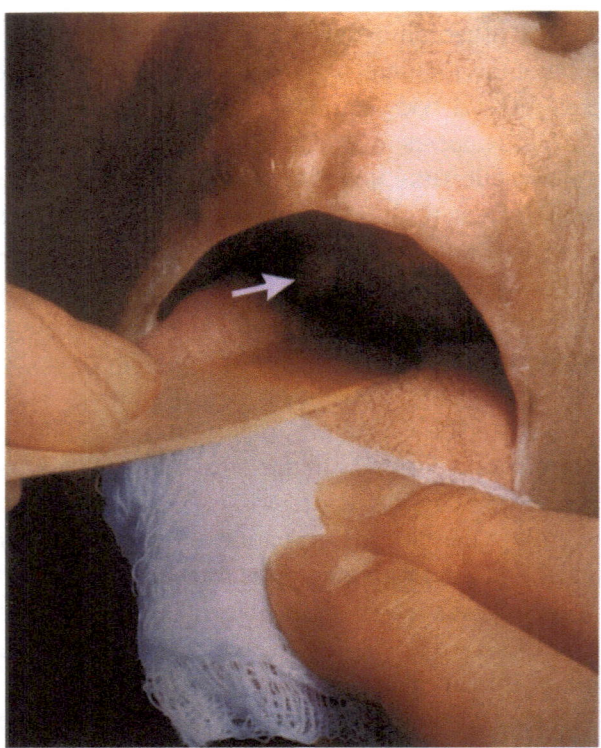

Figure 11.30 Carotid body tumor grew toward the pharynx in this woman. Note the displaced uvula (arrow).

local complications mentioned or invasion of the skull base. Fewer than 10% of these tumors show malignant changes and can metastasize.

Excision of the paragangliomas (Figure 11.31) is done through an extended presternomastoid approach. In large tumors we use nasotracheal intubation and, occasionally, anterior subluxation of the mandible to improve exposure. The hypervascularity of the tumor becomes obvious as soon as the carotid sheath is exposed in the lower neck. The tumor often engulfs the vagus and the CCA. Dissection proceeds upward toward the bifurcation. Following the plane immediately below the adventitia decreases bleeding during the dissection. Bipolar coagulation is used to control the abundant small vessels encountered.

The hypoglossal, vagus, glossopharyngeal, and superior laryngeal nerves should be identified and preserved. Cranial nerve injury is the most common complication of this operation, particularly when dissecting large tumors. Occasionally it is necessary to amputate the ECA origin to mobilize the tumor anterosuperiorly. The distal branches of the ECA are eventually ligated before removing the tumor.

Insertion of a shunt into the ICA guides the dissection of the tumor around this artery. The

intraoperative use of autotransfusion is advisable for large tumors, where a blood loss of several units is expected.

In some cases there is an associated ICA plaque, and here we prefer to dissect the carotid bifurcation branches away from their origin, heparinize the patient, and clamp the vessels. The carotid endarterectomy is done first, and then the tumor is excised. The arteriotomy is closed with a patch, as the elongation of the bulb and ICA from the growth of the tumor in the bifurcation may result in kinking. During dissection of the internal carotid, spasm is frequent and should be relieved by infiltration with papaverine or by internal dilatation.

A number of reports have appeared advising preoperative embolization of carotid body tumors and stating that this technique improves the safety and ease of surgical dissection. We disagree with this contention. We have seen three instances of stroke during embolization of these tumors because the occlusive material escaped into the ICA stream. Furthermore, having operated on several patients who had had preoperative embolization, we have not found that the dissection is any less demanding than in those who did not have preoperative embolization.

a

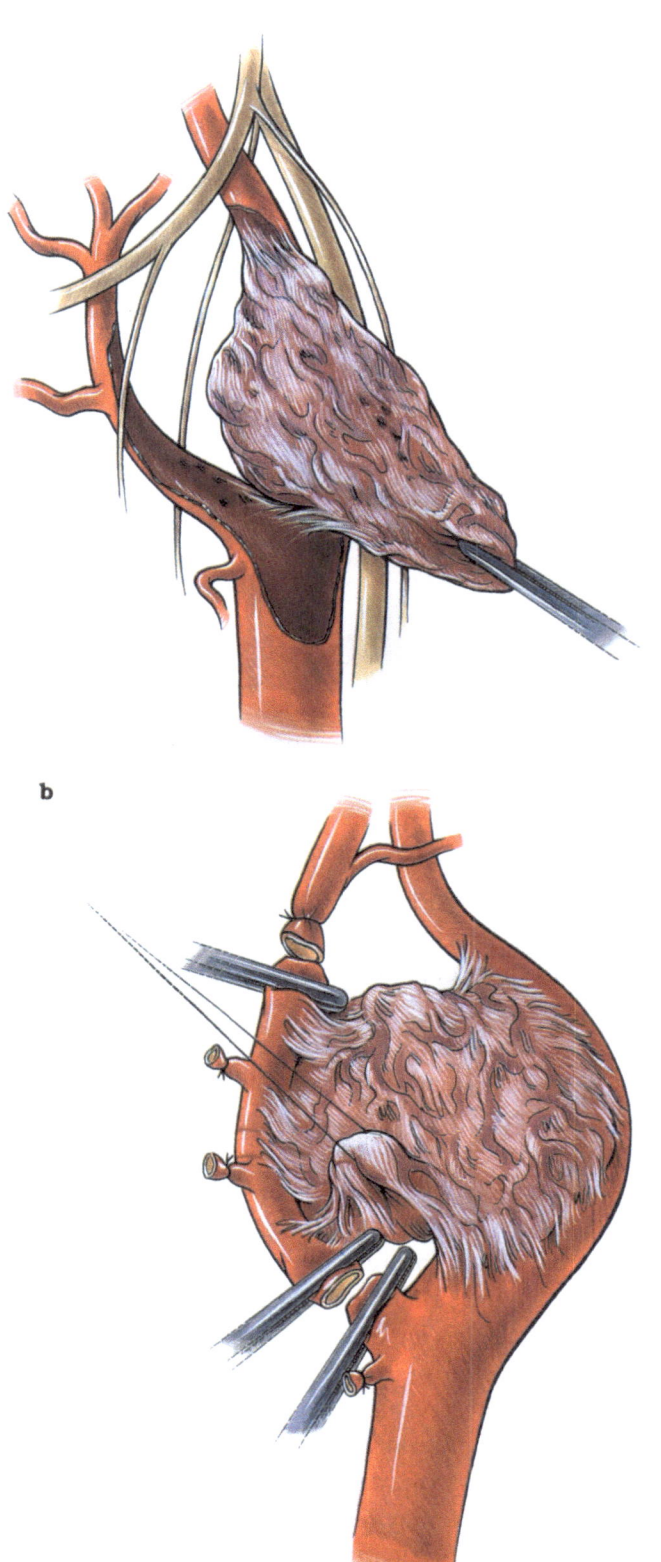

b

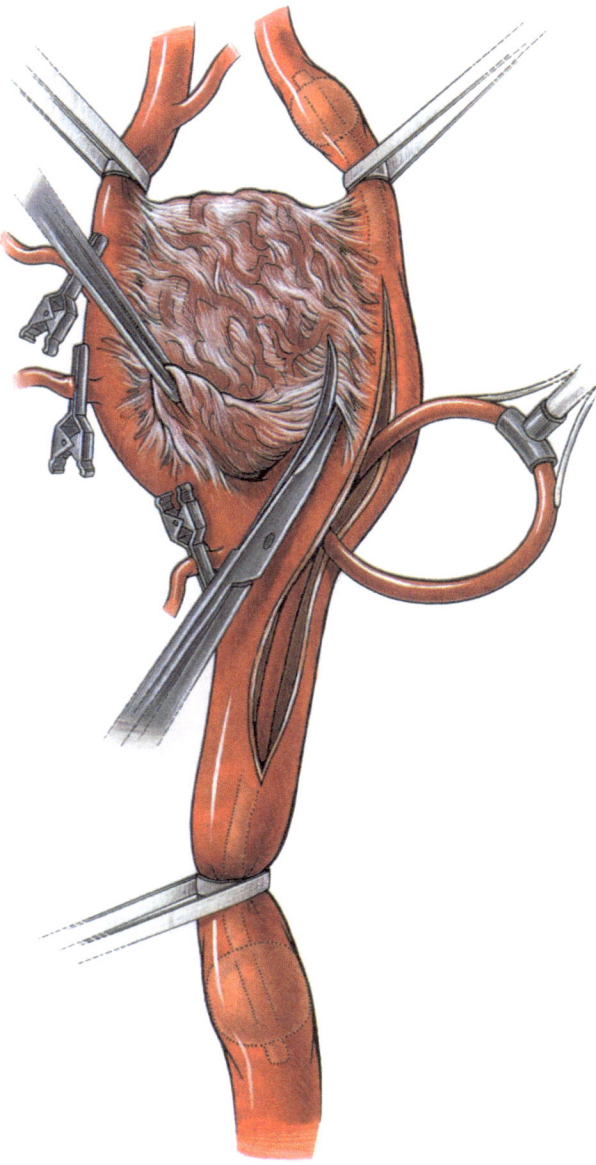

c

Figure 11.31 Three techniques used for resection of a carotid body tumor. (**a**) Subadventitial dissection. (**b**) Transection of the proximal external carotid artery. (**c**) Clamping of the carotid bifurcation and use of an intraluminal shunt.

Figure 11.32 Management of an innominate-tracheal fistula (**a**) with closure of the innominate artery through a midsternotomy (**b**). **Upper Inset:** If there is no suitable stump of innominate artery distally that can be closed safely, a direct subclavian to common carotid artery anastomosis preserves continuity for later reconstruction.

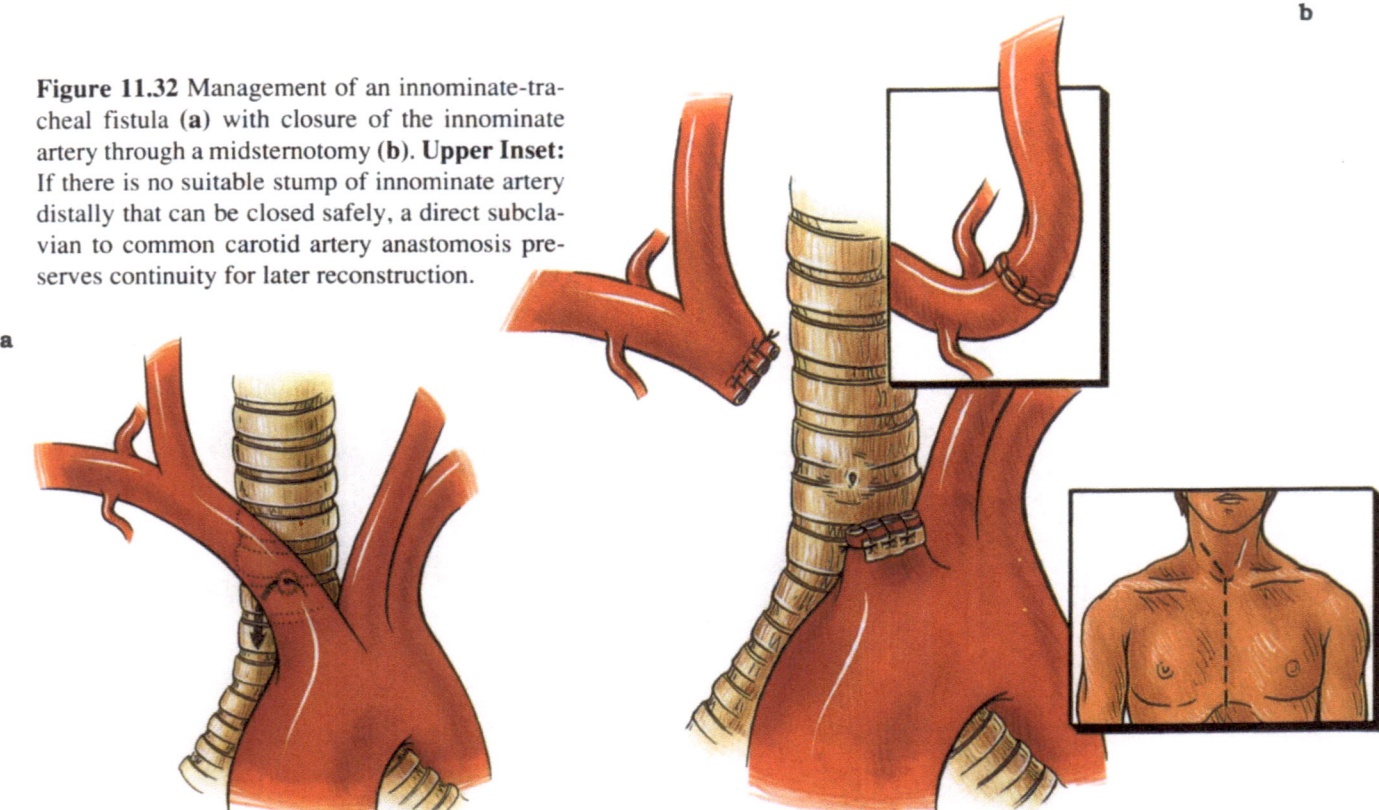

In cases of bilateral carotid tumors, we prefer to start with the smaller one. This practice decreases the chances of recurrent laryngeal nerve damage. Evaluation of vocal cord function is mandatory before the second side is done.

Innominate-Tracheal Fistula

Innominate-tracheal fistulas may complicate tracheostomy, prolonged tracheal intubation, and reconstructive surgery of the trachea. This complication is one of the truly dire surgical emergencies with sudden airway compromise and hemorrhage. Inflating the balloon of the intratracheal tube or digital compression of the IA against the sternum sometimes, but not always, controls bleeding temporarily. An expeditious median sternotomy should be done with digital compression of the IA, which is clamped proximally and distally to stop the bleeding (Figure 11.32). Arterial reconstruction is not advisable in what is always a contaminated field that is likely to later become infected and bleed. Ligation, in contrast,

is usually safe provided the bifurcation of the IA is left undisturbed, leaving a patent right CCA and SA function to be reconstructed at a later date. Patients who survive the acute episode may develop ischemia of the upper extremity or VBI (because of CCA to SA and VA to SA steal), in which case they are reconstructed later by a cross-cervical bypass.

In patients in whom bleeding is minimal and who can be controlled by compression (digital or with an inflated endotracheal tube), one may consider a different approach that allows concomitant revascularization of the IA (Figure 11.33). In these patients the proximal IA and its branches are clamped through a right anterolateral thoracotomy (second or third intercostal space) and a right supraclavicular incision. The latter usually permits ligation of the distal IA with preservation of its branches. Access to the distal IA may be difficult if the artery is short and may require resection of the inner third of the clavicle. Alternatively, the proximal SA and CCA may be divided and anastomosed to each other in the neck. Once the bleeding is controlled, an axilloaxillary crossover bypass through a redcaped clean field provides inflow to both branches of the IA.

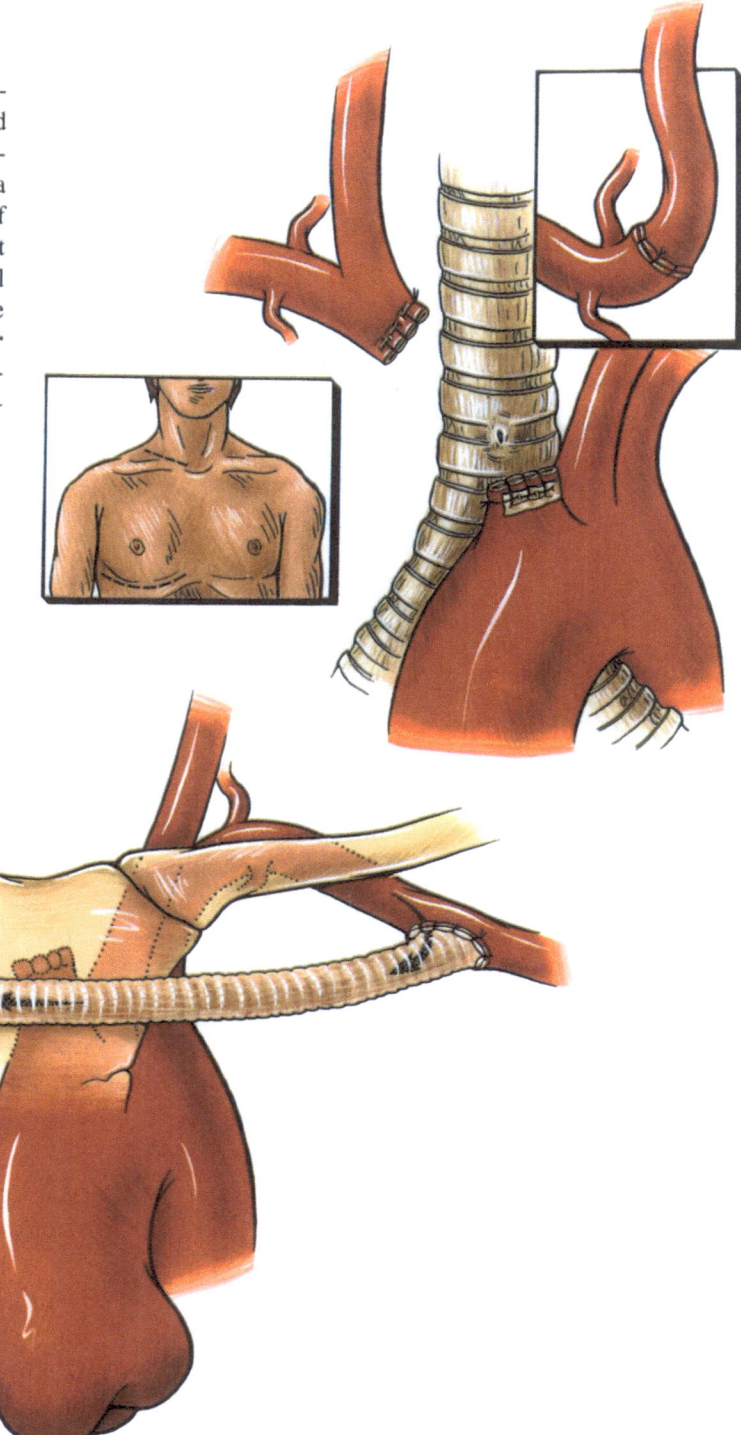

Figure 11.33 Management of a innominate-tracheal fistula through a right supraclavicular and right thoracic incision (**a**) which will then be followed by an immediate reconstruction through a clean field with axillary-axillary bypass (**b**). If distal control of the innominate artery is difficult through the supraclavicular approach the proximal common carotid and subclavian arteries may be divided and anastomosed to each other (**upper right inset**). The axillo-axillary bypass will provide flow to the right vertebral and common carotid arteries.

12   Complications

Stroke

Stroke is a specific and devastating complication of the repair of the arteries addressed in this book. It is generally caused by prolonged ischemia during clamping, embolization from a lesion or repair site, thrombosis of the reconstructed artery, or reperfusion of a previously hypotensive cerebrovascular bed. Other causes of perioperative stroke are mural dissections or bleeding into the neck.

From a practical point of view, it is important to distinguish the stroke that becomes obvious at the conclusion of the operation from the one developing after the patient has awakened neurologically intact. We request an anesthetic technique that aims to have the patient awaken immediately after closure of the neck.

Strokes that occur during the operation are a result of (1) ischemia that developed during the period the artery was clamped or (2) embolization to the brain: (a) during dissection of the atheroma-bearing artery; (b) through a shunt; (c) from an occluding clamp crushing an atheroma; (d) following thrombosis of the operated artery because of a technical error in its repair (including intimal damage during insertion of shunt or intraluminal dilatation).

If one can exclude technical error during the operation as the cause of the stroke (not possible unless an intraoperative arteriogram has been obtained) and can demonstrate a patent artery, the cause of the intraoperative stroke cannot be reversed and should be dealt with by medical therapy. Once the neck is closed, noninvasive assessment is unreliable owing to postoperative swelling and air bubbles in the tissues. The risk of worsening the perfusion of an ischemic and edematous brain far outweighs the remote chances of reversing the stroke with reexploration in search of a local problem not shown on the intraoperative arteriogram. In fact, reexploration of a patient with an intraoperative stroke is advised only when a technical problem identified in the intraoperative arteriogram is suspected to be the cause of a discrete sensorimotor deficit with intact consciousness.

The *early postoperative stroke* is another story. Here the patient awakens lucid and neurologically intact, and a half-hour or longer after awakening develops a sensorimotor deficit that is usually progressive. The problem results from thrombus formation at or near the operative area caused by a kink, an intimal flap, or an irregular/constricting suture line. The thrombus is usually composed of gray-pink, platelet-rich aggregates of loose consistency. For early postoperative stroke some advocate a computed tomographic (CT) scan of the brain without contrast to determine the extent of the infarction and to rule out intracranial bleeding. A brain CT scan is seldom of any use for early detection of discrete ischemic areas. The CT scan can show a small, hemorrhagic infarction, but the likelihood of hemorrhage being the cause of such a delayed postoperative deficit is small. On the other hand, performing arteriography in this situation serves only to delay the remedy, which is immediate reoperation. Our policy is to explore immediately all patients with early postoperative stroke who are not comatose.

Finally, *a stroke may develop two or more days later*, following an apparently normal recovery. Such strokes are often due to reperfusion injury or to thrombosis of the arterial repair. The former is more likely to appear in a patient with extensive occlusive disease involving several trunks of supply; it is probably related to the fragility of the small arteries and the loss of autoregulation from long-standing hypotension. Patients developing new deficits 3 days or more after an operation should have a CT scan without contrast to rule out bleeding. If the CT scan is positive for bleeding or shows a new infarct, or if the patient is obtunded, medical treatment is advised. If the CT scan is negative and the patient is lucid, an arteriogram should be obtained to define the condition of the reconstructed arteries and of other extracranial vessels that may be responsible for the symptoms. If a thrombosis is found, reoperation must be considered, provided the CT scan of the brain is unchanged from the preoperative scan and the patient has a normal level of consciousness.

Thrombosis

Intra- or early postoperative thrombosis of an arterial repair in the neck is often the consequence of a technical flaw. These flaws can be found at any arterial repair: a distal intimal flap, an intramural hematoma, a kink due to additional elongation after endarterectomy or to an improperly measured bypass, or a suture line that constricts the vessel. The incidence of intra- or early postoperative thrombosis can be minimized by the routine use of intraoperative completion arteriography.

In addition to these local technical problems, a bypass or a transposed artery may become compressed externally in its trajectory, or become angulated, or constricted by axial rotation during tunneling. In the neck, autogenous vein grafts are more prone to these problems than are prosthetic materials. Whatever bypass material is used, the surgeon should check the correctness of the length and lay of the bypass before closure.

We have already mentioned the compression and angulation of prosthetic grafts of the SAT in the retrosternal space and thoracic inlet. As the sternal edges are reapproximated, the distance between the midline and the SA is shortened, which may cause kinking of a bypass graft from the ascending aorta to either subclavian artery. Prosthetics arising from the ascending aorta (see Figure 7.7) are often anastomosed to the carotid bifurcation. When the anastomosis is done end-to-end after division of the CCA, some elongation occurs with time that may result in kinking of the ICA above the bulb (Figure 12.1).

Any bypass in the supraclavicular area should take into account the changes that will take place when the head resumes its neutral position or is rotated toward the operative site. Angulation may also develop in vein bypasses to the distal ICA or distal VA as the saphenous vein lengthens when distended by arterial pressure.

Dissection

Intramural dissection by a hematoma can occur at any level where arterial flow insinuates itself into the media of an artery, often as the result of a poorly finished endarterectomy, where a loose medial flap is left into which blood can dissect. During the course of an IA endarterectomy, failure to tack the edge of the aortic intima with a suture may result in dramatic dissection of the arch of the aorta. With carotid endarterectomy a distal dissection is more frequent than a proximal one. A dissection should be suspected if, after opening the ICA to flow, one can see a hematoma with discoloration in its wall. This finding, when verified by intraoperative arteriography, the presence of a thrill, or a jet sound detected by ultraso-

a, b

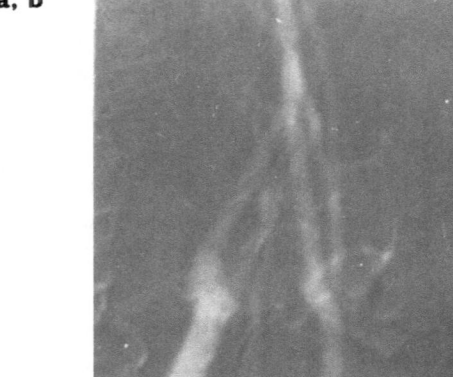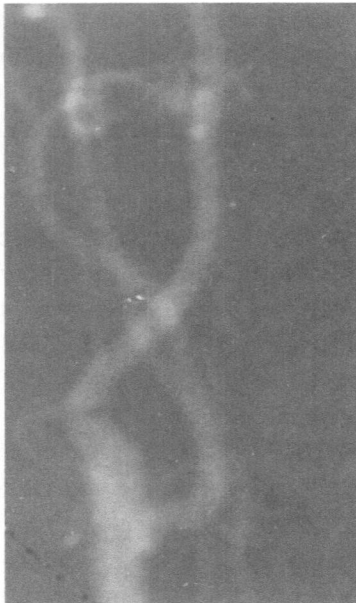

Figure 12.1 In this ascending aorta to carotid bifurcation graft the distal anastomosis is end-to-end. **(a)** Postoperative arteriogram shows a good size and length match. **(b)** One year later elongation in the previously dissected carotid has taken place, and a kink has developed above the internal carotid bulb.

nography, demands immediate reopening and, usually, placement of an interposition vein graft.

Bleeding

Bleeding is a potential problem with any arterial reconstruction. Commonly, bleeding after repair of any artery is caused by too much spacing between stitches or by a suture break with subsequent unraveling of the suture line. Such suture breaks, anecdotally reported by many surgeons, are not necessarily due to improper handling and may instead be a consequence of poor quality control in the production of sutures. The consequences of suture line failure in the arterial territory that concerns us are often serious.

The elastic structure of the aorta and the SA makes their wall particularly vulnerable to tears. The wall thickness/vessel diameter ratio is small in both arteries. During the immediate postoperative period, a tear may result in brisk bleeding with mediastinal tamponade or airway compromise. Incorporation of a Teflon felt strip is recommended when the surgeon is confronted with a thin or friable ascending aorta that

becomes sandwiched between the graft inside and the felt strip outside. Large or cutting needles and any anastomotic tension should be avoided on grafts taking off (usually at right angles) from the SA to avoid tearing it.

Prosthetic patches, particularly those made with polytetrafluorethylene (PTFE) material, often cause annoying bleeding from the needle holes, which prolongs the operation. The use of fine needles that match as closely as possible the diameter of the suture they carry helps with this problem. In some instances heparin may have to be fully reversed to stop needle hole leaks in a patch.

Venous bleeding after carotid endarterectomy is often the result of a venous tie getting loose during a Valsalva maneuver. Venous branches of large caliber and short length, e.g., the anterior facial vein, should be suture-ligated to avoid dislodgement of their occluding ties.

Arterial bleeding after carotid endarterectomy is seen in individuals whose blood pressure has been allowed to rise during the immediate postoperative period. Sometimes no bleeding source is found at reexploration once medical therapy has brought the hypertension under control.

Infection

Infection at the site of a carotid endarterectomy in the absence of a prosthetic graft or patch is a rare event. With vascular repairs of the neck, graft infection is caused by contamination of the field through a breach in operative technique or by the proximity of a pharyngoesophageal fistula or a tracheostomy. Occasionally skin erosion and contamination of a prosthesis occurs in previously irradiated necks that have poor skin and soft tissue coverage.

Infection of a mediastinal prosthesis or patch is a more serious problem. The source of infection is usually a tracheostomy, a skin infection involving the sternum and extending through the midline to the underlying prosthesis, or a breakdown of the skin suture line above the sternum in an irradiated neck. We have already discussed the steps that must be taken to protect and cover the graft in this location in order to minimize the occurrence of this catastrophe. The surgical maneuvers to deal with this situation are discussed in Chapter 13.

Complications Specific to the Surgical Approach

The most frequent complications attending reoperation are discussed in Chapter 13. However, a number of problems may occur with primary operations during exposure of the arteries. With transsternal repairs, faulty closure of the sternum may result in its abnormal mobility. A pneumothorax follows inadvertent entry into the pleural space. Division of the brachiocephalic vein to expose the left SA may result in left internal jugular and subclavian vein thrombosis with swelling, redness, and discomfort. Careless dissection of the bifurcation of the IA or of the isthmus of the aorta may injure a recurrent laryngeal nerve.

With supraclavicular dissections lymph leaks may occur on the right side because of inadvertent injury to accessory thoracic ducts or to an anomalous main right thoracic duct in a patient with a retroesophageal right SA. On the left side the thoracic duct may be double or triple as it empties into the jugulosubclavian confluent, and one of these components may be inadvertently injured. If a leak is observed at operation, every effort should be made to control it before closing. Small lymphoceles usually subside after bowel rest and aspiration. In cases where the parietal pleura has been entered, the resulting chylothorax may require reoperation for more proximal ligature of the thoracic duct.

Paralysis of the hemidiaphragm may follow handling of the phrenic nerve during exposure of the second portion of the SA. Breaking through the parietal pleura during dissection of the SA does not require any specific measures, provided the visceral pleura shows no evidence of air leak. Injury to the sympathetic nerves is most likely to occur during exposure of the proximal VA when the connections between the intermediate and stellate ganglion may be damaged. The resulting Horner syndrome is usually incomplete (mild ptosis, no anhidrosis) and often recedes spontaneously in weeks.

With the anterior approach to the ICA and VA, the vagus, hypoglossal, spinal accessory, superior and inferior laryngeal, and glossopharyngeal nerves are at risk. The steps to avoid injury to these nerves are discussed under the respective techniques for reconstruction of the ICA and VA in Chapters 8 and 9. Before a carotid operation is done on the side opposite to a previous carotid, proximal right subclavian, or left thoracic operation, preoperative laryngoscopy is needed to ensure that an unrecognized vocal cord palsy has not occurred. If it has, a tracheostomy may be required. The greater occipital nerve may be injured or may have to be cut when extending the upper end of a presternomastoid incision. This may result in annoying sensory symptoms in the earlobe.

13   Reoperations

Reoperations present special difficulties and often require innovative solutions. These solutions are different depending on the specific complications that prompt the reoperation: occlusion, infection, and false aneurysm formation. We discuss the problems presented by reoperations in the supraaortic trunks (SAT), internal carotid artery (ICA), and vertebral artery (VA) separately.

Reoperations on the Supraaortic Trunks

Occlusion

Rarely one must perform a thrombectomy for an immediate postoperative occlusion, usually caused by a technical error. In this case the thrombectomy is followed by the surgeon revising the previous technical flaw or choosing a different corrective technique. With chronic occlusion the choices are dictated by the general condition of the patient, the reappearance of previous symptoms, the arteriographic findings, and the type of operation and incision that were used before.

Unless the patient presents a high surgical risk or some other contraindication to surgery, the best way to repair a failed intrathoracic reconstruction is through a second thoracotomy. Reopening the sternum requires care and the use of an oscillating saw. The sternum is pulled upward, using the ends of the previous wire of which only the anterior loop has been cut. When approaching the anterior portion of the aorta, it is often helpful to enter both pleural cavities under the sternal edges to allow the heart and mediastinum to drop into the chest while the sternal edges are lifted.

If the previous operation was an endarterectomy of the IA, a good portion of ascending aorta should be available for insertion of a bypass. If the previous operation was a bypass from the ascending aorta, it is best to use the same site for proximal reimplantation. To accomplish this step, the occluded graft is transected, and using retrograde dissection the previous anastomotic site is isolated by partial exclusion-clamping. The previous anastomosis is then excised and a new bypass inserted.

If the repeat sternotomy must be avoided because of a previous coronary vein graft or an internal mammary artery transposition, or if the patient has become a poor risk since the first operation, the alternative is a crossover cervical bypass. The latter can be done only if there is at least one patent SAT that can be used as a source. If not, the alternative is an atypical reconstruction using other sources of inflow such as the descending thoracic or supraceliac aorta or even the iliac or common femoral arteries, as discussed in Chapter 10.

If the thrombosis has taken place in a previous cervical repair, the repeat operation is normally done again in the neck. The specific choice of operation is dictated by what was done before. For instance, if the failed operation is a carotid-subclavian or subclavian-carotid bypass, the second operation should be an axillary-axillary or carotid-carotid (Figure 13.1) bypass to avoid redissecting the supraclavicular fossa, a step fraught with a substantial rate of complications. A transthoracic approach should be considered in good risk patients in whom failure of the cervical approach (because of disease of the inflow vessel) could have been averted had a transthoracic approach been used in the first place. The same applies to those patients who have occluded previous cervical reconstructions and have developed new lesions in other SATs during the interval.

Infection

Infection is a rare but dreaded complication of operations on the SAT. The usual presentation of an *early infection* is bleeding. The infected artery breaks down at the suture line or a vein graft disintegrates, resulting in a massive hemothorax, a hemomediastinum, or a leaking false aneurysm at the base of the neck. This type of emergency must be dealt with as rapidly as possible without further workup.

Late infection usually presents as a chronic false aneurysm or a periprosthetic abscess. These patients should have an arteriogram not only to show whether there is a false aneurysm or a thrombosed graft but also to help the surgeon decide on a ligature technique versus the need for a remote reconstruction away from the infected vessels. Ultrasonography of the neck and computed tomography (CT) scans of the chest are helpful for outlining the periprosthetic collection and detecting another proximal intrathoracic anastomotic false aneurysm that may not be obvious on the arteriogram. Needle puncture and aspiration are sometimes needed to confirm the diagnosis.

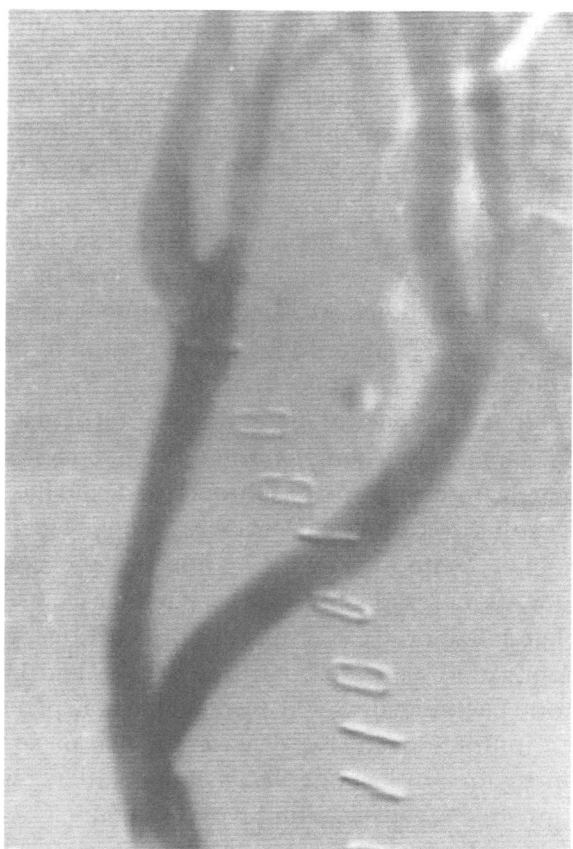

Figure 13.1 Common carotid-to-common carotid retropharyngeal transposition done to revascularize the left carotid bifurcation. A previous left subclavian to carotid graft had failed.

An infected brachiocephalic reconstruction is handled by following the same principles that apply to any infected graft. One needs to obtain proximal control, remove all of the infected material, and, if indicated, perform an alternative arterial reconstruction.

Proximal control is usually obtained through a median sternotomy. If the patient has a ruptured or leaking proximal aneurysm on the ascending aorta, the best approach is to place the patient on cardiopulmonary bypass and deep hypothermia; circulatory arrest is then undertaken immediately before opening the chest in order to avoid exsanguination during the repeat sternotomy incision. In most cases, however, control may be obtained without undue difficulty by using generous lateral clamping of the ascending aorta and pharmacologically induced hypotension. All prosthetic material is removed, and the gap in the ascending aorta is closed with large, interrupted, monofilament sutures buttressing the aortic wall between two fascial bands obtained from the sheath of the rectus abdominalis. If the infected mediastinum needs to be debrided, this step is followed either with continuous lavage through large drains or omentoplasty, with or without primary closure of the sternum. Patients who survive often have residual sternal infection.

In the presence of infection, ligation of just one SAT may result in complications. It is of course safe when the infected graft has thrombosed, and it is the only solution available when there is active bleeding associated with infection. Ligation and excision of one SAT is reasonably safe in patients who have isolated SA or CCA artery reconstructions with patent arteries on the contralateral side and brisk carotid back-bleeding. On the other hand, in patients with multiple occlusive disease the risk of stroke after ligation of just one SAT is high. Patients with an infected reconstruction involving both CCAs or all three SATs must have an alternative surgical reconstruction if a stroke is to be avoided.

This alternative revascularization can be performed in situ at the time of operation using autogenous material such as saphenous vein graft or an arterial autograft. The latter may be fashioned from a superficial femoral artery that is either normal or was occluded and is endarterectomized at the time of the reconstruction. In the rare patient whose infected graft was originally done to correct an occlusion of the IA through a bypass from the ascending aorta to one of the branches of the IA (end-to-side) or through a crossover cervical bypass, the alternative of IA endarterectomy after excision of the infected graft should be entertained. If a patch is needed to close the arteriotomy, it can be fashioned from autogenous vein or artery.

The remote bypasses used to treat infected reconstructions of the SAT include the remote cervical crossover bypasses or bypass from the descending thoracic aorta or the supraceliac aorta, iliac, or femoral arteries (see Chapter 10).

Aneurysms

Late, noninfected aneurysms following reconstruction of the SAT are rare. We have seen only one patient with a false anastomotic aneurysm arising from a prosthetic bypass inserted into the ascending aorta. False aneurysms, however, have been seen at the distal anastomotic site of prosthetic aortocarotid graft, especially when an ICA endarterectomy was performed simultaneously. They have also been seen in carotid-subclavian bypasses, on the subclavian side, probably caused by the notorious fragility of this artery and the mobility of the base of the neck. Late aneurysmal dilatation of vein grafts used for carotid-subclavian bypass has been reported. Noninfected false aneurysms in the carotid anastomosis of a prosthesis are treated by direct reconstruction. To avoid repeated dissection of the supraclavicular fossa, false aneurysms in the subclavian position are best dealt with by exclusion of the SA and use of the CCA to revascularize the VA (transposition) and as a source for a carotid-axillary artery bypass.

Reoperations on the Internal Carotid Artery

Occlusion

Early reoperations, done within 10 days of the initial procedure, do not present technical problems, as the surgeon may follow the same pathway for dissection used for the initial operation. After 2 weeks the reexploration is made more difficult by dense fibrinous adhesions and edema, which makes the tissues and particularly the vessel wall friable. Provided the contraindications outlined in Chapter 12 do not exist in the case of an early occlusion, it is mandatory to reopen the artery, correct whatever errors are found, and close the artery with a patch or bypass it with a venous graft. If a thrombectomy of the distal ICA is required, it must be done with the utmost care because of the possibility of creating a carotid-cavernous fistula or tearing the distal ICA with the intracranial manipulation of the Fogarty catheter. Our preference is to introduce a Fogarty catheter about 8 cm and then retrieve the clot. The distal clot often follows removal of the proximal clot if there is adequate carotid back-pressure. If this method is unsuccessful, a small amount of urokinase is injected into the cleared proximal ICA and the artery is clamped. Twenty minutes later it is allowed to back-bleed and carry the partially dissolved clot with it into the arteriotomy. If this maneuver does not result in back-bleeding, further manipulation should be discontinued and the carotid is ligated. Upon completion of the clot retrieval by back-flow, an intraoperative arteriogram before flow is resumed ensures that no thrombotic material remains in the internal carotid artery.

Late reoperations, done months or years after the original operation for recurrence of disease, present an entirely different challenge. Here the scarring may be firm, the boundaries unclear, and the neurovascular structures bound to one another. The surgeon must obtain safe proximal and distal control before facing unexpected bleeding from having inadvertently entered the carotid artery or the internal jugular vein. The general principle for reoperations applies here: Obtain control of the vessels involved in an area not dissected previously. Once this "terra firma" has been dissected and the pertinent vessels isolated in it, the surgeon can attend to the problem area.

During reoperations, it is not uncommon to find a slightly buckled ICA or ECA in a subcutaneous position or underneath the anterior edge of an atrophied sternomastoid muscle. This possibility should be kept in mind as soon as the subcutaneous plane is entered.

Getting proximal control in a carotid reoperation is usually simple. The incision is carried farther down (to the clavicle if needed) to dissect the CCA below the level dissected at the previous operation. The omohyoid and sternothyroid muscles may have to be transected. The dissection of the carotid artery is then made from below upward. The jugular vein is attached to the CCA but can be separated easily, except around the stump of the previously ligated facial vein. The vagus nerve may present a problem here because at reoperations it is often found on top of, rather than behind, the CCA.

At the top of the incision the surgeon looks for and generally follows two landmarks: the tendinous anterior edge of the sternomastoid and the digastric muscle. The tendinous edge of the sternomastoid muscle is a safe guide for extending the dissection upward, posterior to the ICA up to the mastoid insertion of the muscle. The position of the hypoglossal nerve should be determined next. If dense scarring prevents the surgeon from seeing the nerve, it is safer to go higher, isolate the posterior belly of the digastric by freeing its lower edge and retracting it upward, searching underneath it for previously undissected ICA. The digastric muscle may be cut to improve exposure. The hypoglossal nerve is identified from the top of the field downward. If the posterior loop of the ansa is visible, it can serve as a guide that leads to the main hypoglossal trunk. The vagus nerve is likely to be on top of the ICA at the upper end of the field. If the previous operation has dissected this area, the retrojugular approach described in Chapter 8 is used and the vagus nerve is reflected anteriorly. Once the distal ICA, the hypoglossal and vagus nerves, and the origin of the ECA are identified, the bulb may be dissected if a patching procedure is planned either with or without endarterectomy. If the plan is to perform a bypass to the distal cervical ICA the carotid bifurcation and bulb are not dissected.

The most common problem when dissecting scarred arteries is entering the subadventitial plane, which may lure the surgeon with its ease for dissection. If this error is realized before breaking into the lumen, the adventitia should be closed using a fine vascular suture and the false plane abandoned. Should the lumen of the carotid be entered during dissection, gentle finger pressure is the best move. Assuming that at this moment one does not yet have the necessary proximal and distal control to arrest flow temporarily, it is best to try to repair the arterial wound by anchoring a fine suture immediately above the tip of the controlling finger and running a continuous suture proximally from there under some tension. Alternatively, proximal control may be obtained by digital pressure and distal control by an intravascular balloon catheter. The use of clamps should be avoided other than in the areas chosen for proximal and distal control. Clamps usually result in worse tears than those they are meant to control, and they may damage cranial nerves not yet identified.

Our preferences for reconstruction of restenosing carotid bifurcation disease differ. One of us (E.K.) uses Dacron patching preferentially and reserves grafting (vein or polytetrafluorethylene [PTFE]) for cases where patching is not feasible. The other (R.B.) prefers to do a CCA-to-ICA vein graft for all carotid reoperations, provided a suitable vein is available. Vein grafts behave well in this location and generally provide a good size match to the ICA. The appeal of this technique (see Chapter 8) is that there is no need to dissect the bifurcation or the carotid bulb, which are likely sources of mishaps during reoperations.

When patching a previously operated carotid, the arteriotomy should extend beyond the limits of the first operation. No attempt is made to remove the intima if the restenosis is secondary to intimal hyperplasia. The patch outline must be tailored to the anatomy of the lumen. If, on the other hand, the stenosis is a new atheromatous lesion, a standard endarterectomy should be carried out and closed with a patch. If an internal carotid bypass is planned and the vein is absent or unsuitable, we do not hesitate to use thin-walled 6 mm PTFE, provided the distal anastomosis is proximal to the digastric muscle. Repairing the carotid above this point with this semirigid prosthesis is not advisable because of axial rotation as well as kinking of the junction between the thin-walled carotid and the semirigid graft. An alternative solution is to use an arterial autograft from the superficial femoral artery.

Infection

Early infection is rare, especially in the absence of prosthetic materials, and it usually develops in a nondrained hematoma. Simple wound drainage may suffice if bleeding has not occurred and a prosthetic patch has not been used. On the other hand, if bleeding has taken place or there is a prosthetic patch, one must proceed with ligation of the three branches of the bifurcation and excision of the infected artery or of the previous prosthetic patch and substitution with autogenous tissue. The choice between ligation or

autogenous reconstruction is determined by the extent of the infection and by the status of the other carotid and vertebral arteries.

Late chronic infection may occur in prosthetic patches and calls for removal of the patch and its replacement with an autogenous patch from either saphenous vein or an endarterectomized segment of an occluded superficial femoral artery. In these cases the replacement patch is sutured using polyglycol rather than polypropylene suture. An ICA autogenous venous bypass is also a sound alternative.

Aneurysms

Postoperative aneurysms are rare. Usually it is a false aneurysm arising from a Dacron patch or an aneurysmal dilatation of a wide venous patch (Fig-

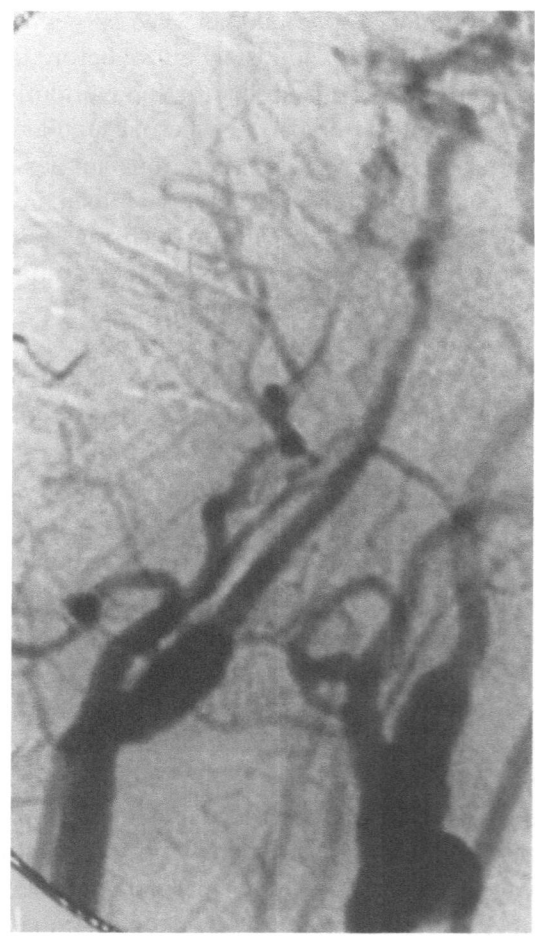

Figure 13.2 False aneurysm (right lower corner) arising from the suture line of a Dacron patch of the carotid bulb.

ure 13.2). In exceptional cases a false aneurysm occurs following failure of the suture line after a primary closure.

It is important to note that all these aneurysms are filled with a large thrombus which may embolize during their dissection. Therefore if the distal ICA cannot be controlled with ease, it is better to heparinize the patient and arrest carotid flow by CCA and ECA clamping. After this step, the dissection is carried out from below upward to obtain control of the ICA. If the proximal ECA is difficult to control externally, the aneurysm can be opened, clamping the ICA and controlling the ECA by balloon occlusion from within the aneurysm.

The continuity of the ICA, after excision of one wall of the aneurysm, is reestablished with a venous or prosthetic graft. The ECA is revascularized by separate grafting, using a constructed bifurcation graft, or by its reattachment to an opening in a 6 mm thin-walled PTFE graft.

Reoperations on the Vertebral Artery

Occlusion

If occlusion is detected early, the operation to correct it should follow immediately because distal extension may occur and preclude salvage of the vessel or, even worse, result in a brainstem stroke. We differ in our approach to the thrombosis of a proximal VA reconstruction. One of us (E.K.) prefers to correct the proximal VA thrombosis by a distal VA bypass. The other (R.B.) favors thrombectomy and correction of the technical problem causing the thrombosis, usually a redundant interposition graft or a faulty anastomosis.

If a distal VA repair thromboses, under no circumstances should blind balloon catheter embolectomy be done in the distal VA, as the risk of a

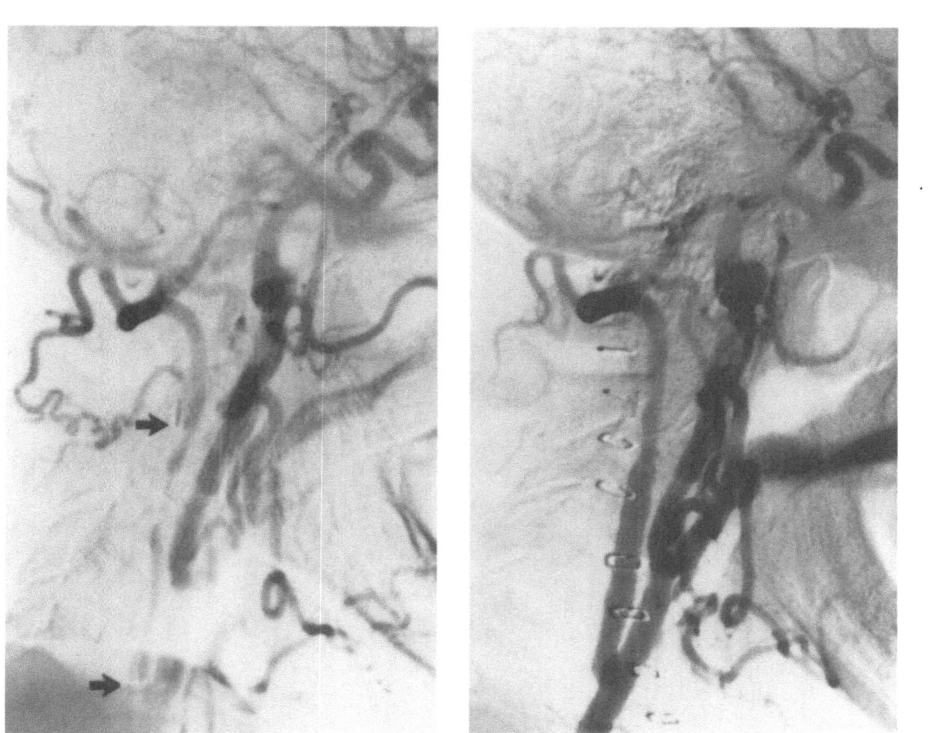

a   **b**

Figure 13.3 Patient with recurrence of symptoms 16 months after an initially successful distal vertebral artery bypass with saphenous vein. (**a**) The graft (between arrows) is nearly occluded by intimal hyperplasia. (**b**) A new vein graft was placed, and symptoms were relieved.

perforation and massive subarachnoid bleeding is probably high. If a proximal reconstruction deteriorates by restenosis or by kinking due to elongation of the VA or the graft, it is best treated by doing a distal VA reconstruction. We have seen two instances of intimal hyperplasia of a vein graft inserted in the distal position that required replacement with a new autogenous graft (Figure 13.3).

Infection

Because most VA reconstructions are done using a transposition technique, infection of a VA reconstruction always presents the problem of preserving the donor vessel whether it is the CCA, ICA, or SA. With infected proximal VA transpositions, the donor CCA is involved. The distal portion of the carotid can be preserved by means of a retroesophageal carotid-carotid bypass using an autogenous graft. This is followed by a distal VA reconstruction. If this procedure is not possible, ligature is the alternative. Infection in a distal VA reconstruction can be handled only by ligature. If the original operation was a transposition to the ICA, unfortunately the latter has to be ligated as well.

Aneurysm

We have never seen a false aneurysm in the territory of a VA operation.

14   Epilogue

Improvements in the surgical reconstruction of the arteries supplying the head depend on the development of more refined methods of selecting patients and safer operations. At present, symptomatic lesions can be corrected with a combined mortality and morbidity of 1 to 2% for the carotid and vertebral arteries and 3 to 5% for the supraaortic trunks. The results of recent randomized studies (North American Symptomatic Carotid Endarterectomy Trial, European Carotid Stenosis Trial) have demonstrated that this surgical risk is lower than the risk posed by the natural history of symptomatic disease of these arteries. The final word on what to do with specific asymptomatic lesions should be suspended until the conclusion of randomized studies that are still in progress.

Diagnostic refinements such as three-dimensional MR arteriography and high-resolution ultrasound imaging will most likely sharpen the anatomic definition of disease and, as a result, the selection of patients. The safety of these operations can also be enhanced through better assessment and management of cardiac risk before and during the operation.

Technically, surgical access to these arteries has been resolved at all levels outside the cranium, although exposure of the distal internal carotid artery in the temporal canal and of the vertebral artery in its predural segment is difficult and carries substantial morbidity.

Transposition techniques are used with increasing frequency, particularly in the vertebral arteries. Eversion techniques in the carotid bifurcation restore anatomic normalcy, correct concomitant elongation, and avoid the need for patching. They have become even safer with the advent of intraoperative digital arteriography, which permits thorough assessment of the repair. In the supraaortic trunks, the use of horizontal ipsilateral or crossover bypasses is declining in favor of cervical transposition techniques for single lesions and direct intrathoracic reconstruction for innominate artery and multiple lesions.

Of the drugs under study, further development of calcium channel blockers targeted to the brain vasculature may reverse some of the relative ischemia that exists in the tissue surrounding a brain infarction and may prevent or decrease the centrifugal extension of the infarction.

Use of the endovascular radiologic techniques in the carotid or vertebral arteries is presently limited. Their use must await the development of a safe trapping device to prevent distal embolization. Furthermore, the thin walls of the upper cervical ICA and the intraspinal VA make them less suitable for the technique of balloon angioplasty than other arteries. On the other hand, precise placement of detachable balloons has already resolved some of the problems encountered in managing lesions that are surgically inaccessible.

As we mentioned in the introduction, repair of the arteries supplying the head was late in coming to the practice of surgery. Nevertheless, it has gained a prominent position in the practice of surgeons who can now operate on these arteries with a record for safety and durability unmatched anywhere else in the arterial tree.

Bibliography

1. Virchow R. Thrombose und Embolie: gefassen Fndung vad septische Injektion in gesammelte Abhandlnngen fur wisseuschaftlichen Medicin. AM Medinger, Frankfort, 1856.
2. Elsching A. Uber den Einfluss des Verschlusses des Arteria Ophthalmica und der Carotis auf das Sehorgan. Albrecht Von Graefes Arch Klin Exp Ophthalmol 1893; 39:51.
3. Abercrombie J. Pathological and Practical Research on Diseases of the Brain and the Spinal Cord. Waugh Innes, Edinburgh 1828.
4. Cohnheim J. Untersuchungen uber die embolischen Processe. A. Hirschwald, Berlin 1872.
5. Chiari H. Uber das Verhalten des Teilungswinkels der Carotis bei der Endarteritis chronica deformans. Verh Dtsch Pathol Ges 1905.
6. Hunt JR. The role of the carotid arteries in the causation of vascular lesions of the brain, with remarks on certain special features of the symptomatology. In Proceedings of the American Neurological Association Meeting 1913; 704.
7. Broadbent WH. Absence of pulsation in both radial arteries, the vessels being full of blood. Read 1875; 165.
8. Takayasu M. A case with peculiar changes of the central retinal vessels. Acta Soc Ophthalmol Jpn 1908; 12:554.
9. Sloan HG. Successful end-to-end suture of the common carotid artery in man. Surg Gynecol Obstet 1921; 33:62.
10. Lefevre MH. Sur un cas de plaie du bulbe carotidien par balle, traite par la ligature de la carotide prim-itie, et l'anastomose bout a bout de la carotide externe avec la carotide interne. Bull Mem Soc Chir 1918; 12:923.
11. Moniz E, Lima A, de Lacerda R. Hemiplegies par thrombose de la carotide interne. Presse Med,1937; 52:977.
12. Fisher M. Occlusion of the internal carotid artery. Arch Neurol Psychiatry 1951; 65:347.
13. Fisher M. Occlusion of the carotid arteries. Arch Neurol Psych 1954; 72:187.
14. Hutchinson EC, Yates PO. The cervical portion of the vertebral artery: a clinico-pathological study. Brain 1956; 79:319.
15. Hutchinson EC, Mane MD, Yates PO. Carotico-vertebral stenosis. Lancet 1956; 2:8.
16. Conley JJ, Pack GT. Surgical procedure for lessening the hazard of carotid bulb excision. Surgery 1952; 31:845.
17. Carrea R, Molins M, Murphy G. Surgical treatment of spontaneous thrombosis of the internal carotid artery in the neck: carotid-carotideal anastomosis. Acta Neurol Latinoam 1955; 1:71.
18. DeBakey ME. Successful carotid endarterectomy for cerebrovascular insufficiency: nineteen-year follow-up. JAMA 1975; 233:1083.
19. Eastcott HHG, Pickering GW, Rob CG. Reconstruction of internal carotid artery in a patient with intermittent attacks of hemiplegia. Lancet 1954; 2:994.
20. Davis JB, Grove WJ, Julian OC. Thrombotic occlusion of the branches of the aortic arch; Martorell's syndrome: report of a case treated surgically. Ann Surg 1956; 144:124.

21. Ehrenfeld WK, Chapman RD, Wylie EJ. Management of occlusive lesions of the branches of the aortic arch. Am J Surg 1969; 118:236.

22. Lin PM, Javid H, Doyle EJ. Partial internal carotid artery occlusion treated by primary resection and vein graft. J Neurosurg 1956; 13:650.

23. Cate WR, Scott HW. Cerebral ischemia of central origin: relief by subclavian vertebral artery thromboendarterectomy. Surgery 1959; 45:19.

24. DeBakey ME, Morris GC, Jordan GL, Cooley DA. Segmental thrombo-obliterative disease of branches of aortic arch. JAMA 1958; 166:998.

25. Bahnson HT, Spencer FC, Quattlebaum JK. Surgical treatment of occlusive disease of the carotid artery. Ann Surg 1959; 149:711.

26. Crawford ES, DeBakey ME, Fields WS. Roentgenographic diagnosis and surgical treatment of basilar artery insufficiency. JAMA 1958; 168:509.

27. Parrot JC. The subclavian steal syndrome. Arch Surg 1964; 88:661.

28. Clark K, Perry MO. Carotid vertebral anastomosis: an alternate technique for repair of the subclavian steal syndrome. Ann Surg 1966; 163:414.

29. Berguer R, Andaya LV, Bauer RB. Vertebral artery bypass. Arch Surg 1976; 111:976.

30. Roon AJ, Ehrenfeld WK, Cooke PB, Wylie EJ. Vertebral artery reconstruction. Am J Surg 1979; 138:29.

31. Matas R. Traumatisms and traumatic aneurysms of the vertebral artery and their surgical treatment with the report of a cured case. Ann Surg 1893; 18:477.

32. Henry AK. Extensile Exposure. Churchill Livingstone, London, 1945.

33. Corkill G, French BN, Michas C, et al. External carotid-vertebral artery anastomosis for vertebrobasilar insufficiency. Surg Neurol 1977; 7:109.

34. Carney AL, Anderson EM. Carotid distal vertebral bypass for carotid artery occlusion. Clin Electroencephalogr 1978; 9:105.

35. Thevenet A, Chaplal PA, Negre E. L'arret circulatoire en hypothermie profonde dans la chirurgie des branches de la crosse aortique. Ann Chir Thorac Cardiovasc 1968; 7:69.

36. Barnett HJM, Plum F, Walton JN. Carotid endarterectomy: an expression of concern. Stroke 1984; 15:941.

37. Warlow C. Carotid endarterectomy: does it work? Stroke 1984; 15:1068.

38. European Carotid Surgery Trialists' Collaborative Group. MRC European carotid surgery trial: interim results for symptomatic patients with severe (70-99%) or with mild (0-29%) carotid stenosis. Lancet 1991; 17:1235.

39. North American Symptomatic Carotid Endarterectomy Trial Collaborators. Beneficial effect of carotid endarterectomy in symptomatic patients with high-grade carotid stenosis. N Engl J fed 1991; 325:445.

40. Wright NL. Dissection study and mensuration of the human aortic arch. J Anat 1969; 1 04:377.

41. Smith D, Larsen JL. On the symmetry and asymmetry of the bifurcation of the common carotid artery. Neuroradiology 1979; 17:245.

42. Adams WE. The Comparative Morphology of the Carotid Body and Carotid Sinus. Charles C Thomas, Springfield, IL: 1958.

43. Heath D, Smith P, Harris P, Winson M. The atherosclerotic human carotid sinus. J Pathol 1973; 110:49

44. Boyd JD. Observations on the human carotid sinus and its nerve supply. Anat Anz 1937; 8:386.

45. Edwards E. Advances in gross anatomy in the 20th century. JAMA 1977; 237:1954.

46. Forster FK, Chikos PM, Frazier JS. Geometric modeling of the carotid bifurcation in humans: implications in ultrasonic doppler and radiologic investigation. J Clin Ultrasound 1985; 13:385.

47. Yates PO, Hutchinson EC. Cerebral infarction: The Role of Stenosis of the Extracranial Cerebral Arteries. Medical Research Council Special Report Series, No. 300. Her Majesty's Stationary Office, London, 1961.

48. Jamieson RW, Smith DB, Anson BJ. The cervical sympathetic ganglia: an anatomical study on one hundred cervicothoracic dissections. Q Bull Northwestern Univ Med School 1952; 26:219.

49. Gillilan LA. Extra and intracranial blood supply to brains of dog and cat. Am J Anat 1976; 146:237.

50. McDonald DA. Blood Flow in Arteries. Edward Arnold, London, 1960.

51. Gosling R, Newman D, Bowden N, Twinn K. The area ratio of normal aortic junctions: aortic configuration and pulse wave reflection. Br J Radiol 1971; 44:850.

52. Motomiya M, and Karino T. Flow patterns in the human carotid artery bifurcation. Stroke 1984; 15:50.

53. Moore WS, Boren C, Malone JM, et al. Natural history of non-stenotic, asymptomatic ulcerative lesions of the carotid artery. Arch Surg 1978; 113:1352.

54. Blaisdell FW, Glickman 1,1, Trunkey DD. Ulcerated atheroma of the carotid artery. Arch Surg 1974; 108:491.

55. Kroener JM, Dorn PL, Shoor PM, Prognosis of asymptomatic ulcerating carotid lesions. Arch Surg 1980; 115:1387.

56. Scotti G, Melancon D, Oliver A. Hypoglossal paralysis due to compression by a tortuous internal carotid artery in the neck. Neuroradiology 1978; 14:263.

57. Lusby RJ, Woodcock JP, Machleder HI et al. Transient ischaemic attacks: the static and dynamic morphology of the carotid artery bifurcation. Br J Surg 1982; 69 (suppl):S41.

58. Meyer WW, Walsh SF, Lind J. Functional morphology of human arteries during fetal and postnatal development. In Schwartz CJ, Werthessen NT, Wolf S (eds): Structure and Function of the Circulation. Plenum Press, New York, 1980.

59. Fisher CM, Adams RD. Observations on brain embolism with special reference to the mechanisms of hemorrhagic infarcts. J Neuropathol Ep Neurol 1951; 10:92.

60. Hollenhorst RW. Significance of bright plaques in the retinal arterioles. JAMA 1961; 1 75:23.

61. Russell RW. Observations on the retinal blood vessels in monocular blindness. Lancet 1961; 2:1422.

62. Boldrey CE, Maass L, Miller E. The role of atlantoid compression in the etiology of internal carotid thrombus. J Neurosurg 1956;13:127.

63. de Kleyn A, Nieuwenhuyse P. Schwindelanfalle und Nystagmus bei einer Bestimmten Stellung des Kopfes. Acta Otolaryngol (Stock)1927; 11:155.

64. Toole JF, Tucker SH. Influence of head position upon cerebral circulation. Arch Neurol 1960; 2:616.

65. Koskas F, Kieffer E. Anatomy of the vertebral artery and spinal mechanics. In: Berguer R, Caplan L (eds): Vertebrobasilar Arterial Disease. Quality Medical Publishing, St. Louis; 1991.

66. Berguer R, Hwang NHC. Critical arterial stenosis: a theoretical and experimental solution. Ann Surg 1974; 180:39.

67. Mann C, Herrick JF, Esses HE, Baldes EJ. Effect on the blood flow of decreasing the lumen of a blood vessel. Surgery 1938; 4:219.

68. Weale F. Surgical Hemodynamics: An introduction to surical haemodynamics. Year Book Medical Publishers, Chicago, 1967.

69. Lusby RJ, Woodcock JP, Machleder HI, et al. Transient ischaemic attacks: the static and dynamic morphology of the carotid artery bifurcation. Br J Surg 1982; 69 (suppl 1):S41.

70. Caplan L, Tettenborn B. Thromboembolic vertebrobasilar ischemia. In: Berguer R, Caplan L (eds): Vertebrobasilar Arterial Disease. Quality Medical Publishers, St. Louis: 1991.

71. Astrup J, Siesjo BK, Symon L. Thresholds in cerebral ischemia: the ischemic penumbra. Stroke 1981; 12:723.

72. Berguer RB, Sieggreen M, Lazo A, Hodakowski GT. The silent brain infarct in carotid surgery. J Vasc Surg 1987; 3:442.

73. Ruotolo C; Kieffer E. Dynamic arteriography. In Berguer R, Caplan L (eds): Vertebrobasilar Arterial Disease. Quality Medical Publishing, St. Louis 1991.

74. Alexander W. The treatment of epilepsy by ligature of the vertebral arteries. Brain 1882; 5:170.

75. Sundt TM, Sharbrough FW, Piepgras DG. Correlation of cerebral blood flow and electroencephalographic changes during carotid endarterectomy. Mayo Clin Proc 1981; 56.533.

76. Cormier JM, Chapelier A. Greffe veineuse carotidienne. In Kieffer E, Natali J (eds.): Aspects Techniques de la Chirurgie Carotidienne. AERCV Publishers, Paris, 1987.

77. Fisch UP, Oldring DJ, Senning A. Surgical Therapy of Internal Carotid Artery Lesions of the Skull Base and Temporal Bone. Otolaryngol. Head Neck Surg 1980, 88:548.

78. Pech A, Mercier D, Thomassin JM, Piligian F. L'abord chirurgical de la partie haute de la carotide interne cervicale. J Français d'Oto-Rhino-Laryngol 1983;32:401-406.

79. Purdue GF, Pellegrini FV, Arena S. Aneurysms of the high internal carotid artery: A new approach. Surgery 1981; 89:268.

Index